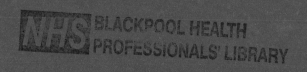

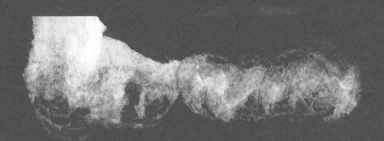

MASTER TECHNIQUES IN ORTHOPAEDIC SURGERY

■

THE ELBOW

Second Edition

THE ELBOW

Second Edition

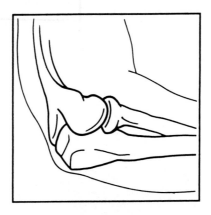

Editor

BERNARD F. MORREY, M.D.
Professor of Orthopedic Surgery
Mayo Medical School
Emeritus Chairman
Department of Orthopedics
Mayo Clinic
Rochester, Minnesota

Illustrators

Jim Postier
Matthew Morrey

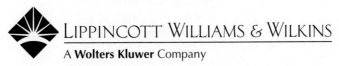

LIPPINCOTT WILLIAMS & WILKINS
A **Wolters Kluwer** Company
Philadelphia • Baltimore • New York • London
Buenos Aires • Hong Kong • Sydney • Tokyo

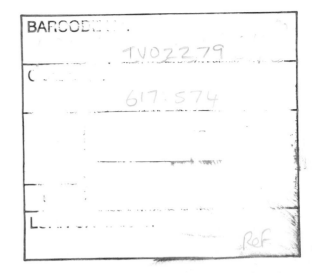

Acquisitions Editor: James Merritt
Developmental Editor: Pam Sutton
Production Editor: Janice Stangel
Manufacturing Manager: Tim Reynolds
Cover Designer: Karen Quigley
Compositor: Maryland Composition

© 2002 by LIPPINCOTT WILLIAMS & WILKINS
530 Walnut Street
Philadelphia, PA 19106 USA
LWW.com

Printed in China

Library of Congress Cataloging-in-Publication Data

The elbow / editor, Bernard F. Morrey ; illustrator, Jim Postier.—2nd ed.
    p.; cm. — (Master techniques in orthopaedic surgery ; [v. 1])
  Includes bibliographical references and index.
  ISBN 0-7817-1991-7
  1. Elbow—Surgery. I. Morrey, Bernard F., 1943- II. Master techniques in orthopaedic surgery (2nd ed.) ; [v. 1]
  [DNLM: 1. Elbow—surgery. 2. Orthopedics. WE 168 M423 1994 v.1]
  RD558.E423 2001
  617.5'74—dc21

          2001029921

---

10 9 8 7 6 5 4 3 2 1

To
My orthopaedic mentors at Mayo Clinic
who introduced me to the intriguing world of elbow surgery.

My colleagues at the Mayo Clinic
who have generously referred to me interesting elbow problems throughout the years;
and particularly Doctor An who has been my "partner"
in investigating the workings of this complex joint.

All orthopaedic surgeons
who have shared their interesting cases with me
so that strides might be made in the diagnosis
and management of this often overlooked joint.

And to our families
who understand and support us in our endeavors.

■

CONTENTS

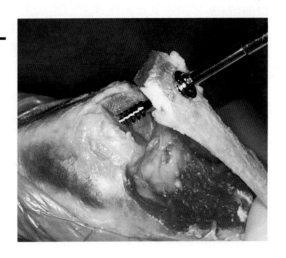

CONTRIBUTORS

Ralph W. Coonrad, M.D.
Associate Professor, Emeritus, Division of Orthopedic Surgery, Duke University; and, Medical Director and Chief Surgeon, Emeritus, Lenox Baker Childrens Hospital, Durham, North Carolina

Jon R. Davids, M.D.
Assistant Consulting Professor, Department of Orthopaedic Surgery, Duke University Medical Center, Durham, North Carolina; and, Medical Director, Motion Analysis Laboratory, Shriners Hospital, Greenville, South Carolina

Neal S. ElAttrache, M.D.
Associate Clinical Professor, Department of Orthopaedic Surgery, University of Southern California School of Medicine; and, Director, Sports Medicine Fellowship, Kerlan-Jobe Orthopaedic Clinic, Los Angeles, California

Avrum I. Froimson, M.D.
Clinical Professor, Department of Orthopaedics, Case Western Reserve University; and, Department of Orthopaedic Surgery, Cleveland Clinic, Cleveland, Ohio

Gerard T. Gabel, M.D.
Department of Orthopaedic Surgery, Baylor College of Medicine, Houston, Texas

Robert N. Hotchkiss, M.D.
Chief, Hand Service, Hospital for Special Surgery; Director, Alberto Vilar Center for Research of the Hand and Upper Extremity; and, Associate Professor of Clinical Surgery (Orthopaedics), Weill Medical College of Cornell University, New York, New York

Frank W. Jobe, M.D.
Clinical Professor, Department of Orthopaedic Surgery, University of Southern California School of Medicine, Los Angeles, California

Jesse B. Jupiter, M.D.
Professor, Department of Orthopaedic Surgery, Harvard Medical School; and, Chief, Orthopaedic Hand Surgery, Massachusetts General Hospital, Boston, Massachusetts

Pierre Mansat, M.D.
Clinical Assistant, Department of Orthopaedics and Traumatology, University Hospital of Toulouse–Purpan, Toulouse, France

Bernard F. Morrey, M.D.
Professor of Orthopedic Surgery, Mayo Medical School; and, Emeritus Chairman, Department of Orthopedics, Mayo Clinic, Rochester, Minnesota

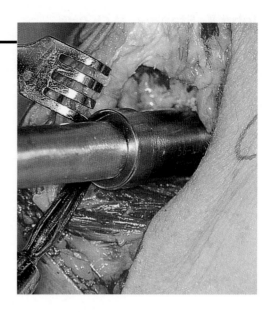

Scott J. Mubarak, M.D.
Clinical Professor, Department of Orthopedics, University of California, San Diego; and, Medical Director of Orthopedic Clinical Program, Department of Orthopedics, Children's Hospital, San Diego, California

Robert P. Nirschl, M.D.
Clinical Professor, Department of Orthopedic Surgery, Georgetown University Medical School, Washington, D.C.; and, Director of Orthopedic Sports Medicine Fellowship Program, Arlington Hospital/Nirschl Orthopedic Sports Medicine Clinic, Arlington, Virginia

Shawn W. O'Driscoll, M.D., Ph.D.
Professor of Orthopedic Surgery, Mayo Medical School, Mayo Foundation, Rochester, Minnesota

Felix H. Savoie III, M.D.
Codirector, Upper Extremity Department, Mississippi Sports Medicine, Jackson, Mississippi

Alberto G. Schneeberger, M.D.
Department of Orthopedic Surgery, Balgrist University of Zurich, Zurich, Switzerland

Morton Spinner, M.D.
Clinical Professor of Orthopaedic Surgery, Department of Orthopaedic Surgery, Albert Einstein College of Medicine, Bronx, New York

Robert J. Spinner, M.D.
Assistant Professor, Departments of Neurologic Surgery and Orthopedics, Senior Associate Consultant, Department of Neurologic Surgery, Mayo Clinic, Rochester, Minnesota

David Stanley, B.Sc., F.R.C.S.
Consultant Orthopaedic Surgeon, Northern General Hospial, N.H.S. Trust, Sheffield, England

John K. Stanley, M.Ch.Orth.
Professor of Hand Surgery, University of Manchester, Manchester, England; and, Consultant Hand Surgeon, Upper Limb Unit, Wrightington Hospital NHS Trust, Lancashire, England

Ian A. Trail, M.D., F.R.C.S.
Honorary Clinical Lecturer, Department of Orthopaedic Surgery, Manchester, England; and, Consultant in Hand and Upper Limb Surgery, Hand and Limb Department, Wrightington Hospital NHS Trust, Lancashire, England

ACKNOWLEDGMENTS

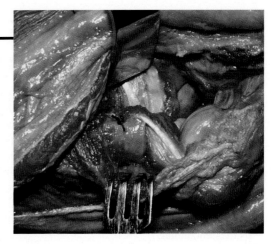

It is with a growing sense of appreciation that I acknowledge the shared contribution of so many of my colleagues in the orthopedic community. Our current understanding of the problems of elbow management has grown steadily over the years, not in small part due to the willingness of the orthopedic community to share experiences with this challenging and capricious joint. It is with a sense of indebtedness that I, therefore, acknowledge the numerous interactions and shared consultations with so many of my associates and colleagues in the orthopedic community. I would particularly acknowledge and recognize my partner, Shawn W. O'Driscoll, for his ongoing stimulus and innovative, creative, and probing thought process. During the preparation of the second edition, I found myself continuing to reflect on the confidence and support of my mentors Dick Bryan, Ron Linscheid, and Jim Dobyns. I wish to specifically recognize the contributions of Doctor An in the biomechanics laboratory as a basis of so much of our original thinking, as well as a source of inspiration and encouragement to continue the process of developing a scientific basis for clinical practice. It is with a great sense of humility and appreciation that I recognize these individuals' genuine commitment to education, to integrity, and to the inquisitiveness that has characterized our Mayo practice and with which I have been fortunate to be associated. I also wish to recognize the tireless efforts of my special colleagues, Bob Adams and Sherry Koperski, who manage the increasing complex logistics of my practice, as well as Donna Riemersma who was also responsible for manuscript preparation.

Finally, the numerous hours and considerable time that is required to prepare such a volume comes at no small expense to one's personal life, therefore, I acknowledge once again with sincere appreciation, the patience and understanding of my wife, Carla.

SERIES PREFACE

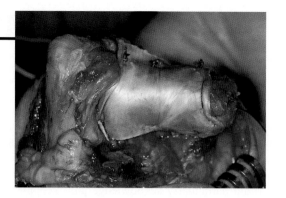

The first volume of the series *Master Techniques in Orthopaedic Surgery* was published in 1994. Our goal in assembling the series was to create easy-to-follow descriptions of operative techniques that would help orthopaedists through the challenges of daily practice. The books were intended to be more than just technical manuals, they were designed to impart the personal experience of the "master orthopaedic surgeons."

Master Techniques in Orthopaedic Surgery has become precisely what we hoped for—books that are used again and again, and are found at home and in the offices of practicing orthopaedists and residents in training. Most importantly, they are recommended by orthopaedists who look to them for practical advice and suggestions concerning the difficult but common problems they encounter.

The series is now entering its second edition phase. You will again find recognized leaders as volume editors, known for their contributions to research, education, and the advancement of the surgical state of the art. Chapter authors have been selected for their experience, operative skills, and recognized expertise with a particular technique. The classic procedures are still included; some techniques have changed as new technology has been incorporated; and new procedures that have been popularized during the last several years have been added.

We are maintaining the same user-friendly format that was so well-received when the series was first introduced—a standardized presentation of information replete with tips and pearls gained through years of experience, with abundant color photographs and drawings to guide you step-by-step through the procedures.

With these new editions, we again invite you into the operating room to peer over the shoulder of the surgeon at work. It is our goal to offer the orthopaedic surgeon seeking an improved proficiency in practice access to the maximum confidence in selecting and executing the appropriate surgery for the individual patient.

PREFACE

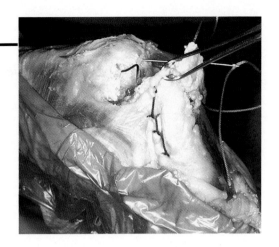

In recent years there has been increasing attention paid to the elbow by the orthopedic community. I believe this is due to a set of converging factors, including the increasingly difficult problems posed by the pathology of this joint with the realization that an emerging set of solutions are becoming available. In this volume the complexity of elbow pathology is addressed by a series of established and innovative solutions, some of which have been developed since the first edition. Advances in surgical techniques have included a better understanding of elbow exposure such as for coronoid fractures. The scientific basis of improved management of complex trauma is based upon a clear definition of the relative contributions of the articular and soft tissue elements of elbow stability. Advances in arthroscopy have been significant both for elective and traumatic conditions and these advances are reflected in the current text. The current techniques for total elbow arthroplasty and longterm follow-up are presented in greater detail along with descriptions of two resurfacing implant designs.

The alternative to total elbow arthroplasty, including interposition with the Achilles' tendon allograft, is discussed in detail. Details on the indications for and broadening use of external fixation is also provided.

Challenging pathology and encouragement by the ongoing communication of my colleagues has resulted in undertaking this edition's preparation with enthusiasm and excitement. I genuinely hope and sincerely believe that this book will be of value to my colleagues and to the orthopedic community, just as it has been to myself and my coauthors.

Bernard F. Morrey, M.D.

PART I

Elbow

1

Limited and Extensile Triceps Reflecting and Exposures of the Elbow

Bernard F. Morrey

Facility with exposures to the elbow characterized by flexibility and extensibility is an essential prerequisite to the execution of the full spectrum of elbow surgery while optimizing function and minimizing complications. In this chapter I emphasize how limited exposures to the elbow can be expanded to address broadened pathology and perform more complex procedures. The review includes three most important exposures from a conceptual standpoint: the Kocher, Mayo, and medial extensile. Virtually all needed exposures can be drawn from one of these three. Details are found in those chapters addressing specific pathology. Although I do not favor and have performed only one olecranon osteotomy for exposure, this technique is relatively easy and commonly performed and hence is detailed in Chapter 4 and is further discussed in Chapter 6.

There are two conceptual incision types: an extensile posterior or limited, specific for purpose exposure (Fig. 1-1). Both proximal and distal limited and focal procedures laterally have been described. Distally, the skin incision is placed over Kocher's interval between the anconeus and the extensor carpi ulnaris and brought proximally over the lateral epicondyle. Proximally, an incision is placed over the lateral column and brought distally past the lateral epicondyle.

For extensile exposures, a straight posterior incision is used. We term this the "universal" incision. For fear of injuring the ulnar nerve, a posterior incision of variable length (12 to 18 cm) is placed just medial or lateral to the tip of the olecranon and not directly over the cubital tunnel. The most extensile exposure is realized with this simple straight posterior skin incision, since both medial and lateral aspects of the triceps mechanism and both collateral ligaments can be exposed through it.

B.F. Morrey, M.D.: Mayo Medical School and Department of Orthopaedics, Mayo Clinic and Mayo Foundation, Rochester, Minnesota.

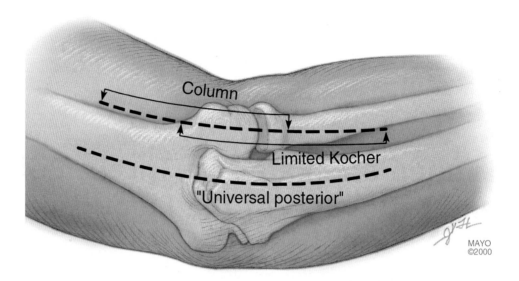

FIG. 1-1. The straight posterior incision is considered "universal" as the entire joint can be exposed through this skin incision. Specific "for purpose" skin incisions such as for the "Column" or limited Kocher are frequently portions of a more extensive incision, such as the extensile Kocher incision.

LIMITED: LATERAL SURGICAL EXPOSURES

The distal lateral approach is indicated in the case of simple excision of the radial head. Landmarks include the lateral epicondyle, radial head, palpate interval between anconeus and extensor carpi ulnaris.

SURGERY

The skin incision is made from the subcutaneous border of the ulna obliquely across the posterolateral aspect of the elbow in line with Kocher's interval and ends at the lateral epicondyle (Fig. 1-2).

The interval between the anconeus and extensor carpi ulnaris is identified and entered (Fig. 1-3). For excision of the radial head, the extensor carpi ulnaris and a small portion of the supinator muscle are dissected free of the capsule and retracted anteriorly (Fig. 1-4). The annular ligament is then identified and entered. Care should be taken to enter the annular ligament approximately 1 cm above the crista supinatoris to avoid injury to the lateral ulnar collateral ligament (Fig. 1-4).

Expanding the Distal Lateral Exposure (7)

Expanding the distal lateral exposure is indicated in reconstruction of the lateral ulnar collateral ligament.

Landmarks include the lateral epicondyle, posterior border of the extensor carpi ulnaris, anterior edge of the anconeus, and the crista supinatoris.

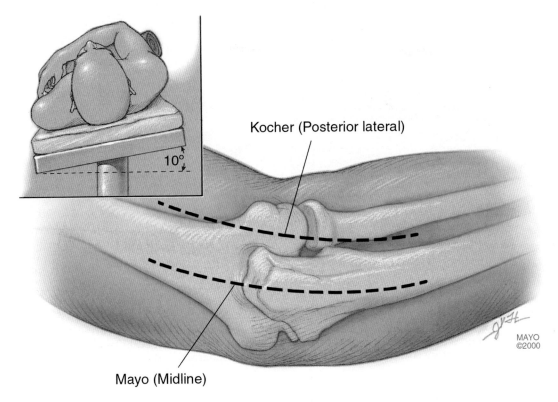

Kocher (Posterior lateral)

Mayo (Midline)

FIG. 1-2. The two most common incisions for extensile exposure of the elbow are a Kocher posterolateral and a straight posterior incision that deviates just medial or lateral to the tip of the olecranon.

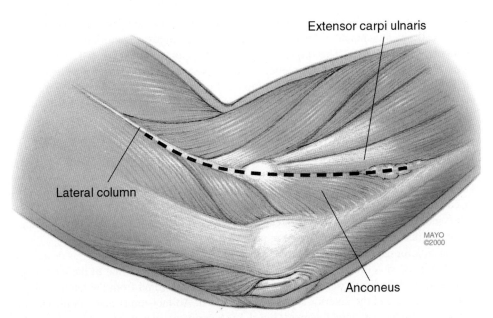

Extensor carpi ulnaris

Lateral column

Anconeus

FIG. 1-3. The interval between the anconeus and the extensor carpi ulnaris is the major landmark for the Kocher incision.

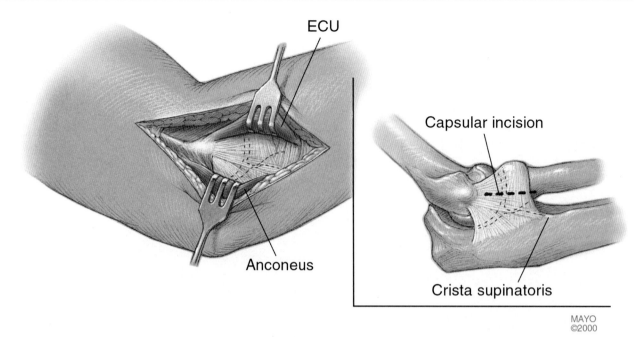

FIG. 1-4. Separating this interval exposes the lateral capsule covering the radial humeral joint. Care must be taken to expose the radial head anterior to the crista supinatoris. (Abbreviation: ECU, extensor carpi ulnaris.)

SURGERY

If the lateral ulnar collateral ligament is to be reconstructed, the skin incision described earlier is simply extended proximally about 3 cm (Fig. 1-3).

After the interval is entered the anconeus is more completely reflected from its ulnar insertion (Fig. 1-5). The lateral collateral ligament complex is identified by first elevating the extensor carpi ulnaris from the annular ligament just distal to the lateral epicondyle (Fig. 1-6). The fleshy attachment of the extensor carpi radialis longus is identified just above the common extensor tendon. This origin is freed from the supracondylar ridge. The dissection then elevates the common extensor tendon and the posterior edge of the extensor carpi radialis brevis from the lateral ligament complex (Fig. 1-7). This is done very carefully to identify and leave intact the lateral collateral ligament complex so that the lateral ulnar collateral ligament can be reconstructed (see Chapter 15).

The Proximal Lateral Exposure (7)

The proximal lateral exposure may be a proximal extension of the distal exposure or a focused proximal approach.

It is indicated for anterior-posterior capsular release for stiff elbow (Column procedure).

Landmarks include the extensor carpi radialis longus, anterior capsule.

If an anterior capsular release is to be performed, a new, limited exposure is described. The skin incision is drawn over the lateral column extending proximal to the lateral epicondyle (Fig. 1-2). The extensor carpi radialis longus is elevated from the lateral column and epicondyle, and the anterior capsule is visualized. An incision is made in the capsule just superior to the collateral ligament (Fig. 1-8). A periosteal elevator is used to elevate the brachialis muscle off the anterior capsule, which can be safely performed, since the arthrotomy provides accurate spatial orientation from lateral to medial across the joint. The procedure then continues as described in Chapter 21.

Note: If an extensile exposure is anticipated, a posterior incision is made. The same deep exposure can be accomplished by extending the posterior lateral skin incision and elevating the lateral skin cutaneous flap.

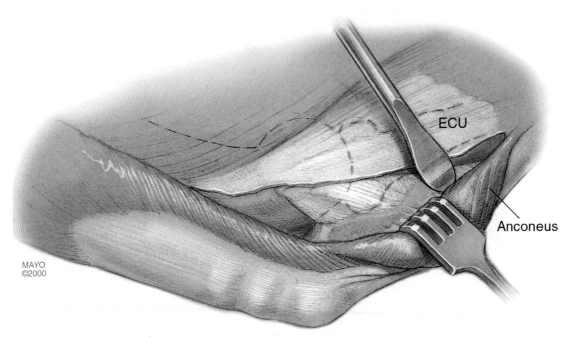

FIG. 1-5. For a more detailed exposure of the lateral ligament complex the anconeus is reflected posterior from its ulnar insertion.

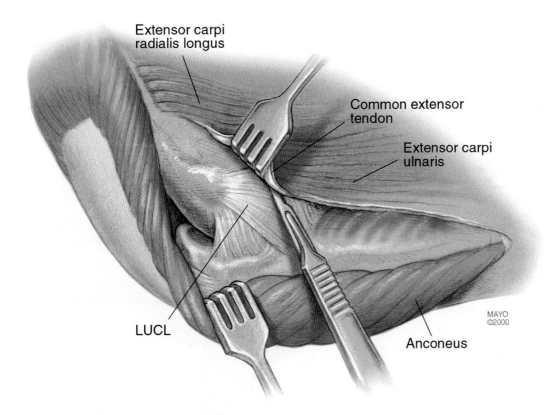

FIG. 1-6. The posterior margin of the extensor carpi ulnaris serves as the interval through which the common extensor muscles may be elevated, exposing the lateral collateral ligament complex. (Abbreviation: LUCL, lateral ulnar collateral ligament.)

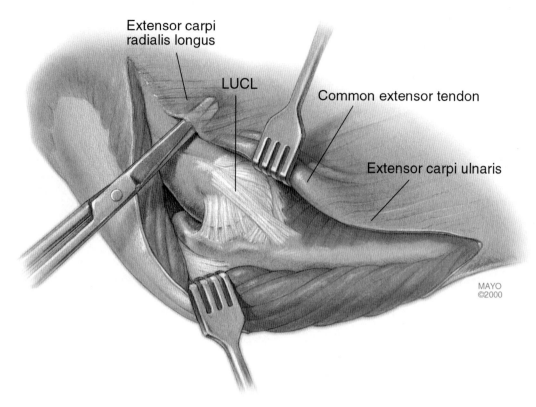

FIG. 1-7. The common extensor tendon may be elevated in continuity with the extensor carpi radialis longus exposing the anterolateral capsule and lateral ulnar collateral ligament.

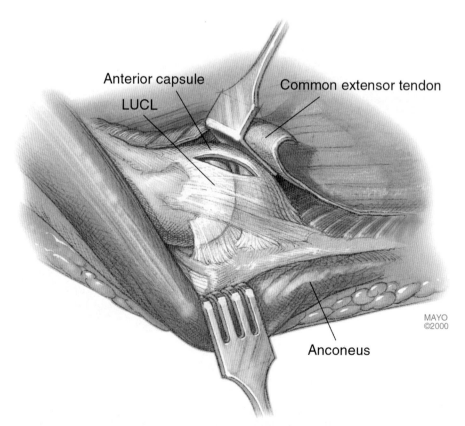

FIG. 1-8. Incision into the capsule provides an orientation that allows exposure of the remainder of the anterior capsule.

EXTENSILE EXPOSURES

The extensile posterolateral exposure (Kocher) (6) is an extension of the limited exposures described earlier involving the release of collateral ligament and capsule.

Extensile exposure to the joint surface is indicated for reconstructive procedures, including open reduction internal fixation, total elbow arthroplasty (resurfacing), and interposition arthroplasty.

Landmarks include the proximal lateral column and the distal Kocher interval.

The triceps may be elevated from the posterior aspect of the humerus by extending the skin incision proximally up the lateral column (Fig. 1-2). This may proceed 6 to 7 cm proximal to the lateral epicondyle without fear of violence to the radial nerve.

Proceed as shown in Fig. 1-5 by completely elevating the anconeus from the ulna. The triceps is easily elevated from the posterior humerus in the normal situation, and even in posttraumatic contractures it can be elevated with a periosteal elevator without much additional difficulty (Fig. 1-9). The lateral collateral ligament is released from the humeral origin as a separate structure or if prior surgery has caused scarring, with the common extensor tendon complex. The anterior capsule is then incised. A varus stress is applied to the elbow, which opens like a book hinging on the medial ulnar collateral ligament (UCL) and common flexor muscles (Fig. 1-10). The triceps remains attached to the ulna.

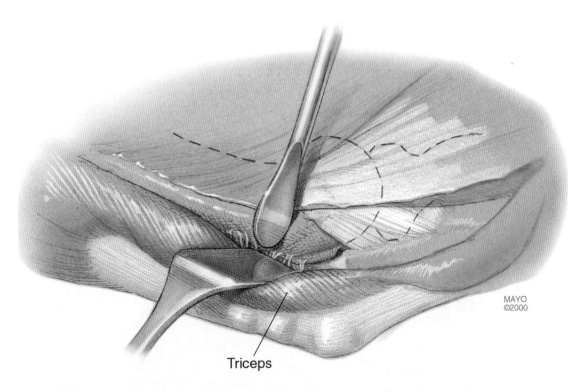

Triceps

FIG. 1-9. The lateral margin of the triceps may be readily separated from the posterior aspect of the lateral column.

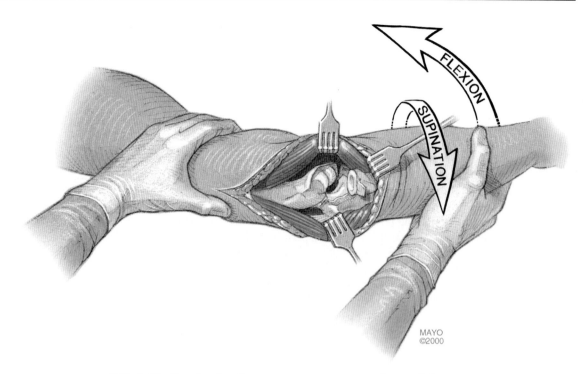

FIG. 1-10. By releasing the common extensor tendon and the anterior capsule as well as the triceps and anconeus posteriorly, a varus stress to the elbow allows it to hinge on the medial collateral ligament and flexor pronator group, providing an extensile exposure to the joint.)

MAYO MODIFIED KOCHER EXTENSILE POSTERIOR-LATERAL EXPOSURE

The triceps attachment is further released from the olecranon and the triceps mechanism is reflected from lateral to medial (Fig. 1-11).

This procedure is indicated in ankylosis release, resurfacing arthroplasty, open reduction with internal fixation (ORIF) lateral column, distal humerus.

Landmarks include the triceps insertion at the olecranon.

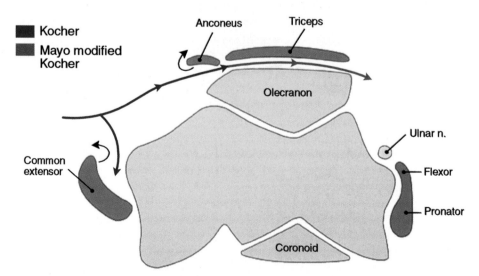

FIG. 1-11. The Kocher approach is extended by releasing the triceps attachment along with the mobilized anconeus muscle.

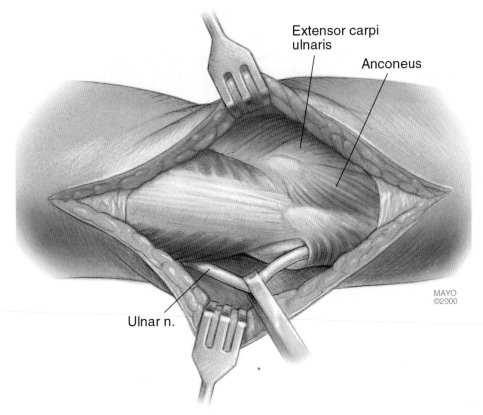

Extensor carpi
ulnaris

Anconeus

Ulnar n.

MAYO
©2000

FIG. 1-12. The brachial fascia is excised at the margin of the medial aspect of the triceps exposing the ulnar nerve. This may be done through a Kocher incision by subcutaneous dissection.

If more extensile exposure is required than has been obtained with the previous steps (Figs. 1-9 and 1-10), a medial skin flap is elevated and the ulnar nerve is identified (Fig. 1-12). It is protected or translocated according to the merits of the case and after the release has proceeded according to the steps shown in Figs. 1-5, 1-8, and 1-9. The triceps and anconeus muscle sleeve is reflected from the tip of the olecranon by releasing Sharpey's fibers (Fig. 1-13). The entire extensor mechanism, including anconeus, is thus reflected from lat-

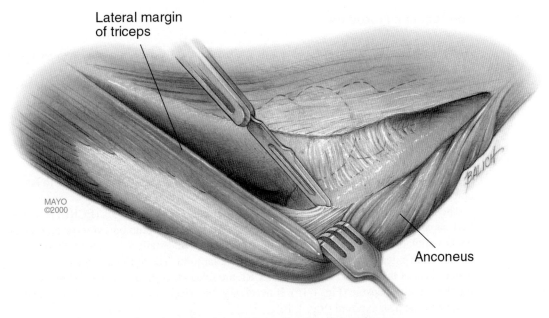

Lateral margin
of triceps

Anconeus

MAYO
©2000

FIG. 1-13. The triceps is released from the tip of the olecranon.

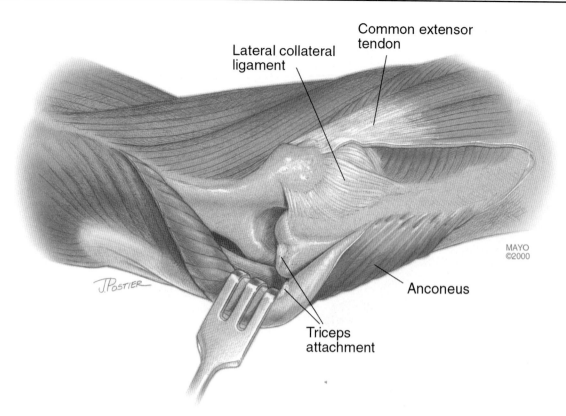

FIG. 1-14. The entire extensor mechanism may be translated from the lateral to the medial aspect of the joint.

eral to medial (Fig. 1-14). After the triceps has been reflected and the posterior capsule released, the lateral collateral ligament may be detached from the humerus, depending upon the goal of the specific procedure and the additional exposure required. By flexing the elbow and removing the tip of the olecranon, the articular surface and the entire posterior humerus can be exposed.

LIMITED EXPOSURE PROXIMAL PORTION OF KOCHER INCISION

The "Column Procedure"

Note: As a similar exposure has been described for the medial joint, this approach will henceforth be referred to as the "lateral column."

It is indicated in the case of anterior-posterior capsular release or removal of coronoid or olecranon osteophytes.

SURGERY

A 6- to 7-cm incision is made over lateral column, 2 cm distal and 4 cm proximal to lateral epicondyle.

The lateral epicondyle is exposed. The extensor carpi radialis longus (ECRL) is identified, as are the muscle fibers immediately proximal to the common extensor tendon. A hockey stick incision is performed laterally and extended distally in line with the fibers of the common extensor tendon over the radiocapitellar joint. The muscular attachment of the distal fibers of the brachial radialis and ECRL are released from the lateral column, exposing the extensor capsule (Fig. 1-15). If necessary, the triceps may be elevated and the posterior capsule also exposed (Fig. 1-16).

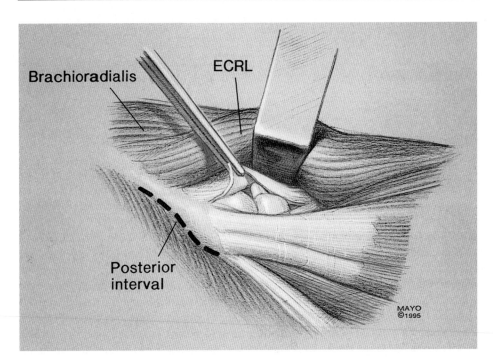

FIG. 1-15. Limited exposure to the anterior capsule realized by elevating the humeral origin of the ECRB and distal fibers of the brachioradialis.

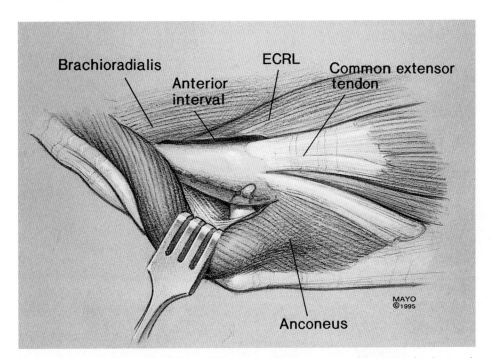

FIG. 1-16. By elevating the triceps from the posterior aspect of the lateral column, the posterior capsule and olecranon may be exposed.

POSTERIOR-MEDIAL EXPOSURE

The extensile Mayo approach of Bryan-Morrey (1) is indicated in the case of ankylosis release, semiconstrained total elbow arthroplasty, ORIF medial column, distal humeral fractures.

SURGERY

A 14-cm skin incision is made just medial to the tip of the olecranon. The dissection is carried to the medial aspect of the triceps 6 cm proximal and 4 cm distal to the tip of the olecranon. The ulnar nerve is identified, and if a femoral translocation is carried out, it is released from the margin of the triceps and elevated from its bed (Fig. 1-17). The cubital tunnel retinaculum is split and the nerve is released to the first motor branch. A subcutaneous pocket is developed, the intermuscular septum is removed (Fig. 1-18), and the nerve is translated anteriorly. The triceps is released from the entire posterior aspect of the distal humerus. The forearm fascia and ulnar periosteum are elevated from the medial margin of the ulna. The Sharpey fiber attachment of the triceps to the olecranon is released by sharp dissection (Fig. 1-19). The distal forearm fascia and ulnar periosteum are elevated from the ulna. The lateral margin of the proximal ulna is then identified and the anconeus is elevated from its ulnar bed (Fig. 1-20). The extensor mechanism and capsule continues to be reflected from the margin of the lateral epicondyle (Fig. 1-21). If a medial column fracture has occurred, the tip of the olecranon is removed and the fracture may be addressed. For semiconstrained total elbow arthroplasty the lateral and medial collateral ligaments are released and the extensor mechanism is reflected lateral to the epicondyle. The elbow is flexed and the tip of the olecranon is removed to expose the joint (Fig. 1-22).

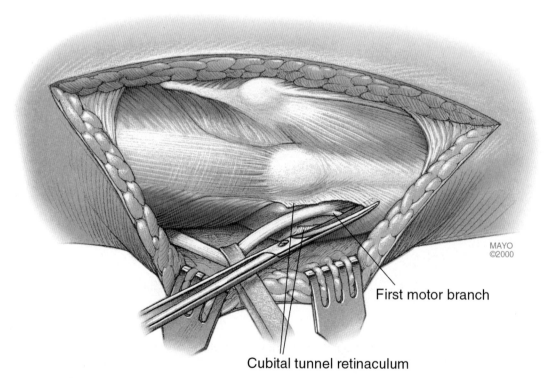

MAYO
©2000

First motor branch

Cubital tunnel retinaculum

FIG. 1-17. Through a posterior skin incision, the ulnar nerve has been identified and dissected from its bed at the margin of the triceps. The cubital tunnel retinaculum has been released with further dissection to the first motor branch. It is translocated anterior to the medial epicondyle to a subcutaneous pocket.

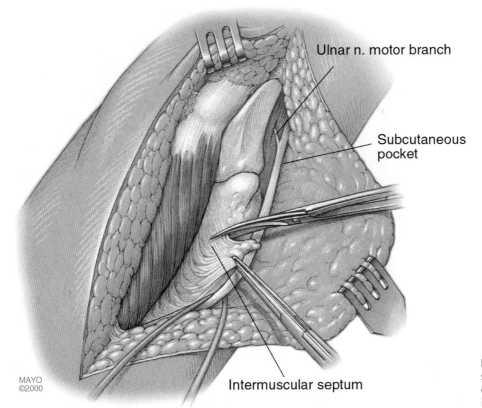

Ulnar n. motor branch

Subcutaneous
pocket

Intermuscular septum

MAYO
©2000

FIG. 1-18. The intermuscular
septum is removed to avoid
compression on the nerve with
its new anterior course.

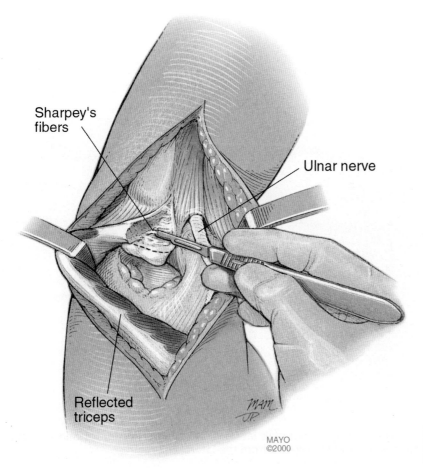

Sharpey's
fibers

Ulnar nerve

Reflected
triceps

MAYO
©2000

FIG. 1-19. Incontinuity elevation of the
insertion of the triceps from the olecranon.

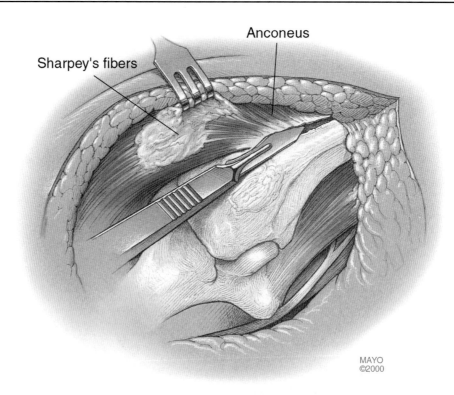

FIG. 1-20. The forearm fascia and ulnar periosteum has been elevated from the ulna distally, the triceps from the posterior aspect of the humerus proximally, and the insertion in the triceps is further reflected from its insertion into the tip of the olecranon. Further reflection laterally allows identification of the anconeus, which is then elevated from its ulnar insertion.

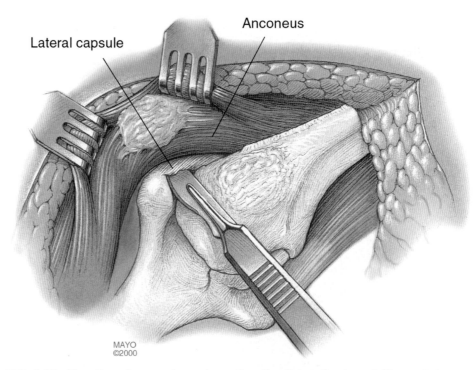

FIG. 1-21. The dissection continues laterally, allowing reflection of fibers of the extensor mechanism and the capsule from the lateral column.

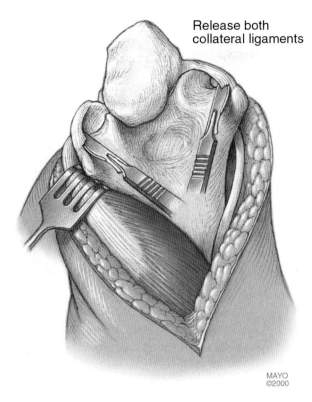

Release both
collateral ligaments

MAYO
©2000

FIG. 1-22. By subluxing the extensor mechanism lateral to the lateral condyle, the lateral ulnar collateral ligament may be released. For total elbow arthroplasty the medial collateral ligament is also released, allowing complete exposure of the ulnohumeral joint.

The Triceps

In every instance in which the triceps has been completely reflected either from lateral to medial (Fig. 1-14) or from medial to lateral (Fig. 1-21) it is always securely reattached to the olecranon with a crisscross type of suture. Drill holes about 3 cm in length are placed in a cruciate fashion in the olecranon from proximal to distal (Fig. 1-23A). A third transverse hole is drilled through the olecranon to secure a second stabilizing suture (Fig. 1-23B). The margin of the triceps is first grasped with an Alis clamp and brought over the olecranon (Fig. 1-24A). A No. 5 nonabsorbable suture is introduced with a straight needle from distal lateral to proximal medial for the modified Kocher and from distal medial to proximal lateral for the Mayo exposure. The suture is first brought through the tip of the olecranon and passes through the triceps tissue at its anatomic attachment site with the elbow in 90 degrees (Fig. 1-24A). A Bunnell type of crisscross suture is then placed in the triceps tendon, after which the suture enters the opposite hole in the olecranon now being passed from proximal to distal. After the suture has emerged from the second hole in the olecranon it is brought back over the top of the ulna through the soft-tissue distal expansion of the extensor sleeve (Fig. 1-24B). Care is taken to tie this stitch off to the side of the subcutaneous border of the ulna to avoid irritation or skin erosion. The second suture is placed transversely across the ulna, again, beginning on the side from which the triceps reflection began (Fig. 1-25). It is simply brought back across the triceps tendon in a transverse fashion to snugly stabilize the triceps insertion against the olecranon. All sutures are tied with the elbow in 90 degrees of flexion, again with the knots off the subcutaneous border.

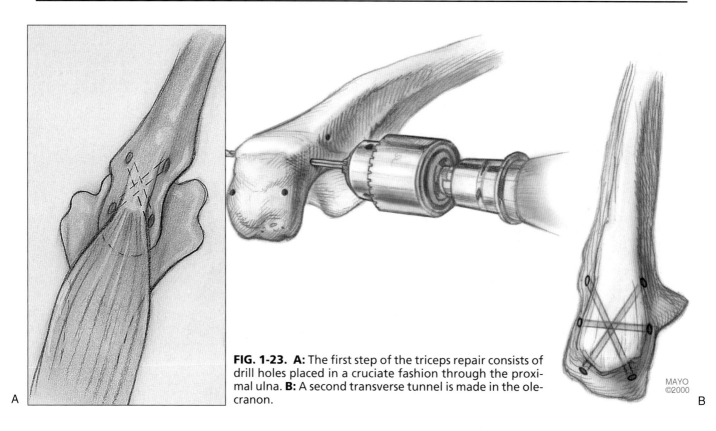

FIG. 1-23. A: The first step of the triceps repair consists of drill holes placed in a cruciate fashion through the proximal ulna. **B:** A second transverse tunnel is made in the olecranon.

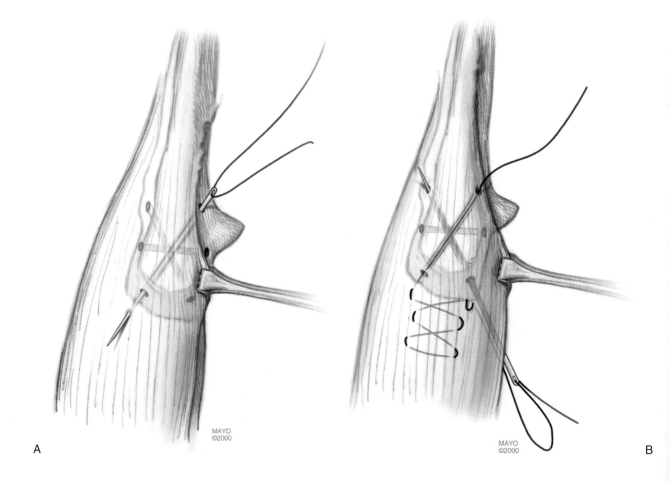

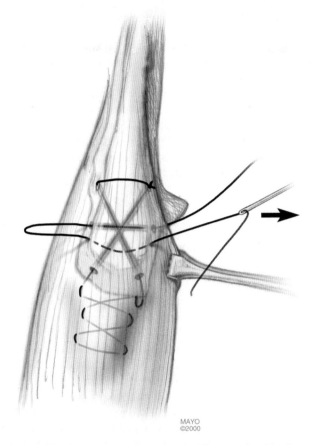

MAYO
©2000

FIG. 1-25. A transverse suture is then typically placed across the proximal ulna, further securing the triceps mechanism to its ulnar insertion.

Closure

For both medial and lateral exposures, if an interval has been entered it is reapproximated. On the lateral side, a running-0 absorbable suture is used to close Kocher's interval. The common extensor and common flexor muscles are reattached. If needed, two holes are placed in the supracondylar ridge and the ECRL, and the remaining portion of the common extensor tendon are reattached directly to bone.

Skin closure is with staples, although sometimes a subcuticular stitch is used, particularly in females. The aftercare varies dramatically, depending upon the pathology being addressed, and this is discussed in the appropriate chapter. It is worthy of note, however, that I typically splint the elbow in extension with an anterior splint. This protects the incision and may help reduce the tendency to develop flexion contracture.

FIG. 1-24. A: The triceps is reduced and a No. 5 nonabsorbable suture begins from distal to proximal, starting on the side of the reflected extensor mechanism, thus medially for the Mayo approach and laterally for the extensile Kocher approach. **B:** The suture is crisscrossed in the triceps tendon and then brought back through the other drill hole in the ulna. The suture is tied to the margin of the ulna, taking care to avoid the subcutaneous border.

MEDIAL EXTENSILE EXPOSURES (5)

Comment: It is suggested the medial extensile exposure now be termed the *medial column approach,* as it is analogous to that of the lateral side (Hotchkiss R, Personal Communication, April 1999).

The procedure is indicated if there is access to the coronoid with intact radial head and anterior capsule release, ulnar nerve dissection is required, there is a need to preserve the posterolateral ulnohumeral ligament complex, anterior and posterior access to the joint is needed, or conversion to triceps-sparing exposure of Bryan-Morrey anticipated.

It is less desirable if there is need of excision of heterotopic bone on the lateral side or access to radial head is needed.

SURGERY

The patient is usually supine, supported by a hand or elbow table. The patient's head may require support, and a roll is placed under the scapula.

The deep exposure may be accessed through a midline posterior incision or a posterior medial incision. The key to this exposure is identification of the medial supracondylar ridge of the humerus, the medial intermuscular septum, the origin of the flexor pronator muscle mass, and the ulnar nerve (Fig. 1-26).

The subcutaneous skin is elevated and the medial intermuscular septum is identified. Anterior to the septum, running just on top of the fascia (and not in the subdermal tissue), the medial antebrachial cutaneous nerve is identified and protected. It may occasionally be necessary to divide this nerve to gain full exposure and adequately mobilize the ulnar nerve, especially in revision surgery. If the patient has had previous surgery, the ulnar nerve is usually most easily identified proximally before proceeding distally. If a previous anterior transposition was performed, the nerve should be carefully identified both proximally and distally before proceeding.

The surface of the flexor pronator muscle mass origin is visualized by elevating and sweeping the subcutaneous tissue laterally as a flap with the medial antebrachial cutaneous nerve.

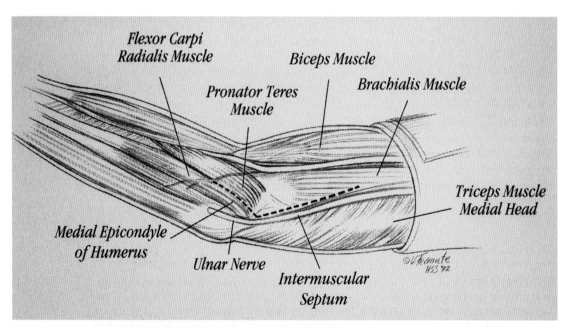

FIG. 1-26. Landmarks for the medial extensile exposure include the medial epicondyle, intramuscular septum, and ulnar nerve.

The medial intermuscular septum is identified anteriorly and posteriorly and then released for a distance of about 5 cm proximally (Fig. 1-27).

Locate the medial supracondylar ridge and begin elevating the anterior muscle with a periosteal elevator. Subperiosteally elevate enough of the anterior structures of the distal humeral region to allow the placement of a wide retractor. The median nerve, brachial artery, and vein are superficial to the brachialis muscle and are not identified. The flexor pronator muscle mass is divided in line with its fibers, leaving a portion of flexor carpi ulnaris tendon attached to the epicondyle (Fig. 1-28). A small cuff of fibrous tissue of the origin can be left on the supracondylar ridge as the muscle is elevated to facilitate reattachment when closing. The muscle is elevated from the capsule encountering the brachialis muscle laterally. A proximal, transverse incision in the lacertus fibrosis may also be needed to adequately mobilize this layer of muscle. The muscle is elevated from the capsule as the dissection proceeds laterally and distally, exposing the entire anterior capsule (Fig. 1-29). At this stage the pathology is addressed. If necessary the posterior capsule may be exposed by elevating the triceps from its lateral distal humeral attachment (Fig. 1-30).

We have found that the described surgical exposures to the elbow are sufficient, so virtually all the reconstructive procedures can be adequately performed. All may be executed after a posterior skin incision (Fig. 1-31). The surgeon should be aware that the classic extensile approach described by Kocher implies that the anterior capsule has been incised and the lateral collateral ligament has been released (6). The Mayo (R. S. Bryan) modification of the Kocher approach consists of reflection and release of the extensor mechanism from the tip of the olecranon in a fashion similar to that described for the Mayo approach (1) (see Fig. 1-11). This permits much better exposure of both humeral and ulnar articular surfaces. However, if reflected, the triceps must be securely reattached to bone. Further, when the Mayo modified Kocher release has been performed, the ulnar nerve must be exposed and released as necessary to avoid compression with varus angular forearm manipulation.

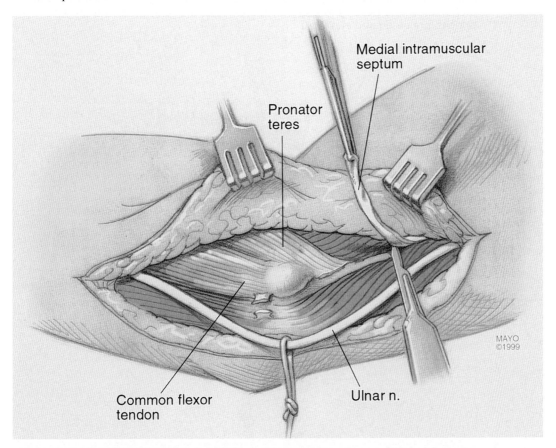

FIG. 1-27. The dissection is carried to the intramuscular septum, which is released.

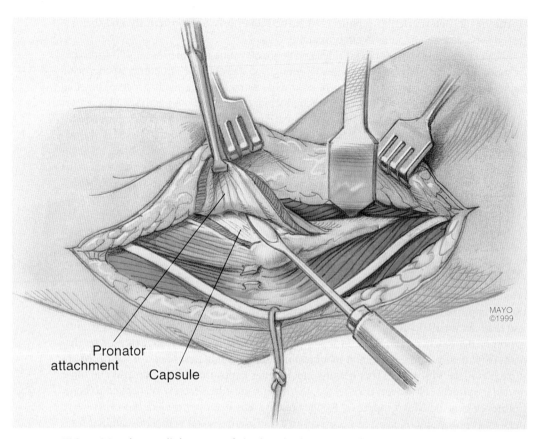

FIG. 1-28. The medial aspect of the brachialis is identified and elevated from the distal humerus. The flexor and pronator muscle mass are identified. The pronator component is released and elevated.

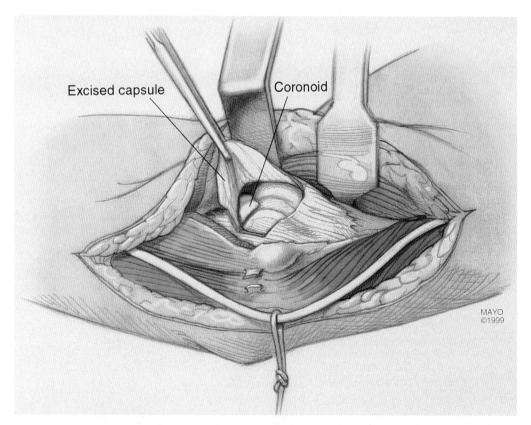

FIG. 1-29. The entire sleeve of soft tissue is elevated from the capsule.

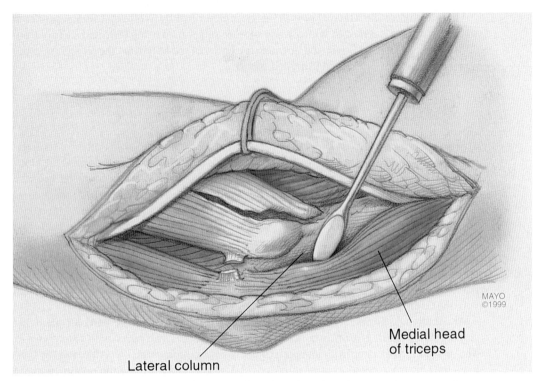

FIG. 1-30. The posterior column is exposed by elevating the triceps and anconeus from the posterior aspect of the lateral column.

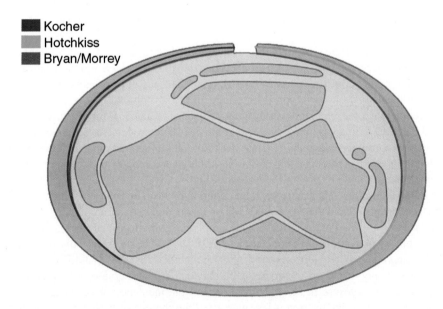

FIG. 1-31. The posterior skin incision allows ready exposure of the medial and lateral aspects of the joint by mobilization of the cutaneous flaps medially and laterally.

Modification of the Mayo approach has been described by Wolfe and Ranawat (12) in which the triceps is removed with a wafer of bone rather than being reflected sharply from the olecranon. Finally, conversion or extension between the Mayo and the Hotchkiss experience is readily accomplished if needed.

RESULTS

There have been limited attempts to document the efficacy of one or the other of the various types of triceps-sparing approaches. In the original description we compared the clinical result of the Mayo approach to that of the triceps splitting or transverse release of the triceps attachment (1). There were no triceps disruptions after approximately 75 procedures done with the triceps being released in continuity (Mayo approach) compared with an approximately 20% complication rate when the triceps was released transversely. Wolfe and Ranawat (12) have also observed no instances of triceps insufficiency with their modification of this approach. The use of the Mayo medial exposure was also shown to have improved triceps strength after total elbow arthroplasty (8). This manner of exposing the elbow was found to be associated with approximately 20% greater extension strength than with the Campbell (Van Gorder) type of exposure.

An additional consideration in those with rheumatoid arthritis is the thin olecranon that compromises healing if an osteotomy is carried out (3). The transverse osteotomy of McAusland is associated with an approximately 5% nonunion rate (7). Although for fractures the chevron osteotomy may improve these results and decrease the nonunion rate, I personally have not had the clinical need to osteotomize the olecranon in the last 14 years, and this should be avoided if the olecranon has been thinned.

COMPLICATIONS

One beauty of the previously described exposures is that they are relatively free of complication. Today most problems are related to the pathology rather than to the surgical approach.

Difficult ankylosis release procedures are associated with a significant amount of swelling as often occurs in patients undergoing total elbow arthroplasty. Wound healing is generally not a problem, however, and is related to the presence of prior incisions and the magnitude of the dissection, as is typical for release of the stiff elbow.

The infection rate after total elbow arthroplasty has been reduced at our institution from a high of 11% in 1970 to approximately 3% over the last 10 years (8). This reduction is coincident with adopting the Mayo approach to the elbow, but other technique changes have occurred in this period, including using antibiotic-impregnated cement and splinting the elbow in extension.

Injury to the ulnar nerve appears to be more common in those instances in which the ulnar nerve is not exposed and the elbow is flexed on the medial collateral ligament, as with the classical extensile Kocher approach (2,11). Simply exposing the ulnar nerve, although it decreases this complication, does not completely obviate it. The theoretical disadvantage of the Mayo approach, which allows translocation of the ulnar nerve, is that this maneuver devascularizes the nerve and the dissection itself may cause ulnar nerve irritation. Having used this particular exposure in more than 500 cases, the incidence of permanent ulnar nerve injury with motor dysfunction is less than 1%. I am therefore comfortable exposing and moving the ulnar nerve in a subcutaneous pocket as an essential and integral part of the Mayo triceps-sparing approach.

Although posterior interosseous nerve palsy is known to occur with some approaches to the radial nerve (4,10), the complication is virtually unheard of when the joint is exposed through Kocher's interval.

Triceps disruption is very uncommon with either the Mayo modified extensile Kocher exposure or the Mayo medial-to-lateral type of approach.

The incidence of triceps disruption therefore is less than 1% in our experience (9). If, however, the triceps should become disrupted after either of the procedures described earlier, if adequate tissue is present, it may be reattached as described for the primary procedure. If the remaining tissue is inadequate, triceps power is restored by either an anconeus slide or an Achilles tendon allograft reconstruction (see Chapter 11).

RECOMMENDED READINGS

 1. Bryan RS, Morrey BF. Extensive posterior exposure of the elbow: a triceps-sparing approach. *Clin Orthop* 1982;166:188.
 2. Ewald FC, Jacobs MA. Total elbow arthroplasty. *Clin Orthop* 1984;182:137.
 3. Inglis AE, Ranawat CS, Straub LR. Synovectomy and debridement of the elbow in rheumatoid arthritis. *J Bone Joint Surg* 1971;53A:652.
 4. Kaplan EB. Surgical approaches to the proximal end of the radius and its use in fractures of the head and neck of the radius. *J Bone Joint Surg* 1941;23:86.
 5. Kasparyan NG, Hotchkiss RN. Dynamic skeletal fixation in the upper extremity. *Hand Clin* 1997;13:643–663.
 6. Kocher T. *Text-book of operative surgery,* 3rd ed. London: A and C Black; 1911.
 7. Morrey BF. Surgical exposures of the elbow. In: Morrey BF, ed. *The elbow and its disorders*. Philadelphia: WB Saunders; 1985.
 8. Morrey BF, Askew LJ, An KN. Strength function after elbow arthroplasty. *Clin Orthop* 1988;234:43–50.
 9. Morrey BF, Bryan RS. Complications of total elbow arthroplasty. *Clin Orthop* 1982;170:204–212.
10. Strachan JH, Ellis BW. Vulnerability of the posterior interosseous nerve during radial head resection. *J Bone Joint Surg* 1971;53B:320.
11. Trancik T, Wilde AH, Borden LS. Capitellocondylar elbow arthroplasty. Two to eight year experience. *Clin Orthop* 1987;112:175.
12. Wolfe SW, Ranawat CS. The osteo-anconeus flap: an approach for total elbow arthroplasty. *J Bone Joint Surg* 1990;72A:684.

2

Arthroscopy of the Elbow

Shawn W. O'Driscoll and Felix H. Savoie III

Arthroscopy is probably the area of greatest growth and advance in the treatment of elbow disorders in recent years. It is now being performed by an ever-increasing number of surgeons for a wide variety of conditions (2,4,5,9,11,16,17,19,24,28,30,32,35). It is useful both for diagnosis and treatment, but the techniques are demanding, and potentially devastating neurovascular injuries are a concern (4,9,17,28,34). As elbow arthroscopy assumes a greater role in the diagnosis and management of elbow problems, definite indications are still emerging. Here we present the emerging techniques. Great caution must be exercised in expanding one's competency.

INDICATIONS/CONTRAINDICATIONS

Diagnostic Arthroscopy

Diagnostic arthroscopy does not substitute for a careful history and physical examination and routine investigation. The indications for diagnostic arthroscopy in general are (a) undiagnosed pain with abnormalities on clinical or radiographic examination, (b) suspected loose body, (c) snapping (or clicking, locking, clunking, etc.), (d) the need to obtain a biopsy, (e) contracture of spontaneous onset, (f) evaluation of valgus instability in overhead athletes, and (g) suspicion of an intraarticular benign tumor such as an osteoid osteoma. Patients with pain but no abnormalities on careful clinical examination, radiographs, or other investigations rarely are diagnosed by arthroscopy. Absence of physical or other findings is a relative contraindication, unless it is being performed to prove that no intraarticular pathology exists.

S.W. O'Driscoll, M.D., PH.D.: Orthopedic Surgery, Mayo Medical School, Mayo Foundation, Rochester, Minnesota.

F.H. Savoie III, M.D.: Upper Extremity Department, Mississippi Sports Medicine, Jackson, Mississippi.

Therapeutic Arthroscopy

Until recently the major indications for operative arthroscopy were (a) removal of loose bodies, (b) synovectomy, (c) debridement of the joint surface or adhesions, and (d) excision of posterior osteophytes causing impingement, as occurs in athletes and in early osteoarthritis. More recently, release of contractures and osteocapsular arthroplasty for osteoarthritis have become increasingly common. With release of contractures one must consider the risk of neurovascular injury. The ability to distend the capsule, which is so essential for displacement of the nerves away from the portals, is greatly reduced in stiff elbows (8). Endoscopy has also been used to treat olecranon bursitis (25) and lateral epicondylitis (14).

PREOPERATIVE PLANNING

One cannot overstate the necessity for a careful history and physical examination. Standard anteroposterior (AP) and lateral radiographs are usually sufficient, although oblique views are sometimes helpful. Magnetic resonance imaging (MRI) and computed tomography (CT) scans offer little help and are rarely indicated. Arthrography is not necessary.

A very important point is to determine preoperatively whether or not the ulnar nerve subluxates or dislocates anteriorly. If it does, as is the case in 16% of the population, it is at risk for injury when the anterior medial portal is established.

Loose bodies are to be suspected in a patient with mechanical symptoms, including locking, catching, or snapping, and are often seen in association with degenerative changes such as osteophytes on the olecranon and coronoid or osteochondritis dissecans. They do not cause flexion contractures; those patients almost always have associated posterior-impinging osteophytes on the olecranon and in the olecranon fossa, as part of an early degenerative process.

Standard AP and lateral radiographs are obtained routinely, and oblique views are sometimes helpful. Unfortunately, as many as 30% of loose bodies are not detected on plain radiographs (24). Thus it is wise to evaluate the entire elbow thoroughly at the time of arthroscopy so that none are missed. Patients undergoing arthroscopy for removal of anterior loose bodies should all be arthroscoped posteriorly as well. Especially in degenerative conditions, one will often find loose bodies "that are not loose" (i.e., that are stuck in the soft tissues and only minimally mobile).

Surgery

In no other joint is portal anatomy as critical as in the elbow. The proximity of the neurovascular structures demands accurate portal placement. Although many portals have been described, there are nine primary working portals about the elbow. A thorough knowledge of anatomy and of the approximate location of these portals is essential to avoid complications.

On the medial side there are two useful portals. The proximal anteromedial portal as described by Poehling et al. is favored by most prone arthroscopists (30). It allows full access to the anterior aspect of the elbow joint with minimal risks of neurovascular structures. The essential at-risk structure in utilizing these portals is the ulnar nerve. It is therefore mandatory that one stay anterior to the intermuscular septum in establishing this portal. It is usually located 2 cm above the medial epicondyle and approximately 1 to 2 cm anterior to the intermuscular septum (Fig. 2-1).

The standard anteromedial portal is located approximately 2 cm anterior and 2 cm distal to the medial epicondyle. The median nerve, brachial artery, and ulnar nerve are all at risk in utilizing this portal (1). It also allows full access to the anterior aspect of the elbow (Fig. 2-2).

On the lateral side, there are actually four portals that may be utilized in anterior com-

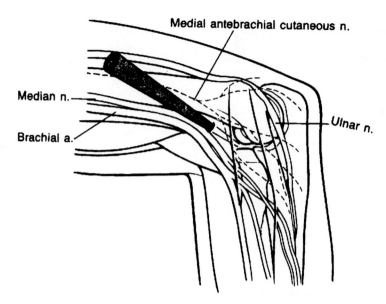

Figure 2-1. Proximal anteromedial portal.

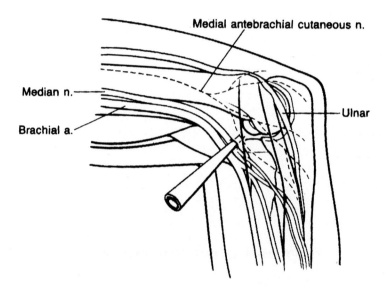

Figure 2-2. Standard anteromedial portal.

partment arthroscopy of the elbow. The standard anterolateral portal is usually described as being 1 cm distal and 3 cm anterior to the lateral epicondyle. This portal, initially described by Andrews and Carson, courses in close proximity to the posterior interosseous nerve (Fig. 2-3) (2).

The midanterolateral portal is located approximately 2 cm directly anterior to the lateral epicondyle. Although this portal provides less risk to the radial nerve, it still may come in close proximity to the radial nerve. This portal is useful in debriding the anterior aspect of the radial head during radial head excision (Fig. 2-4).

The proximal anterolateral portal is utilized by many authors as a diagnostic portal. Described separately by Day and by Field et al., this portal provides a maximum safety buffer by utilizing the brachialis muscle as a cushion to protect the radial nerve (7,33). It is useful primarily in diagnostic anterior compartment arthroscopy of the elbow and in lateral epicondylectomy and capsular release procedures (Fig. 2-5).

The straight lateral or soft spot portal can be used in anterior compartment arthroscopy as well. Although somewhat difficult to enter, an incision is made directly over the radial

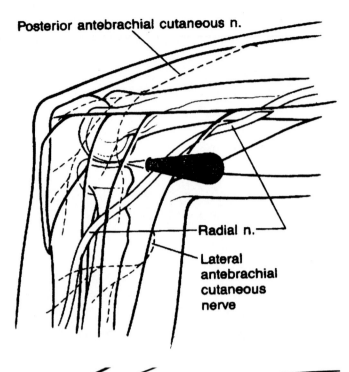

Figure 2-3. Standard anterolateral portal.

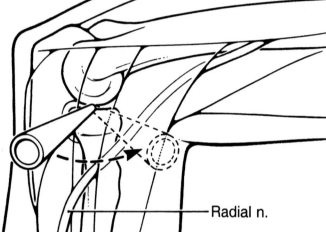

Figure 2-4. Standard anterior midlateral portal.

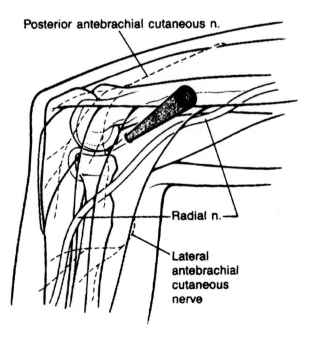

Figure 2-5. Proximal anterolateral portal.

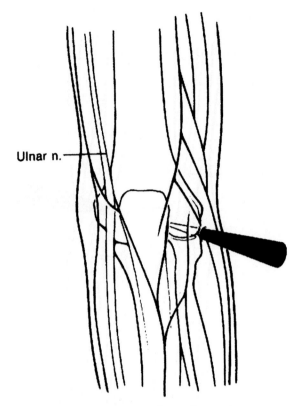

Figure 2-6. Midlateral portal.

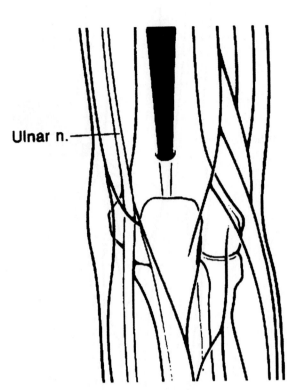

Figure 2-7. Posterior central portal.

capitellar articulation and the soft tissues are immobilized to allow the cannula to enter the anterior aspect of the elbow (Fig. 2-6).

Posteriorly, there are three portals primarily utilized in posterior elbow compartment arthroscopy. The straight posterior or posterocentral portal is located approximately 3 cm above the tip of the olecranon (Fig. 2-7). This is primarily used in visualizing the medial and lateral compartments as well as the olecranon fossa. It is also used for instrumentation in ulnohumeral arthroplasty, olecranon spur excision, and debridement of medial gutter and elevation of the triceps in arthrofibrotic patients.

The superior posterolateral portal can be located anywhere from the level of the tip of the olecranon to 3 cm proximal to this area in the posterolateral gutter. It is established outside the triceps tendon and is useful in debriding the olecranon fossa and in visualizing the fossa during ulnohumeral arthroplasty. This is also useful in debriding the lateral gutter and in visualizing both the tip of the olecranon and the posterolateral gutter (Fig. 2-8).

The more inferior posterolateral portal is located in the posterolateral gutter at the level of the radiocapitellar articulation. Also known as the soft-spot portal (Fig. 2-9), it allows complete access to the posterolateral gutter and is useful in debriding posterolateral plica, osteochondritis dissecans of the capitellum, and in excising the radial head.

Loose-Body Removal

Loose-body removal has been considered the prime indication for elbow arthroscopy. Success rates have been consistently reported in the 90% range or better (4,18,20,22,27).

The lateral decubitus position is preferred (Fig. 2-10).

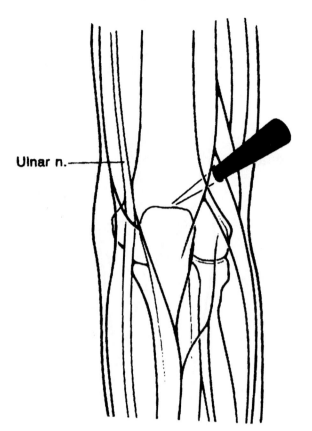

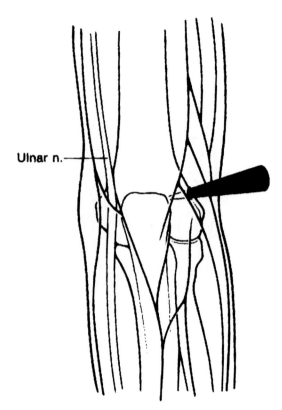

Figure 2-8. Proximal posterolateral portal.

Figure 2-9. Distal posterolateral portal.

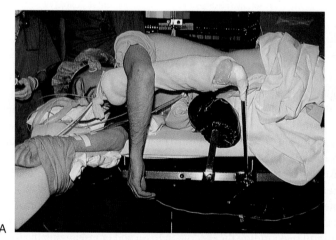

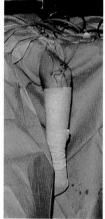

Figure 2-10. A: The patient is placed in the lateral decubitus position with the arm resting on a padded bolster. The arm hangs free with the elbow flexed to 90 degrees. **B:** The forearm and hand are wrapped with an elastic bandage. This combination of forearm wrapping and tourniquet application limits the intraoperative swelling to the region of the elbow and permits rapid diffusion of any accumulated fluid from the elbow region.

Technique

Instruments and their use are important considerations in loose-body removal (Fig. 2-11). Loose bodies are removed with various-sized graspers that have teeth. Those that are smooth on their outside surface, without irregular surfaces or corners, work best, as they do not catch on the soft tissues as they exit the elbow. Always grasp loose bodies so that they

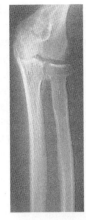
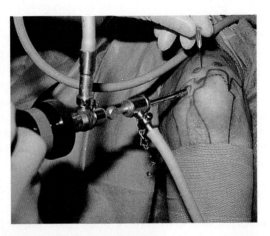
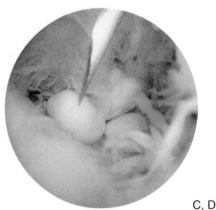

A, B   C, D

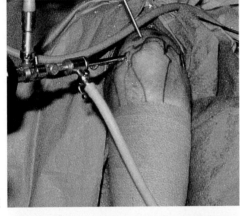
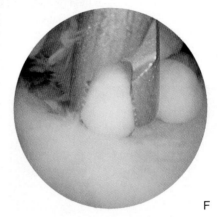

E   F

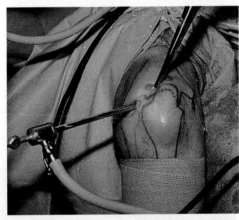
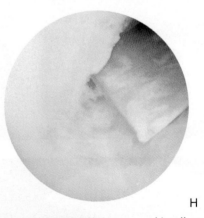

G   H

Figure 2-11. A typical case example illustrating many of the techniques used in elbow arthroscopy. **A,B:** Radiographs of a patient with synovial osteochondromatosis. **C,D:** Technique for posterior compartment surgery and establishing the appropriate position of the portal. The arthroscope is directed to the posterior compartment, where loose bodies are seen. A needle is introduced in the precise position that one estimates to be ideal for the portal to be established. **E,F:** After establishing the portal with a knife under direct vision, a grasping instrument is inserted to remove the loose body. The remaining loose bodies are similarly removed. **G,H:** The area of synovial osteochondromatosis that is adherent to the posterior aspect of the humerus at the edge of the olecranon fossa is osteotomized with a small, curved osteotome under direct vision. This is quicker and more efficient than using a bur or a small biting instrument, which tends to make the risk rather tedious. If the osteotomized piece is large, it can be fragmented for removal.

can be pulled out longitudinally, rather than obliquely or transversely, which often requires that they be rotated into position for the grasper. Grasp them very firmly. Rotate them fully so as to confirm they are not still attached to soft tissue prior to extraction. Observe the fragment until it exits the capsule so that it can be recovered if lost from the jaws of the grasper. Check each one after extraction, to confirm a fragment has not broken off in the soft tissues. Rotate the loose body in the soft tissues to "work it out." Large loose bodies in the anterior elbow can be pushed out with the sheath of the scope (uncouple and back the scope itself out of the sheath a few millimeters to avoid damaging the lens) while pulling it with the grasper. Finally, don't hesitate to enlarge the portal somewhat rather than risk losing the fragment in the soft tissues.

Debridement

Debridement, or ectomy surgery, in the elbow is used for radial head excision, excision of olecranon or coronoid spurs, arthroscopic ulnohumeral arthroplasty, or olecranon fenestration and in lateral epicondylitis.

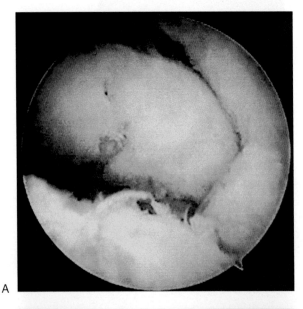

A

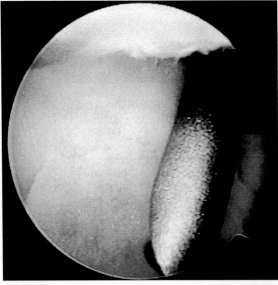

B

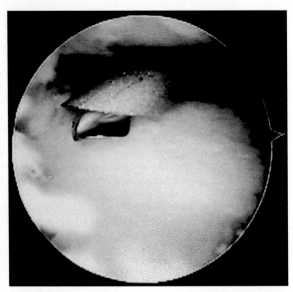

C

Figure 2-12. A: Arthritic radial head. **B:** Anterior debridement of an arthritic radial head. **C:** Coplaning through a posterior soft portal of the radial head.

In radial head excision the arthroscope is placed in the proximal medial portal and the midlateral portal is used for instrumentation (Fig. 2-12A). The anterior aspect of the radial head is resected to prevent penetration of the anterior capsule. *Penetration of the anterior capsule in this area will result in damage to the posterior interosseous nerve.* It is essential that during arthroscopic radial head excision the anterolateral capsule not be violated by the shaver; otherwise, significant neurologic complications will occur. Once a majority of the anterior aspect of the radial head has been excised (Fig. 2-12B), the inflow is placed in this anterolateral portal and a soft-spot portal is utilized to bring the shaver from the posterior into the anterior compartment. This shaver is then used to plane the posterior aspect of the radial head until it is even with the resected anterior margin (Fig. 2-12C). In cases of radiocapitellar impingement this planing is continued for distances of approximately 6 mm. In cases in which there is proximal radial ulnar joint involvement, this is continued until the proximal radial ulnar joint is completely free of the remaining proximal radial head.

Synovectomy

Synovectomy is a challenging version of the debridement operation. The very idea of attempting a total arthroscopic synovectomy may provoke anxiety. First, the radial nerve lies right against, or within a few millimeters of, the anterolateral joint capsule (Fig. 2-13). Second, the ulnar nerve lies adjacent to the capsule in the posteromedial gutter. Add to these perils the fact that diffuse proliferative synovitis such as that seen in rheumatoid arthritis can obliterate one's view of the joint.

To ensure accurate visualization start working in an area that does not place structures at risk (e.g., the olecranon fossa). The initial work can be done with poor visualization if both the scope and the shaver are in the fossa. Then work toward the medial gutter. Small pituitary rongeurs are useful for beginning to clear the gutter. The synovium is grasped without fully closing the jaws, so as not to pull out the capsule or ulnar nerve. As the view enlarges, a 3.5 shaver can be used, with the side cutting opening facing away from the nerve (toward the scope) and gravity outflow without suction. In the anterior elbow, we use a third portal, such as the proximal anterolateral portal, to place a retractor. A Howarth blunt periosteal elevator that is easy to place and broad enough to be effective in retracting the anterior capsule is inserted. Start working with the shaver against the distal humerus and

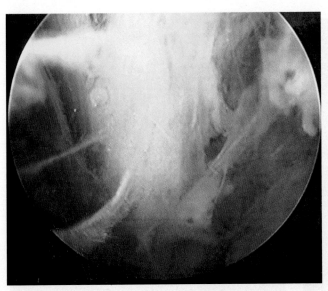
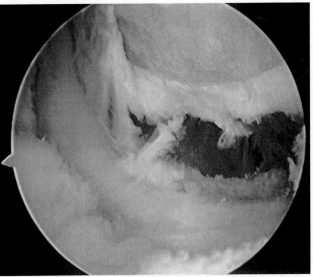

A   B

Figure 2-13. Visualization of the radial (**A**) and ulnar nerves (**B**) reveal their proximity to the capsule and vulnerability to injury.

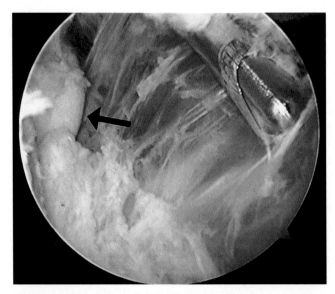

Figure 2-14. Removal of tissue from the capsule is performed without suction. *Arrow* identifies the radial head.

progress from proximal to distal and from medial to lateral. Again, by having the shaver connected only to gravity outflow and with the opening facing away from the capsule (Fig. 2-14), one can sweep across the capsule and remove the synovium without perforating the capsule. Capsular release is usually required not just to restore motion, but to eliminate the pain at the limits of motion.

At the completion of the procedure the wounds are sutured, the tourniquet and elastic bandage are removed, and the swelling around the elbow is manually compressed to decrease it. Moving the elbow passively through an arc of motion several times assists in this regard.

Olecranon Spur Excision

In excision of an olecranon spur, care must be taken not to damage the triceps tendon or to involve the ulnar nerve. The arthroscope is placed in the superior posterolateral portal and

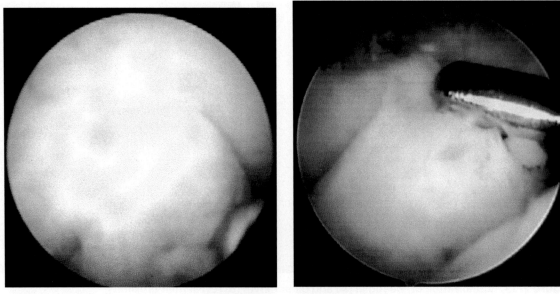

Figure 2-15. A: Olecranon spur. **B:** Shaver in place.

the shaver in the posterior central portal. The spur is evaluated and the margin of excision is delineated (Fig. 2-15A). The shaver is then used to resect the spur using a medial-to-lateral direction of movement (Fig. 2-15B). It is important that the suction be left off when working along the medial gutter to prevent injury to the ulnar nerve. Bony excision is continued until the spur and deformity are excised (Fig. 2-15C). It is essential that extensive resection of the olecranon tip be avoided to prevent worsening onset of instability symptoms.

Ulnohumeral Arthroplasty

Olecranon fenestration, or ulnohumeral arthroplasty, may allow increased motion in the arthritic elbow (32). Initially pioneered by Outerbridge and Kashiwago and refined by Morrey, this procedure has been adapted to arthroscopy with successful results (6). In this procedure, the arthroscope is placed in the proximal posterolateral portal and the instrumentation is placed in the posterior central or straight posterior portal. The olecranon fossa is evaluated (Fig. 2-16A) and a pilot hole is made in the center of the olecranon fossa (Fig. 2-16B). This pilot hole delineates the adequate orientation of the excision as well as the thickness of the olecranon fossa. The shaver is then introduced into this pilot drill hole for a distance of approximately 2 cm or until the tip of the coronoid and the tip of the olecranon recede on flexion and extension, respectively (Fig. 2-16C).

Lateral Epicondylitis

Baker has pioneered the use of the arthroscope in the management of lateral epicondylitis. In these patients, concomitant damage is also often noted to the capsule and to the posterolateral aspect of the elbow. In this initial view, the fenestrations of the capsule as a result of the chronic inflammation of lateral epicondylitis may be noted (Fig. 2-17A). The straight lateral portal is utilized to excise the capsule, allowing visualization of extensor carpi radialis brevis tendon and the contained Nirschl lesion (Fig. 2-17B). The shaver is then used to resect this lesion and abrade the bone (Fig. 2-17C). Occasionally, a cautery device may be used to further elevate this area and allow better access to the lateral epicondyle. Any concomitant calcification should be removed as well. Once the entire degenerative lesion has been excised and the epicondyle is abraded, the arthroscopic portion of the procedure is completed (Fig. 2-17D).

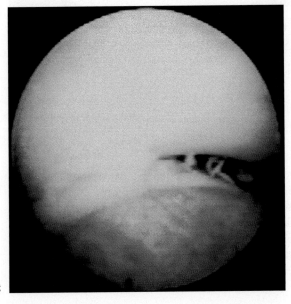

C

Figure 2-15. C: Spur excised.

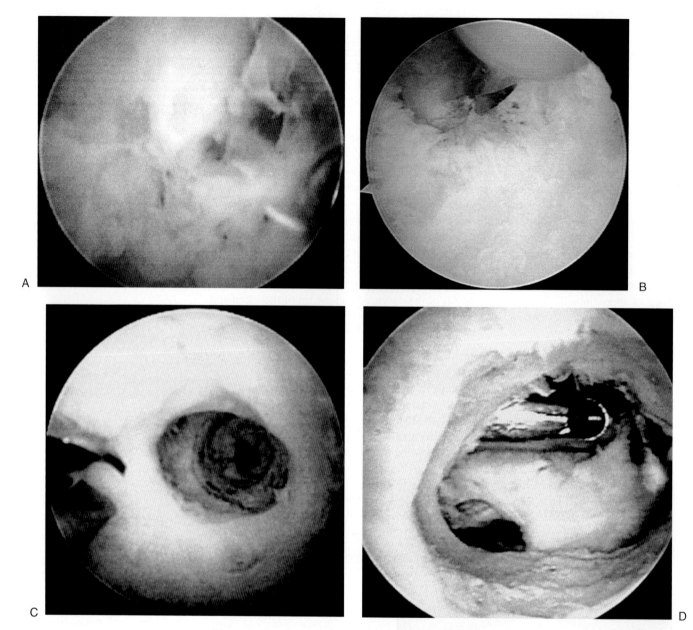

Figure 2-16. A: Olecranon fossa. **B:** Cannulated drill placed in olecranon fossa. **C:** Pilot drill hole. **D:** Completed ulnohumeral arthroplasty; shaver introduced through the anterior portal.

Osteocapsular Arthroplasty

One of the most rewarding arthroscopic interventions is osteocapsular arthroplasty for osteoarthritis (23,26). This procedure involves four components: (a) removal of all loose bodies, including those that are not loose but are stuck in the synovium; (b) removal of all osteophytes in the ulnohumeral articulation, including those on the olecranon, coronoid, and medial trochlea and in the three fossae—olecranon, coronoid, and radial; (c) total synovectomy; and (d) anterior and posterior capsulectomy, with posteromedial and posterolateral capsulectomy for those patients lacking significant degrees of flexion. In patients

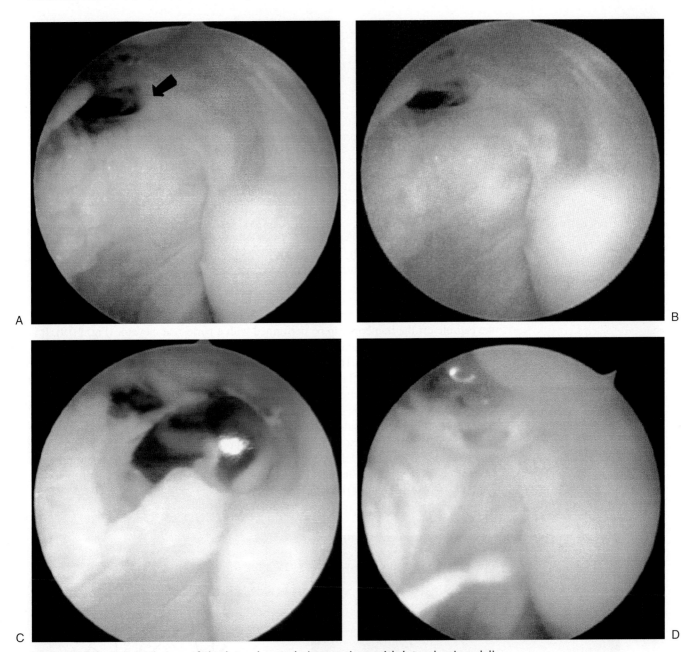

Figure 2-17. **A:** Initial view of the lateral capsule in a patient with lateral epicondylitis. Note rent in capsule (*arrow*). **B:** The angiofibrotic dysplasia or degenerative lesion of the tendon of the extensor carpi radialis brevis tendon or so-called Nirschl lesion as visualized arthroscopically. **C:** Excision of the lesion with a shaver placement during excision. **D:** Completed excision and abrasion of the lateral epicondyle.

with preexistent ulnar neuritis or neuropathy and those with severe loss of flexion, the ulnar nerve is transposed subcutaneously as well (Fig. 2-18).

This is an extensive operation, requiring substantial skill and experience. The respective loose body and synovectomy components of the operation are as described earlier. The osteophyte removal is accomplished with a combination of instruments, principally burrs. Osteotomes can be useful, but removal of the osteotomized fragment can be tedious because of sharp edges and soft-tissue attachments. The shaver (rather than burr) can be used once the bone has been cut into and trabecular bone has been exposed. A shaver is less likely than is a burr to wrap up soft tissue, which puts nerves at risk.

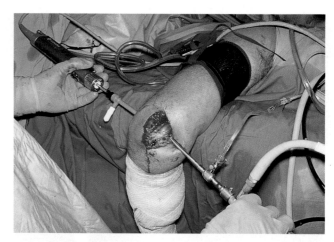

Figure 2-18. Open exposure of the ulnar nerve; translocation performed after the scope procedure.

Capsular release can be performed in one of three sequential stages. Blunt stripping of the capsule off the humerus can be performed with a periosteal elevator (Fig. 2-19). It is probably associated with minimal risk. However, it does not seem to be as effective as capsulotomy or capsulectomy. This is best and most safely performed with a hand instrument such as a wide duck-billed basket punch biopsy (Fig. 2-20). The anterior capsule is most safely cut across its midsection, starting from medial and working toward the lateral side. The plane of dissection between the capsule/scar and brachialis is more obvious medially than laterally. Finally, capsulectomy can be performed after the previous two stages have been completed. This is best performed with a shaver using no suction, but with the outflow on the shaver simply left open to let drainage fall to the floor. One should progress from proximal medial to distal medial, then from proximal lateral to distal lateral. This last region is the site of greatest risk of nerve injury.

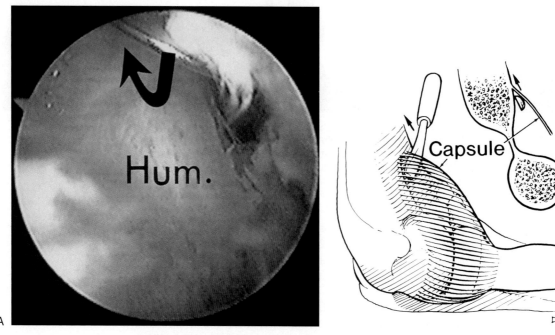

Figure 2-19. A,B: The capsule is stripped from the distal humerus by blunt pressure, if possible.

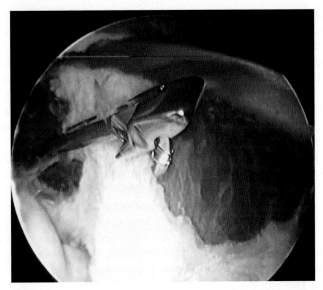

Figure 2-20. Capsulectomy with a blunt basket forceps.

In summary, to most effectively and safely perform these more complex osteocapsular procedures, one should proceed in a logical manner. First, establish the view and place one or two retractors into the joint. Second, clean up the joint by performing a synovectomy. Debride the capsule of any loose scar tissue so that it has the appearance and texture of a structure. Remove the osteophytes and clean up the bone debris. Strip the capsule off the humerus if not already done. (It is useful to do this earlier if the joint is quite tight.) Cut the capsule with the duckbill basket biopsy punch. Excise the capsule with the shaver. Then incise and resect the capsule just anterior to the medial and lateral collateral ligaments. By following this stepwise sequence, one can progress as far as one's skill permits with the least likelihood of complications.

POSTOPERATIVE MANAGEMENT

A compressive dressing is wrapped around the elbow, and the patient is instructed to start using the elbow as tolerated. It is kept elevated when not in use for the first day to decrease swelling. If the procedure was performed for improving motion or for the treatment of arthritis, an indwelling catheter is inserted for brachial plexus block anesthetic if the neurologic examination is normal in the recovery room, and the patient is started on a full range of motion on a continuous passive motion (CPM) machine the same day. All circumferential dressings must be removed to avoid skin damage during CPM. Only an elastic sleeve is used to hold the absorbent dressing in place.

In general, debridement surgery of whatever type follows a similar postoperative course. Soft dressings are placed on the arm, and the patient is asked to begin immediate motion. In cases of stiffness, CPM can be utilized for the first 3 to 10 days.

Wrist curls without weights, elbow flexion, and extension exercises are started at 1 week, and resistive exercises begin at 2 to 3 weeks. If necessary, formal strengthening is initiated by 3 to 4 weeks postoperatively. The patient is allowed to resume normal activities as tolerated usually 3 to 12 weeks after surgery.

RESULTS

O'Driscoll and Morrey evaluated the diagnostic and therapeutic usefulness of arthroscopy (24). A diagnostic arthroscopy was considered beneficial if a patient's outcome was positively influenced by the procedure; that is, the correct final diagnosis was (a) changed from that of the preoperative diagnosis, which was proved to be incorrect, (b) was established when the diagnosis could not be made preoperatively, or (c) was expanded or confirmed when the preoperative diagnosis was incomplete or uncertain. The procedure was said to be of therapeutic benefit to the patient if it was (a) completely successful and obviated the need for any further surgery, (b) partially successful in that the patient was clinically improved and needed no further surgery, or (c) adjunctive in that an important part of the operation was performed arthroscopically and the arthroscopy directed the surgical intervention in an important manner. Of the 71 consecutive arthroscopies in that series, approximately three-fourths of the patients who undergo arthroscopy of the elbow benefit (24). The distribution according to type of benefits was as follows: 31% diagnostic benefit, 24% both diagnostic and therapeutic benefit, and 17% therapeutic benefit only.

Those patients with pain and abnormal clinical or radiographic findings but for whom the diagnosis remains obscure or unknown can be diagnosed by arthroscopy in most cases. Those with suspected loose bodies usually are confirmed to have cartilaginous loose bodies or some other mechanical cause for their symptoms. Undiagnosed painful snapping of the elbow can be associated with loose bodies, radiohumeral plicae, posttraumatic arthritis, primary degenerative arthritis, dense soft-tissue adhesions (e.g., following radial head excision), and posterolateral rotatory instability. Patients with spontaneous onset of contracture typically are found to have a form of inflammatory arthritis, or osteoid osteoma, as in a series of our own cases (unpublished data). Valgus instability can be diagnosed with the arthroscopic valgus stress test described by Andrews (3,6).

Until recently the ideal indication for operative arthroscopy has been considered to be removal of loose bodies, with greater than 90% success rates reported (4,22,24). Currently, it has become our impression that treatment of osteoarthritis by osteocapsular arthroplasty, which includes excision of loose bodies and osteophytes from the olecranon and coronoid, as well as from each respective fossa, and capsular release may be one of the most gratifying procedures, as it is usually so predictably effective and beneficial in terms of both pain relief and restoration of motion (Fig. 2-21).

Redden and Stanley reported 12 of 12 patients with osteoarthritis and loose bodies to benefit from arthroscopic removal of osteophytes and loose bodies (31). They performed a fenestration of the distal humerus through the olecranon fossa to the coronoid fossa. They did not notice any improvement in elbow range of motion, presumably because they did not release the capsular contractures.

Little data exist regarding arthroscopic synovectomy. This is due to the fact that not until recently did we become comfortable with the technical challenges and execution of the procedure. Satisfactory pain relief is obtained in about 75% to 90% of cases. Range of motion is improved, particularly if one is careful to remove the contracted capsule and scar tissue around the elbow.

The role of radial head excision is not clear. Theoretically, the risk of late deterioration to increased biomechanical loading of the ulnohumeral articulation will occur if the radial head is excised. The radial head should probably be left in unless the preceding indications are present, as its role in stability would be greater in a rheumatoid elbow, which has already suffered bone loss and soft-tissue damage.

Lee and Morrey reported on 14 synovectomies in 11 patients with rheumatoid arthritis (15). They had a 93% early success, which declined to 57% by 3.5 years, but concluded that the decline might have been due to limitations of the arthroscopic technique. Those procedures were not total synovectomies and did not include capsular releases. Current experience in our institution suggests that both of these factors are important. Further follow-up will be necessary to ascertain the long-term benefit. Also, the role of arthroscopic synovectomy in more advanced stages of disease and joint destruction remains to be determined. Our experience indicates that a percentage of patients will benefit regardless of the stage of disease.

Arthroscopic capsular release for contracture of the elbow is being performed more frequently now. It has been shown by several authors to be effective (12,29), but complica-

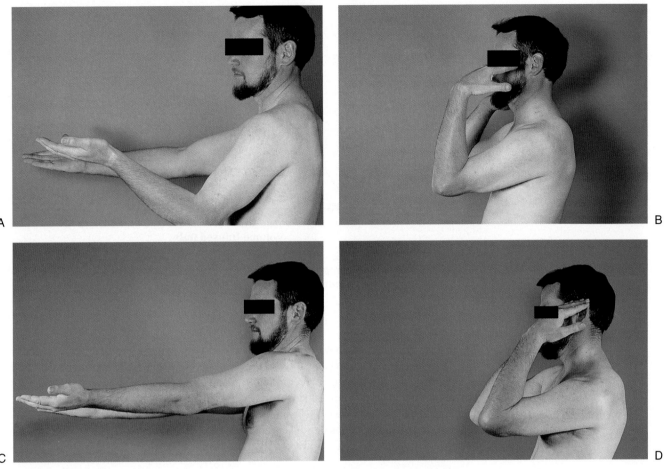

Figure 2-21. A–D: Pre- and postoperative motion after arthroscopic debridement.

tions such as nerve transection have been reported (10,12). Although the safety of this procedure remains to be confirmed, it seems likely that the decreased morbidity and increased surgical access to remove all contracted tissue may bring this procedure into the mainstay of treatment of the stiff elbow (21). The relative importance of capsulotomy versus capsulectomy is yet to be clarified.

COMPLICATIONS

In a review of almost 500 consecutive elbow arthroscopies at Mayo by Kelly et al., complications occurred in 11% (13). They include the following:

- Persistent drainage from the portals.
- Deep infection.
- Minor contractures, usually related to the nature of the underlying condition (such as inflammatory arthritis).
- Transient palsies caused by extravasation of local anesthetic, direct blunt trauma, compression by the tourniquet or forearm wrapping, or the use of the indwelling catheter postoperatively.

Permanent nerve injury. Although we have not experienced any permanent nerve or vascular injuries, the risk of injury to these structures is real, and transections of all three major nerves have been reported. The anterolateral and the anteromedial portals are most

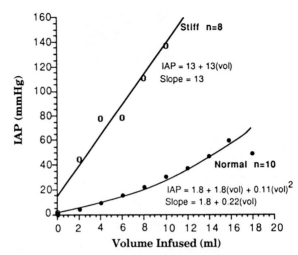

Figure 2-22. Intraarticular pressure (IAP) versus infusion volume: comparison of stiff and normal elbows. The capacity is greatly reduced in the stiff elbow.

likely to be associated with nerve injury because of the proximities of the radial, posterior interosseous, ulnar, and median nerves to these portals (2,16,17,28). These injuries are best avoided by careful technique and constant vigilance. The distances between these nerves and all the portals are increased substantially by flexing the elbow to 90 degrees and distending the joint with saline (28). Displacement of the nerves anteriorly away from the portals is accomplished by capsular distention with 15 to 25 mL of saline, but the average intracapsular capacity of stiff elbows is only 6 mL (Fig. 2-22).

RECOMMENDED READINGS

1. Adolfsson L. Arthroscopy of the elbow joint: a cadaveric study of portal placement. *J Shoulder Elbow Surg* 1994;3:53.
2. Andrews JR, Carson WG. Arthroscopy of the elbow. *Arthroscopy* 1985;1:97.
3. Andrews JR, Timmerman LA. Outcome of elbow surgery in professional baseball players. *Am J Sports Med* 1995;23:407–413.
4. Boe S. Arthroscopy of the elbow: diagnosis and extraction of loose bodies. *Acta Orthop Scand* 1986;57:52–53.
5. Clarke R. Symptomatic, lateral synovial fringe (plica) of the elbow joint. *Arthroscopy* 1988;4:112–116.
6. Field L, Altchek D. Evaluation of the arthroscopic valgus instability test of the elbow. *Am J Sports Med* 1996;24:177–181.
7. Field LD, Altcheck DW, Warren RF, et al. Arthroscopic anatomy of the lateral elbow: a comparison of three portals. *Arthroscopy* (in press).
8. Gallay SH, Richards RR, O'Driscoll SW. Intraarticular capacity and compliance of stiff and normal elbows. *Arthroscopy* 1993;9:9–13.
9. Guhl J. Arthroscopy and arthroscopic surgery of the elbow. *Orthopedics* 1985;8:1290–1296.
10. Haapaniemi T, Berggren M, Adolfsson L. Complete transection of the median and radial nerves during arthroscopic release of post-traumatic elbow contracture. *Arthroscopy* 1999;15:784–787.
11. Jackson D, Silvino N, Reiman P. Osteochondritis in the female gymnast's elbow. *Arthroscopy* 1989;5:129–136.
12. Jones GS, Savoie FH III. Arthroscopic capsular release of flexion contractures (arthrofibrosis) of the elbow. *Arthroscopy* 1993;9:277–283.
13. Kelly E, O'Driscoll S, Morrey BF. Complications of elbow arthroscopy. *J Bone Joint Surg* 2001;83A:25–34.
14. Kuklo TR, Taylor KF, Murphy KP, et al. Arthroscopic release for lateral epicondylitis: a cadaveric model. *Arthroscopy* 1999;15:259–264.
15. Lee BPH, Morrey BF. Arthroscopic synovectomy of the elbow for rheumatoid arthritis. *J Bone Joint Surg* 1997;79:770–772.
16. Lindenfeld TN. Medial approach in elbow arthroscopy. *Am J Sports Med* 1990;18:413–417.
17. Lynch G, Meyers J, Whipple T, et al. Neurovascular anatomy and elbow arthroscopy: inherent risks. *Arthroscopy* 1986;2:191–197.
18. McGinty J. Arthroscopic removal of loose bodies. *Orthop Clin North Am* 1982;13:313–328.
19. Morrey BF. Arthroscopy of the elbow. *Instr Course Lect* 1986;35:102–107.

20. O'Driscoll S. Elbow arthroscopy: loose bodies. In: Morrey B, ed. *The elbow and its disorders.* Philadelphia: WB Saunders; 2000:510–514.
21. O'Driscoll S. Elbow arthroscopy: the future. In: Morrey B, ed. *The elbow and its disorders.* Philadelphia: WB Saunders; 2000:522.
22. O'Driscoll SW. Elbow arthroscopy for loose bodies. *Orthopedics* 1992;15:855–859.
23. O'Driscoll SW. Arthroscopic treatment for osteoarthritis of the elbow. In: Weiss A-PC, ed. *The orthopedic clinics of North America, arthroscopy of the upper extremity.* Philadelphia: WB Saunders; 1995:691–706.
24. O'Driscoll SW, Morrey BF. Arthroscopy of the elbow: diagnostic and therapeutic benefits and hazards. *J Bone Joint Surg* 1992;74A:84–94.
25. Ogilvie-Harris DJ, Gilbart M. Endoscopic bursal resection: the olecranon bursa and prepatellar bursa. *Arthroscopy* 2000;16:249–253.
26. Ogilvie-Harris DJ, Gordon R, MacKay M. Arthroscopic treatment for posterior impingement in degenerative arthritis of the elbow. *Arthroscopy* 1995;11:437–443.
27. Ogilvie-Harris DJ, Schemitsch E. Arthroscopy of the elbow for removal of loose bodies. *Arthroscopy* 1993;9:5–8.
28. Papilion J, Neff R, Shall L. Compression neuropathy of the radial nerve as a complication of elbow arthroscopy: a case report and review of the literature. *Arthroscopy* 1988;4:284–286.
29. Phillips BB, Strasburger S. Arthroscopic treatment of arthrosibrosis of the elbow joint. *Arthroscopy* 1998;14:38–44.
30. Poehling G, Whipple T, Sisco L, et al. Elbow arthroscopy: a new technique. *Arthroscopy* 1989;5:222–224.
31. Redden JF, Stanley D. Arthroscopic fenestration of the olecranon fossa in the treatment of osteoarthritis of the elbow. *Arthroscopy* 1993;9:14–16.
32. Savoie FH, Nunley PD, Field LD. Arthroscopic management of the arthritic elbow: indications, technique, and results. *J Shoulder Elbow Surg* 1999;8:214–219.
33. Stothers K, Day B, Regan WR. Arthroscopy of the elbow: anatomy, portal sites and a description of the proximal lateral portal. *Arthroscopy* 1995;11:449–457.
34. Thomas M, Fast A, Shapiro D. Radial nerve damage as a complication of elbow arthroscopy. *Clin Orthop* 1987;215:130–131.
35. Woods G. Elbow arthroscopy. *Clin Sports Med* 1987;6:557–564.

PART II

Trauma

3

Closed Reduction and Percutaneous Pinning of Supracondylar Fractures of the Distal Humerus in the Child

Scott J. Mubarak and Jon R. Davids

Supracondylar fracture of the distal humerus is the most common and problematic elbow fracture that occurs in children. This fracture represents between 55% and 80% of all children's elbow fractures. It occurs from a fall usually from a height greater than 2 feet. In a review of 391 supracondylar fractures admitted to Children's Hospital in San Diego over an 8-year period, 29% of the injuries occurred in falls from school playground equipment (5) (Fig. 3-1).

INDICATIONS/CONTRAINDICATIONS

Classification

Appropriate treatment is determined by the type of fracture. Extension-type supracondylar fractures of the humerus have been classified into three types. We have subcategorized these types as follows (Fig. 3-2).

Type IA: Nondisplaced Often the fracture line is difficult to see. The diagnosis of nondisplaced fracture is made by the clinical examination, which reveals tenderness, both medially and laterally, over the distal humeral condyles. Though radiographs may show no cortical disruption, a posterior fat pad sign is often present (16). With this fracture the diagnosis may not be confirmed until 3 weeks after injury, when radiographs will show callus formation. The preferred treatment of a nondisplaced supracondylar fracture of the humerus is a long-arm cast, elbow flexed to 90 degrees for 3 weeks.

S.J. Mubarak, M.D.: Department of Orthopedics, University of California, Children's Hospital, San Diego, California.

J.R. Davids, M.D.: Department of Orthopaedic Surgery, Duke University Medical Center, Durham, North Carolina.

49

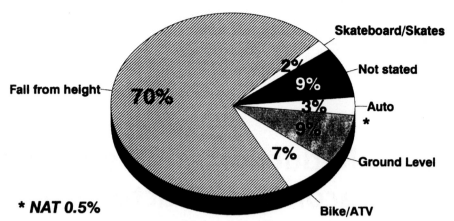

Figure 3-1. Etiology of 393 displaced supracondylar fractures treated at Children's Hospital, San Diego, 1984 to 1992.

Type IB: Minimally Displaced/Medial Compression The minimally displaced fracture must be evaluated carefully to avoid underestimating the degree of deformity, which can lead to subsequent cubitus varus (4). If the radiographs reveal compression (torus) or collapse of the medial column, closed reduction may be required. The carrying angle of the contralateral, uninvolved elbow should be carefully checked. Children with little physiologic valgus (10 degrees or less; i.e., cubitus rectus) are at particular risk for developing an unsightly cubitus varus deformity.

With the preceding findings, the medial torus fracture should be evaluated further. Because of pain and guarding, the child's elbow cannot be fully extended and the carrying angle of the injured side cannot be determined without a general anesthetic. In the operating room, these minimally angulated fractures can be more fully examined, and, if necessary, a closed reduction and percutaneous pinning using one or two 0.062 smooth K-wires via a lateral approach can be performed (Fig. 3-3).

Type IIA: Hyperextension/Posterior Cortex Intact On the lateral radiograph, fractures with extension of the humeral/capitellar relationship of more than 20 degrees will require reduction (Fig. 3-4). Again, clinical evaluation of the uninjured elbow, especially noting hyperextensibility, will help define the need for further examination of the child's injured arm under anesthesia.

Type IIB: Displaced/Angulated with Osseous Contact The displaced/angulated with osseous contact fracture demonstrates both rotational and hyperextension deformity radiographically, but some cortical contact remains, usually on the posterior side.

Both types IIA and IIB of supracondylar fractures will need general anesthesia and closed reduction in the operating room. Type IIB is more difficult to reduce than IIA and requires correction of the angulation and rotation. If there is minimal swelling and a normal neurocirculatory status, this can be done semielectively if the child has recently eaten. Closed reduction and percutaneous pinning using two lateral pins is our treatment of choice for type II fractures (Fig. 3-5).

Type III: Completely Displaced Ninety-eight percent of completely displaced fractures are an extension type, with the proximal fragment anterior to the distal fragment. Only 2% are the flexion type with anterior displacement of the distal fragment (12). In 70% of the cases, the distal fragment is displaced posteromedially with respect to the proximal fragment (12). Medially displaced fractures, when incompletely reduced, will lead to cubitus varus deformity.

The following conditions indicate treatment by closed reduction and percutaneous pinning, which offers advantages in types II and III injuries as well as in type IB injuries with medial collapse:

1. It provides immediate stability of the fracture fragments.

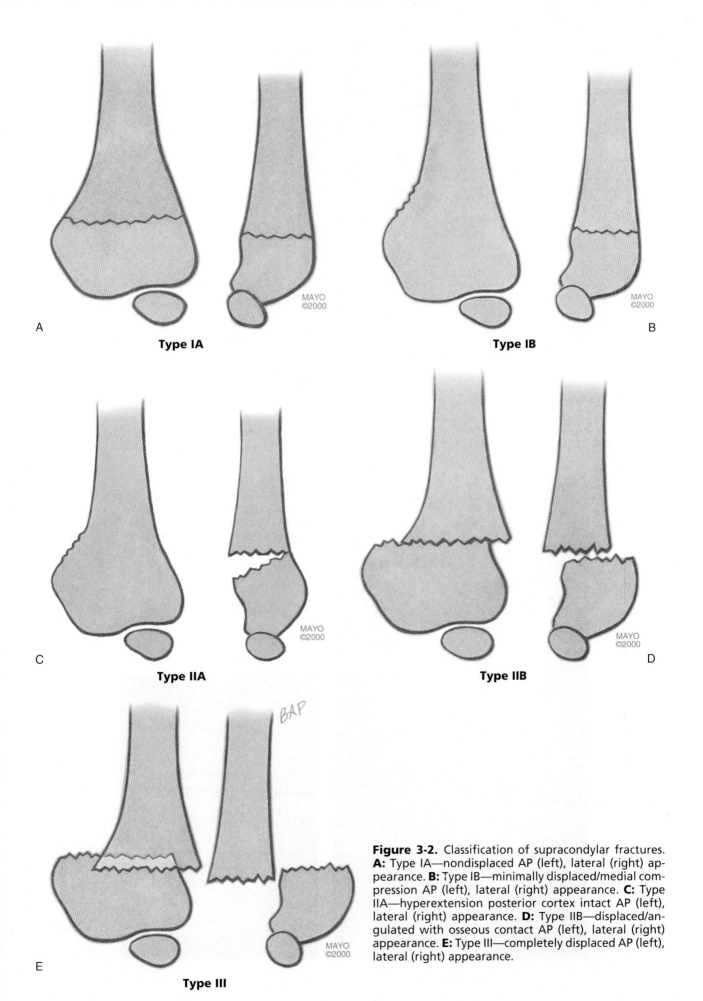

Figure 3-2. Classification of supracondylar fractures. **A:** Type IA—nondisplaced AP (left), lateral (right) appearance. **B:** Type IB—minimally displaced/medial compression AP (left), lateral (right) appearance. **C:** Type IIA—hyperextension posterior cortex intact AP (left), lateral (right) appearance. **D:** Type IIB—displaced/angulated with osseous contact AP (left), lateral (right) appearance. **E:** Type III—completely displaced AP (left), lateral (right) appearance.

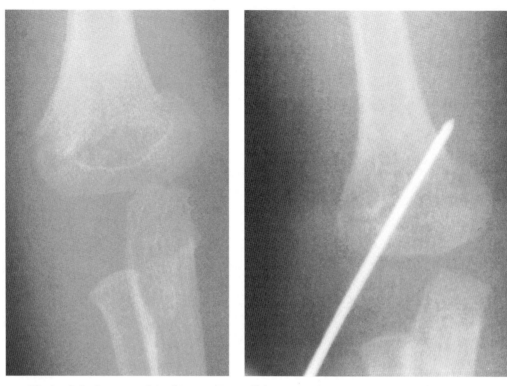

Figure 3-3. Supracondylar fracture IB: medial compression. Examination in the operating room confirmed the varus alignment (**A**). Closed reduction and percutaneous pinning with a single K-wire from the lateral approach was utilized to maintain the reduction (**B**).

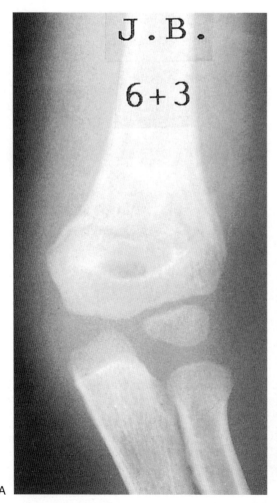

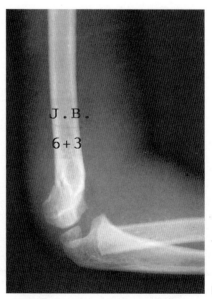

Figure 3-4. Supracondylar fracture IIA. The AP view shows only the slightest suggestion of a fracture line (**A**). The lateral view shows extension of the humeral/capitellar relationship of more than 20 degrees (**B**).

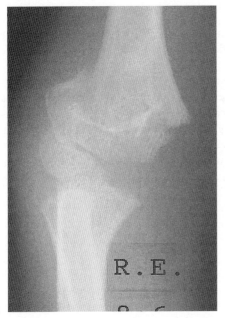
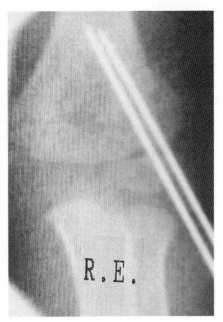
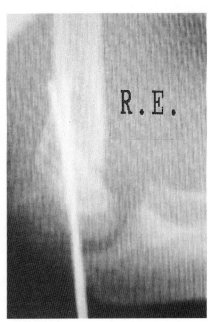

A   B, C

Figure 3-5. Supracondylar fracture IIB. Displaced, angulated, and rotated fracture (**A**). Closed reduction and percutaneous pinning with two K-wires from the lateral approach were performed (**B**). Lateral radiograph demonstrates reduction of the humeral/capitellar relationship (**C**).

2. It allows evaluation of the carrying angle after reduction and pinning. Any varus component can be appreciated immediately and corrected. This is difficult to do with traction or casting techniques.
3. It is simple and cost-effective. The hospital stay is less than 24 hours.
4. It addresses concerns about vascular safety. If there are difficulties with arterial occlusion, closed reduction and stabilization of the fracture fragment will restore the pulse in nearly 90% of cases (15). In the rare case of significant arterial injury, vascular exploration and repair are greatly facilitated by immediate fracture stabilization.

Contraindications for closed reduction and percutaneous fixation include the following:

1. *Severe swelling.* If the swelling is so severe that adequate reduction is impossible by closed means, then open reduction and pin fixation are performed.
2. *Open fracture.* Usually, the proximal fragment will perforate the skin anteriorly through the brachialis muscle, creating a grade I open fracture. These are best treated by an anterior debridement of the fracture fragment, with reduction and internal fixation of the fracture fragments. Care must be taken not to injure the anterior neurovascular structures during the fracture reduction and stabilization.
3. *Irreducible fracture.* In markedly displaced type III fractures, the proximal humeral shaft will occasionally buttonhole into the brachialis muscle and even dimple the skin anteriorly in the cubital fossa (2). Closed reduction may not be possible because of interposed periosteum and muscle, and open reduction is necessary. We prefer an initial lateral approach but will not hesitate to add a medial incision to facilitate gentle reduction of the fracture fragments and then pinning with 0.062 smooth K-wires.
4. *Late diagnosis or loss of reduction.* If the fracture is more than a week old, callus formation will usually preclude closed reduction and percutaneous pinning. Open reduction and internal fixation are generally required. We will perform this on displaced fractures that are more than 6 weeks old, as it is possible to define the fracture margins, remove the callus, and then obtain a near anatomic reduction. Late valgus osteotomy of the distal humerus is reserved for significant cases of cubitus varus and is used as a reconstructive procedure.

Other general concerns before surgery include the following:

1. *Anesthesia.* If the child cannot undergo general anesthesia because of having recently eaten or having experienced multiple injuries, temporary splinting is utilized until the following day.
2. *Technical difficulty.* Percutaneous pinning of the distal humerus in a child can be difficult, even in a stable type IB minimally angulated fracture. The technique should be done by one with expertise using this procedure. By treating supracondylar fractures by this protocol, experience may be rapidly gained on the more stable patterns so that the more difficult type III fractures can also be handled.
3. *Concern about nerve function.* Iatrogenic ulnar nerve palsy can occur following pinning, so concern about the status of this nerve must be resolved before the technique is performed.

PREOPERATIVE PLANNING

Allow the child to remain in the parent's lap and try to perform a careful neurocirculatory evaluation before multiple examinations by other physicians or attempts at blood drawing have occurred. Examine the uninjured arm to assess the carrying angle and hyperextension. Assess the radial pulse, capillary refill, and volar and dorsal compartments. Pinprick examination for sensation is poorly tolerated by most children and is rarely used. We prefer light touch and two-point discrimination to evaluate sensation. The most common nerve injured with a displaced extension-type supracondylar fracture is the anterior interosseous nerve. This purely motor branch of the median nerve is best evaluated by active flexion on the distal interphalangeal joint of the index and thumb.

Standardized radiographic examination of the injured elbow should include anteroposterior (AP), lateral, and both oblique views of the distal humerus. AP and lateral views of the contralateral, uninjured elbow are essential for evaluating Baumann's angle and to recognize minimal displacement of an ossific center. Clinical and radiographic evaluation of the entire forearm on the injured side is essential, as there was a 6% incidence of ipsilateral distal radius fractures with displaced supracondylar fractures in our series (5).

In cases that present with absent or diminished distal pulses, prompt closed reduction will usually restore the vascular integrity. After reduction, if the pulses remain absent to palpation and Doppler evaluation, and the forearm appears ischemic, percutaneous stabilization is performed before surgical exploration of the brachial artery. Preoperative angiography is not utilized, as it simply prolongs the time to the operating room and can increase the period of vascular compromise and ischemia (10,15).

SURGERY

Closed Reduction Percutaneous Pinning

With closed reduction percutaneous pinning the patient is under general anesthesia and is positioned on the operating table with the injured arm placed on a radiolucent arm board. A bed sheet is positioned around the child's torso, so that the anesthesiologist can provide countertraction when reduction of the extremity is carried out by the orthopaedic surgeon. The child's head needs to be braced with tape or a bolster to prevent it from moving off the operating table when traction is applied (Fig. 3-6).

Preoperative radiographs of the injured extremity, along with the films of the contralateral elbow, are evaluated. If an adequate AP radiograph has not been obtained because of the marked displacement and overriding of the fracture fragments, a traction AP and lateral radiograph can be obtained once the child is asleep to more fully evaluate the fracture pattern and to rule out intraarticular involvement (T-condylar fracture pattern).

The image intensifier is placed at the head of the operating table so that the C-arm is free to rotate under the arm board in both an AP and a lateral position without rotating the patient's arm (Fig. 3-6).

The child's arm is now prepped and draped. The surgeon and operative personnel use protective lead aprons and sterile gowns. Longitudinal traction is first applied by the orthopaedic surgeon and countertraction is provided by the anesthesiologist with the previously placed sheet about the patient's trunk (Fig. 3-7). The image is viewed in the AP projection and any translation of the distal fragment is corrected by varus or valgus manipulation (Fig. 3-8). Once adequate length and alignment have been obtained on the AP view, the traction is continued while gentle pressure is applied posteriorly over the olecranon and the elbow is gradually flexed. This pressure is increased at 30 to 40 degrees of flexion to reduce the distal fragment onto the anterior fragment. The elbow is hyperflexed to approximately 130 degrees and held in about neutral to slight pronation, while the image intensifier is rotated to obtain a lateral view of the elbow (Fig. 3-9).

If the reduction has been accomplished and a normal humeral-to-capitellar relationship obtained, percutaneous pinning can be carried out (Fig. 3-10). If an oblique spike of bone is viewed, a rotational malalignment is present and re-reduction may be necessary. Next, while maintaining the elbow in the hyperflexed position, two smooth 0.062 K-wires are inserted through the capitellum (lateral approach) across the fracture site (Fig. 3-11). Even in a minimally displaced fracture, this may be a difficult task in the hands of an inexperienced surgeon. When combined with an unstable fracture and marked soft-tissue swelling, this maneuver may be extremely difficult and frustrating. After the first pin is inserted, the lateral image will demonstrate its placement across the distal humerus. A second K-wire is added for stability through the lateral condyle.

Once the two pins are across the fracture on the lateral projection, the elbow can safely be extended and an AP view can be obtained to demonstrate satisfactory reduction and correct positioning of the pins (Fig. 3-12). It is imperative that both of these pins engage the far cortex. If the reduction is not acceptable at this point, pin removal and repeat closed reduction are necessary. An excellent lateral view of the distal humerus can now be obtained

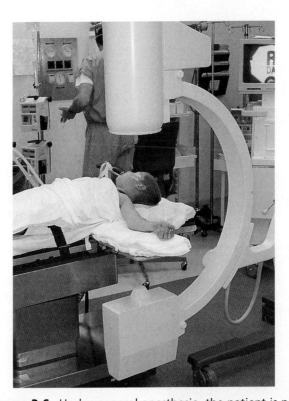

Figure 3-6. Under general anesthesia, the patient is positioned on the operating room (OR) table with a wooden arm board and a sheet is placed under the patient's axilla for the anesthesiologist to provide countertraction. The image intensifier is placed at the head of the OR table. In this position, a lateral image can be obtained without rotating the arm.

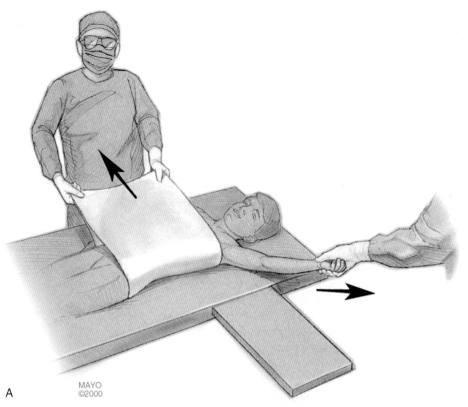

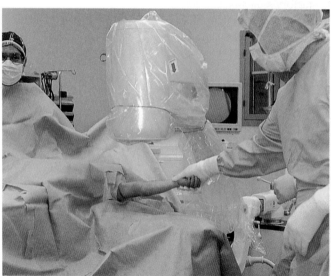

Figure 3-7. The arm is prepped and draped. Longitudinal traction is applied by the operating surgeon and countertraction from the anesthesiologist utilizing the previously placed sheet in the patient's axilla (**A**). The image is brought into position for an AP view (**B**).

A

B

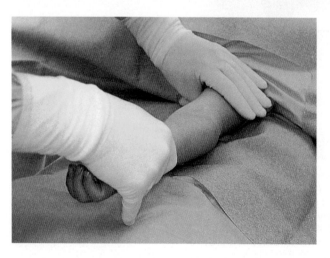

Figure 3-8. Under image control, any translation is corrected by varus or valgus pressure.

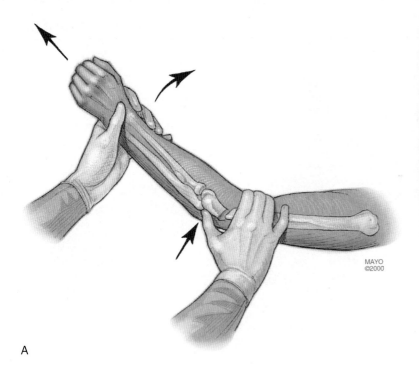

A

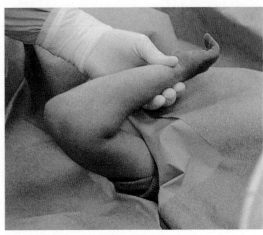

B

Figure 3-9. Once adequate length and alignment have been obtained on the AP view, the traction is continued while gentle pressure is applied posteriorly over the olecranon and the elbow is gradually flexed (**A**). The elbow is held in maximum flexion of around 130 degrees and in neutral to slight pronation (**B**).

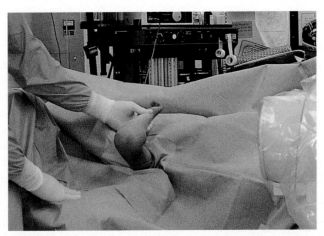

Figure 3-10. A lateral image is now obtained. If the reduction has been accomplished and a normal humeral-to-capitellar relationship obtained, percutaneous pinning can be carried out.

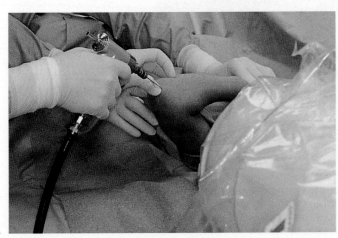

A

Figure 3-11. While maintaining the elbow in the hyperflexed position (**A**). *(continued)*

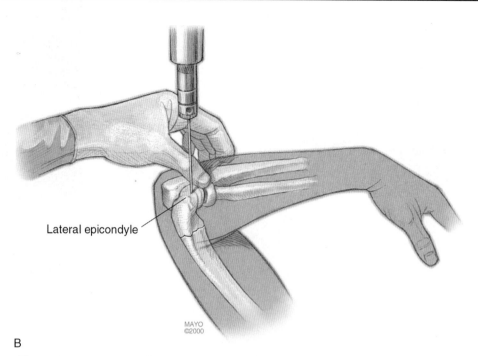

B

Figure 3-11. *Continued.* Two K-wires (0.062) are inserted through the capitellum (lateral approach) across the fracture site under image control (**B**).

by externally rotating the arm, with the image intensifier still maintained in the AP position (Fig. 3-13). If one attempts to do this before pin fixation of the fracture fragments, rotational malalignment can occur. At this point, a medial pin can be inserted for a type III supracondylar fracture. The orthopaedic surgeon should massage the swelling out of the medial side around the epicondyle and place his thumb over the ulnar nerve to protect it while inserting the 0.062 K-wire. Extending the elbow to about 50 degrees will reduce the likelihood of the ulnar nerve subluxing anteriorly, which sometimes occurs with hyperflexion. A 5-mm incision over the medial epicondyle with blunt dissection down to bone/cartilage will allow direct visualization if the surgeon is unable to palpate the nerve due to swelling or inexperience.

The surgeon can now triangulate this third smooth K-wire on the previously placed lateral pins. The medial pin will provide greater stability and prevent loss of the reduction

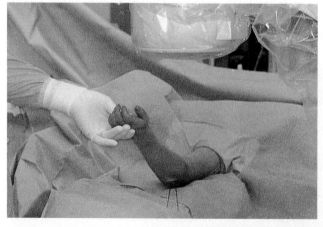

Figure 3-12. Once the two K-wires are across the fracture on the lateral projection, the elbow can safely be extended and an AP view obtained to demonstrate satisfactory reduction and correct positioning of the K-wires. If reduction is unsatisfactory, pin removal and closed reduction must be reattempted.

while the cast is being applied (18). For types I and II fractures, we use only the two parallel or divergent lateral pins. This avoids the risk to the ulnar nerve. These inherently more stable fracture patterns do not require the medial pin. The K-wires are carefully bent to 90 degrees outside of the skin (Fig. 3-14). We leave 1 inch of K-wire extending out to prevent pin migration under the skin and to facilitate removal in the outpatient clinic 3 weeks later.

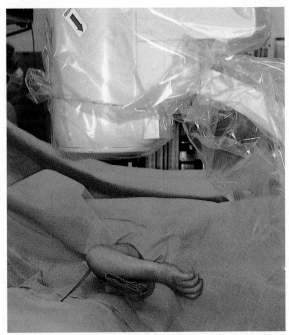

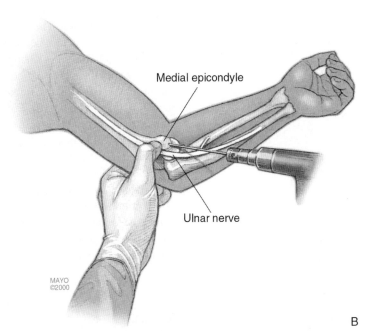

Medial epicondyle

Ulnar nerve

MAYO
©2000

A

B

Figure 3-13. An excellent lateral view can be obtained by externally rotating the arm at this point (**A**). A medial pin can be inserted for type III supracondylar fractures. The surgeon extends the patient's elbow and inserts the pin while protecting the ulnar nerve with the surgeon's thumb (**B**). The surgeon triangulates on the previously placed lateral pins when inserting this third K-wire. This K-wire will prevent loss of reduction for these more unstable fractures. For type II fractures, we use only the two lateral parallel or divergent K-wires.

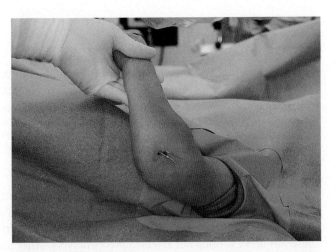

Figure 3-14. The pins are bent to a 90-degree angle, leaving 1 inch extending to prevent migration under the skin. Felt, soft roll, and a long-arm cast that is split are then applied. The patient is observed in the hospital for 24 hours. The patient will be rechecked in 1 week and the pins removed with radiographs out of plaster at 3 weeks.

If there is an angulated or displaced distal radius fracture, closed reduction and single cross-pin fixation through the radial styloid before closed reduction and pinning of the supracondylar fracture provide the most effective treatment in our experience.

POSTOPERATIVE MANAGEMENT

Felt and soft roll are applied. Radiographs are obtained before cast application. The patient is then placed in a long-arm fiberglass cast, which is positioned at approximately 80 degrees of elbow flexion. The cast is univalved and spread, and the patient is observed in the hospital overnight before being discharged.

A collar-and-cuff type of sling prevents the child from using this extremity. Dangling the extremity with the elbow casted in this position (i.e., less than 90 degrees flexion) may result in movement of the cast that can cause the pins to be pulled out prematurely and the fracture reduction to be lost. For this reason the patient is seen 1 week after discharge for clinical as well as radiographic evaluation. At 3 weeks following injury, the cast is removed for radiographs. In nearly all cases, there is sufficient callus formation to allow for pin removal and gentle mobilization of the elbow. A light dressing is applied to the pin sites, and the patient utilizes a sling for about a week. Bathing is permitted at this time to encourage early range of motion and prevent stiffness.

The child is then checked at 6 weeks for a clinical evaluation and at 6 and 12 months for clinical and radiographic evaluation. Very occasionally, growth plate injury can occur with this fracture, and it is important to recognize this problem early. Physical therapy has not been necessary in any of our patients when mobilization was begun 3 weeks after the injury.

RESULTS

At our institution, all the children with type II and type III injuries are treated by the preceding protocol. The results have been extremely satisfying, with nearly anatomic reduction in all cases and perioperative hospital stays of less than 24 hours. Range of motion returns to normal in 95% of the children within 3 months. Cubitus varus has rarely occurred and is usually of minimal magnitude. Only one child originally treated by this protocol has required subsequent valgus osteotomy.

COMPLICATIONS

Early and late complications of supracondylar fracture of the distal humerus are well recognized. Acute vascular compromise with subsequent compartment syndrome can result in Volkmann's contracture if not treated appropriately. The most common late complication is fracture malunion leading to a cubitus varus deformity.

Nerve Injury

The incidence of nerve damage from the injury itself is reported to be around 10% (5,12,17). The most commonly injured nerve in a displaced supracondylar fracture is the anterior interosseous branch of the median nerve. Some series do not recognize this because this nerve is often not assessed preoperatively. After injury to the median nerve, the most likely nerves injured, in decreasing frequency, are the radial and ulnar nerves. On the other hand, in our experience, most ulnar neuropathies are iatrogenic, secondary to pin placement. Also, in all our cases and in those reviewed in the literature, the ulnar neuropathy cleared from 1 to 6 months after pin removal (6,12,17). If an ulnar neuropathy is first appreciated after reduction and a three-pin technique has been utilized, we recommend immediate removal of the medial pin. With a two-cross-pin technique, we would not recommend removal of the medial pin until 3 weeks after the injury to avoid loss of reduction.

Arterial Injury

In approximately 10% of the cases of displaced supracondylar fracture, the radial pulse will be absent at presentation. In greater than 90% of these cases (10,15), the pulse will return with closed reduction and pinning of the fracture under general anesthesia.

All authors writing on this subject agree that the fracture should be reduced and stabilized by percutaneous pinning or, if necessary, even open reduction and fixation. At this point, nearly all authors recommend in the presence of an absent radial pulse and with forearm and hand ischemia exploration of the artery at the fracture site. Shaw et al. explored three cases and documented intimal tears with thrombus obstructing the brachial artery lumen. In two patients, the injured segment was excised and replaced by a saphenous bone graft; prophylactic fasciotomy was also performed. One patient that was explored was noted to have brachial artery entrapment that was treated by appropriate release. Schoenecker et al. recommend brachial artery exploration if Dopplerable pulses did not return within 30 minutes after fracture reduction (14). They would consult a vascular surgeon to aid their exploration. Three of seven patients explored demonstrated interluminal damage or transsection and required saphenous bone graft. Four others demonstrated kinked or entrapped artery at the fracture site, necessitating mobilization of the vessel with reestablishment of the pulses. Garbuz et al. explored five radial arteries and found a similar ratio of luminal damage or laceration and kinking of the brachial arteries (7). The one patient who was treated with ligation had symptoms of long-term claudication. Eight of eleven patients who initially had an absent pulse developed a return of the pulse after the closed reduction. In three children the radial pulse did not return, but no further treatment was required, as the forearm and hand remained pink without any further neurologic deficits.

The Vancouver study group reviewed the pulseless pink hand in 13 patients following closed reduction and percutaneous pinning of the supracondylar fracture (13). They recommended, as noted earlier, segmental pressure monitoring, color flow duplex scanning, and magnetic resonance angiography (MRA) as a noninvasive, safe technique for evaluating brachial artery patency and collateral circulation around the elbow. The vascular injuries were found in all 13 patients studied. Four patients had thrombus and/or intimal tear. These patients underwent vein patch graft angioplasty. Urokinase infusion was used intraarteriorly in four patients, and open thrombectomy was used in one. However, at follow-up study with MRA, these patients showed a high rate of asymptomatic reocculsion and residual stenosis of the brachial artery. Thus they called into question the need for vascular reconstruction of intimal tears when the patient has a pink hand and MRA or other studies demonstrate adequate collateral circulation. They strongly recommend that these patients be observed with a vascular surgeon.

Compartment Syndromes

Compartment syndromes have become an extremely rare complication, since the popularization of immediate closed reduction and percutaneous pinning by Flynn et al. (6). In the review from our institution, only one compartment syndrome has been encountered, and this was recognized early and treated appropriately by volar compartment fasciotomy at the time of reduction and pinning (5).

In any patient if the compartments are palpated and determined to be tense, intracompartmental pressures should be obtained for the volar, dorsal, and hand compartments (8). If the pressures are elevated above 30 mm Hg, fasciotomy should be carried out. The brachial, radial, and ulnar arteries should be explored at the time of decompression.

We prefer a single longitudinal curvilinear incision for decompression of the volar forearm. This incision allows an easy approach to the antebrachial fascia and the transverse carpal ligament as well as to the neurovascular structures of the forearm and the mobile wad. The incision is nearly identical to McConnell's combined exposure of the median and ulnar neurovascular bundles, as described by Henry (9). A straight longitudinal incision is used for the dorsal compartment of the forearm.

Pin Tract Infection

Pin tract infection is rarely a problem if pins are removed at 3 weeks. Oral antibiotics are often used if there is drainage or hypertropic granulation at the pin sites.

Posttraumatic Cubitus Varus

Posttraumatic cubitus varus is extremely rare following adequate reduction and pinning of supracondylar fracture of the humerus. When it does occur, this deformity causes cosmetic concerns and may result in secondary fractures and late ulnar nerve palsy (1,3,11).

Authors' Recommendations

If ischemia is present with a displaced supracondylar fracture, the patient should be taken immediately to the operating room for a closed reduction and percutaneous pinning.

After fracture reduction and stabilization, the circulation should be reassessed. If the forearm and hand are ischemic and there are no palpable pulses by Doppler, a vascular surgeon should be notified, and exploration of the artery and fracture should be performed as previously noted by multiple authors. In nearly one-third of the cases explored, as documented in the literature, the artery is kinked around the fracture site and can be freed up. Often there is associated spasm that may respond to local treatment. The majority of the pathology noted in such cases, however, requires repair of the brachial artery, repair of the damaged lumen, removal of thrombus, and possible saphenous vein graft. All attempts should be made to restore that circulation rather than ligating the brachial vessel.

If the hand is pink, and certainly if a Dopplerable pulse is present, the patient should be observed very closely, and no exploration is recommended. In most cases, the Dopplerable pulse will return in the first 12 hours. If no pulse returns and there is no associated nerve injury, we would observe the patient rather than undergo further studies and possible exploration. However, if there is an overlying median nerve injury that may mask forearm and hand ischemia of the compartments, consideration should be made for further noninvasive vascular studies, MRA, and possible brachial artery exploration with the aid of a vascular surgeon.

At our center, the limb reimplant surgeons (usually hand surgeons) are the most helpful in exploring and repairing the small vessel of the child's brachial artery. In these circumstances after brachial artery repair if the period of ischemia is more than 4 hours, prophylactic fasciotomy of the forearm should be considered.

ILLUSTRATIVE CASE

A 7-year-old boy fell off the monkey bars, sustaining a severely displaced type III fracture. Radiographs showed posterior translation and soft-tissue swelling (Fig. 3-15A). Using the technique described earlier, a closed reduction and percutaneous pinning were successfully performed using two lateral pins and one medial pin (Fig.3-15B). Three weeks later, maintenance of the reduction is confirmed (Fig. 3-15C) and the pins were removed.

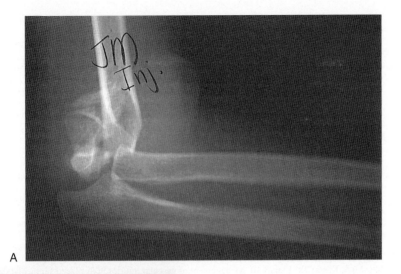

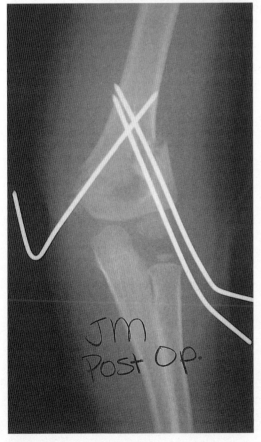

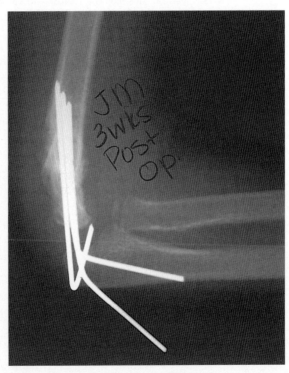

Figure 3-15. Completely displaced supracondylar type III fracture (**A**); AP view (**B**), and lateral view (**C**) after two lateral pins and one medial pin were inserted (at the time of pin removal 3 weeks postoperatively).

RECOMMENDED READINGS

1. Abe M, Ishizu T, Shirai H, et al.. Tardy ulnar nerve palsy caused by cubitus varus deformity. *Surg [Am]* 1995;20:5–9.
2. Archibeck MJ, Scott SM, Peters CL. Brachialis muscle entrapment in displaced supracondylar humerus fractures: a technique of closed reduction and report of initial results. *J Pediatr Orthop* 1997;17:298–302.
3. Davids JR, Maguire MF, Mubarak SJ, et al. Lateral condylar fracture of the humerus following post-traumatic cubitus varus. *J Pediatr Orthop* 1994;14:466–470.

4. DeBoeck H, DeSmet P, Penders W, et al. Supracondylar elbow fractures with impaction of the medial condyle in children. *J Pediatr Orthop* 1995;15:444–448.
5. Farnsworth CL, Silva PD, Mubarak SJ. Etiology of supracondylar humerus fractures. *J Pediatr Orthop* 1998;18:38–42.
6. Flynn JL, Matthews JG, Benoit RL. Blind pinning of displaced supracondylar fractures of the humerus in children: sixteen years experience with long-term follow-up. *J Bone Joint Surg* 1974;56A:263–272.
7. Garbuz DS, Leitch K, Wright JG. The treatment of supracondylar fractures in children with an absent radial pulse. *J Pediatr Orthop* 1996;16:594–596.
8. Gelberman RH, Zakaib GS, Mubarak SJ, et al. Decompression of forearm compartment syndromes. *Clin Orthop* 1978;134:225.
9. Henry AK. *Extensile exposure,* 2nd ed. Edinburgh: Churchill Livingstone; 1973.
10. Millis MB, Singer IJ, Hall JE. Supracondylar fracture of the humerus in children: further experience with a study in orthopedic decision-making. *Clin Orthop* 1984;188:90–97.
11. Oppenheim WL, Clader TJ, Smith C, et al. Supracondylar humeral osteotomy for traumatic childhood cubitus varus deformity. *Clin Orthop* 1984;188:34–39.
12. Pirone AM, Graham HK, Krajbich JI. Management of displaced extension-type supracondylar fractures of the humerus in children. *J Bone Joint Surg* 1988;70A:641–649.
13. Sabharwal S, Tredwell SJ, Beauchamp RD, et al. Management of pulseless pink hand in pediatric supracondylar fractures of the humerus. *J Pediatr Orthop* 1997;17:303–310.
14. Schoenecker PL, Delgado E, Rotman M, et al. Pulseless arm in association with totally displaced supracondylar fracture. *J Pediatr Orthop* 1996;10:410–415.
15. Shaw BA, Kasser JR, Emans JB. Management of vascular injuries in displaced supracondylar humerus fractures without arteriography. *J Orthop Trauma* 1990;4:25–29.
16. Skaggs DL, Mirzayan R. The posterior fat pad sign in association with occult fracture of the elbow in children. *J Bone Joint Surg* 1999;81A:1429–1433.
17. Webb AJ, Sherman FC. Supracondylar fractures of the humerus in children. *J Pediatr Orthop* 1989;9:315–325.
18. Zionts LE, McKellop HA, Hathaway R. Torsional strength of pin configurations used to fix supracondylar fractures of the humerus in children. *J Bone Joint Surg* 1994;76A:253–256.

4

The Surgical Management of Intraarticular Fractures of the Distal Humerus

Jesse B. Jupiter

Intraarticular fractures of the distal humerus have a well-deserved reputation of being very difficult to manage, with a poor prognosis. Nonetheless, techniques that afford rigid fixation have improved the overall results of the management of this difficult fracture.

INDICATIONS/CONTRAINDICATIONS

It has become evident as the techniques and implants designed for stable fixation have improved that most intraarticular fractures of the distal humerus are best treated by open reduction and internal fixation. Operative reduction affords the opportunity to accurately reduce the disrupted trochlea and restore its congruous relationship to the olecranon, thereby ensuring the intrinsic stability of the humeral/ulnar relationship (1–8,10). Even the more complex distal humeral fractures such as those associated with comminution, open fractures, or ipsilateral fractures of the limb are now equally effectively treated by surgical means.

It is well recognized that the surgical anatomy of the distal humerus can prove treacherous as the fragile articulations are supported by a meager amount of subchondral bone and virtually no soft tissue. When faced with such a fracture in the elderly, the ability of the bone to support stable fixation with screws and plates proves to be problematic. In such cases, the surgeon must determine his or her ability to provide stable fixation or consider alternative treatment such as total elbow arthroplasty.

PREOPERATIVE PLANNING

The common pitfalls of surgical intervention should be carefully considered preoperatively. Because of the complex architecture of the distal humerus, routine radiographs will often fail to provide the true extent of the intraarticular fracture. An anteroposterior (AP)

J.B. Jupiter, M.D.: Department of Orthopaedic Surgery, Harvard Medical School; and Massachusetts General Hospital, Boston, Massachusetts.

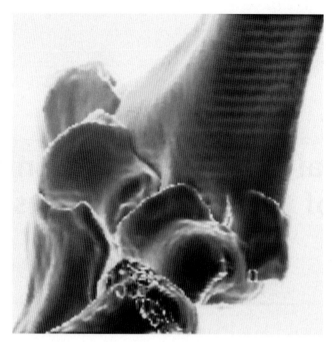

Figure 4-1. A low comminuted distal humerus fracture is accurately depicted in a three-dimensional CT reconstruction.

radiograph obtained with traction on the forearm once anesthesia has been induced will reveal a more accurate representation of the fracture anatomy. Although standard CT scanning or MRI evaluations are of questionable value, the three-dimensional CT reconstructions have added substantially to the preoperative understanding of some comminuted distal intraarticular fractures (Fig. 4-1). Severe comminution of the supracondylar columns should alert the surgeon to the availability of a bone graft and, in the elderly patient, the possible need for total elbow arthroplasty.

SURGERY

Since the operative procedures can be lengthy, in most cases general endotracheal anesthesia is preferred. The patient is placed in the lateral position with the involved limb supported over bolsters, keeping it off the chest wall (Fig. 4-2). A prone position with the arm over the side of the table is an effective means of helping to release the fracture. Either position permits ready access to the iliac crest for autogenous bone graft. A sterile pneumatic arm tourniquet offers the possibility of a wider sterile field and the ability to reapply the tourniquet as needed.

Technique

My preference has been to utilize the transolecranon approach, particularly for comminuted fractures. Through a straight, longitudinal skin incision (Fig. 4-3), the osteotomy is made in a shallow V or chevron fashion in the center of the olecranon sulcus (Fig. 4-4). This area has in fact the smallest zone of articular cartilage in the olecranon. The location will be best identified by elevation of the anconeus muscle off the olecranon to directly visualize the articular surface. A sponge is placed from lateral to medial and used as a countertraction, as the osteotomy is created with a thin-bladed oscillating saw (Fig. 4-5) and completed with a thin-bladed osteotome.

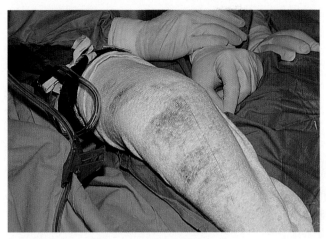

Figure 4-2. The patient is placed in the lateral position. A sterile pneumatic tourniquet is preferred.

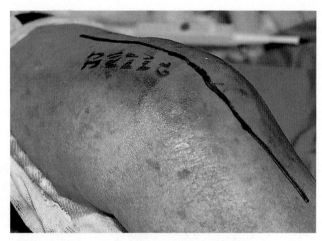

Figure 4-3. A straight longitudinal skin incision is used.

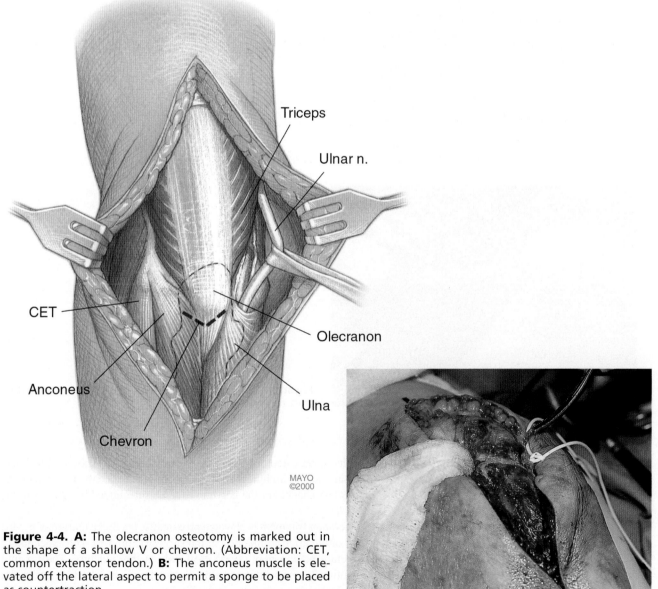

A

Figure 4-4. A: The olecranon osteotomy is marked out in the shape of a shallow V or chevron. (Abbreviation: CET, common extensor tendon.) **B:** The anconeus muscle is elevated off the lateral aspect to permit a sponge to be placed as countertraction.

B

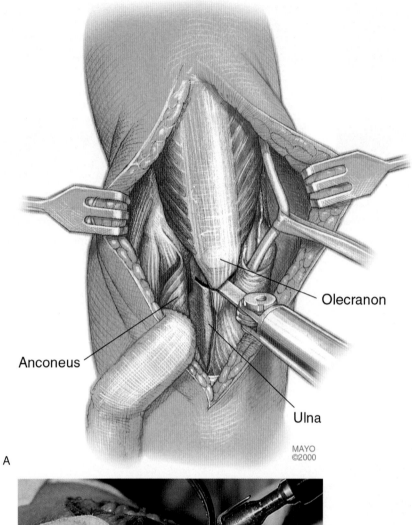

Olecranon

Anconeus

Ulna

MAYO
©2000

A

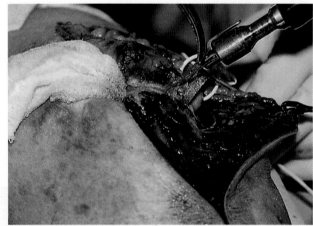

B

Figure 4-5. A,B: A thin-bladed oscillating saw is used to start the osteotomy.

Before creating the olecranon osteotomy, the ulnar nerve should be exposed. The fascia over the flexor carpi ulnaris is longitudinally split over 6 cm to enhance the nerve's mobility. In doing this there is less chance for the nerve to become surrounded by fibrosis in the cubital tunnel.

The osteotomized olecranon fragment is elevated proximally, leaving a margin of triceps tendon on either side to suture upon completion of the surgery (Fig. 4-6). The exact nature of the intraarticular fracture pattern may reveal itself only at this juncture. The fracture hematoma should be cautiously removed using a small dental pick or pulsed lavage, as the articular fragments may lack soft tissue or bony attachments.

Once the fracture anatomy is confirmed, the goal is to reduce the articular fragments onto the bony columns of the distal humerus, initially holding the reduction with provisional Kirschner wire fixation (Fig. 4-7).

In some instances, the intraarticular fracture of the trochlea may be found to be present in both the sagittal and coronal planes (Fig. 4-8). In these cases, the Herbert screws have been of particular use, as the threads can be buried under the articular surface (Fig. 4-9). An alternative to the Herbert screw is the fine-threaded Kirschner wires. If a defect exists in the subchondral bone, one should plan to support the articular fragment with autogenous cancellous bone graft.

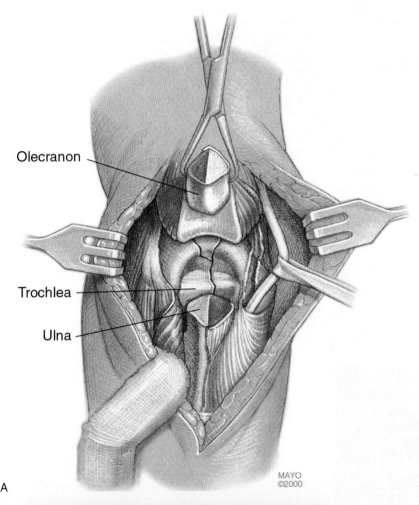

Olecranon

Trochlea

Ulna

MAYO
©2000

A

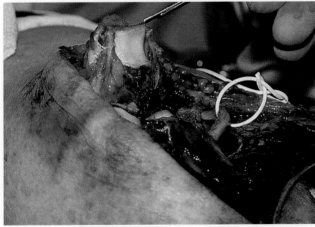

B

Figure 4-6. A,B: The osteotomized proximal olecranon fragment is elevated proximally. Note the ulnar nerve has been isolated and mobilized and protected with the rubber loop.

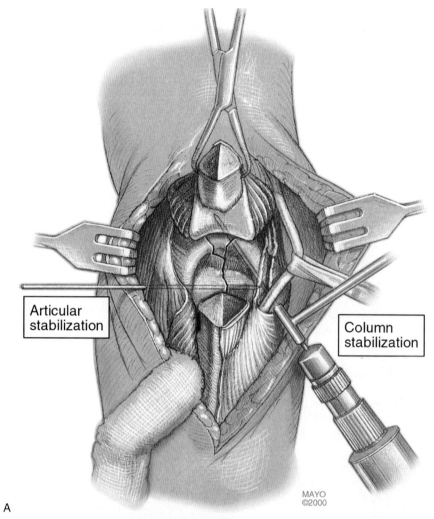

Articular stabilization

Column stabilization

MAYO
©2000

A

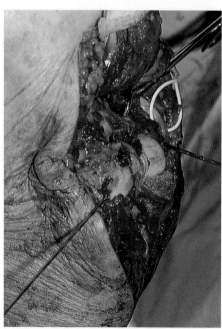

B

Figure 4-7. A,B: The fracture is reduced and provisionally secured with Kirschner wires.

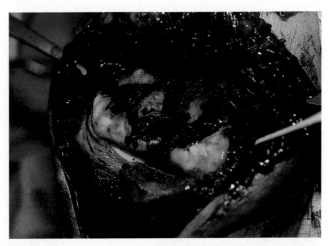

Figure 4-8. Intraarticular fractures of the trochlea occurring in the coronal plane are especially difficult to secure.

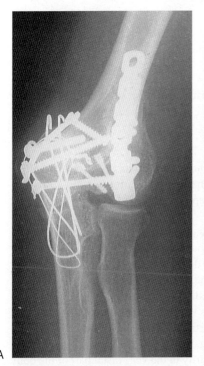
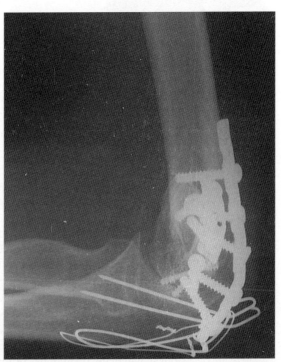

A   B

Figure 4-9. Reduced and fixed fracture in the AP (**A**) and lateral (**B**) projection. The Herbert screw may be used for articular fragments.

Definitive skeletal fixation in most of these fractures begins with interfragmentary screw fixation of the sagittal fracture of the trochlea. One or two 3.5-mm cortical or 4.0-mm cancellous screws will be sufficient to provide a firm hold of the fragments. In those cases in which comminution is present in the sagittal plane, these screws should not be placed as interfragmentary screws; rather, they should be placed without "overdrilling" the near cortex to prevent overcompressing the fragments, which will tend to narrow the trochlea, thus threatening the intrinsic stability of the trochlea/olecranon relationship (Fig. 4-10). With certain fracture patterns the surgeon may find that the articular reconstruction may be facilitated by securing one of the articular components directly to one of the bony columns of the distal humerus. This would be followed by restoration of the remaining articular element to this stable skeletal and articular unit.

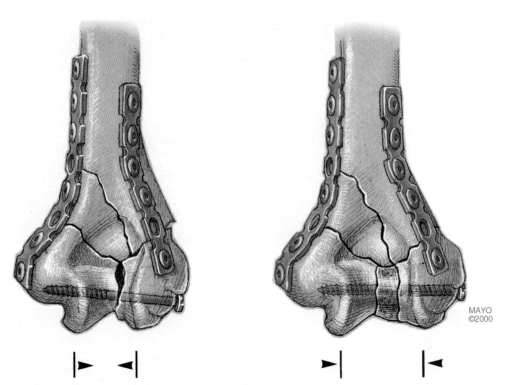

Figure 4-10. When intraarticular comminution exists, a full-threaded, not a lag, screw is best placed without compressing the fragments.

Caution must be exercised with regard to the presence of either the tip or the head of the screws in the cubital tunnel. In such cases, the ulnar nerve is best further mobilized by releasing the distal part of the medial intermuscular septum to allow the nerve to sit more freely in the subcutaneous tissues.

Stable fixation of the articular fragments to the humeral bony columns is preferentially accomplished with strategically placed plates. Mechanical strength will be enhanced by placing the plates and respective screws as close to 90 degrees to each other as possible. For most T or Y fractures that split the bony columns of the distal humerus well proximal to the olecranon fossa, the plates can be applied to the medial ridge of the medial column and along the posterior aspect of the lateral column. The topographical anatomy of the distal humerus is most amenable to this, as the articular cartilage of the capitellum does not extend onto the posterior part of the distal humerus (Fig. 4-11).

There are occasions in which the fracture lies primarily in the very distal part of the bony columns below the level of the medial epicondyle. In such cases a plate applied along the ridge of the medial bony column would be ineffective in supporting the articular fragments. In these cases, several options exist for the surgeon. Using 3.5-mm reconstruction plates, the plate can be contoured to bend around and "cradle" the medial epicondyle (Fig. 4-12). The very distal screws can be directed into the medial epicondyle and angulated from each other to afford an "interlocking" relationship between the screws. An alternative to this is to direct the distal screw proximally to secure fixation into the lateral column (Fig. 4-13).

Yet another option is to place a plate directly onto the lateral aspect of the lateral skeletal column (Fig. 4-14). This would require elevation of the origin of the brachioradialis and wrist extensor muscles, which can be sutured back into place. This placement provides an opportunity to gain a further hold on the trochlea fragments through a screw placed transversely from the most distal screw hole into the trochlea (Fig. 4-15). Defects beneath the plate should be reconstructed with autogenous iliac crest graft.

At this juncture the elbow should be put through a range of motion in order to visually control the stability of the internal fixation. If motion of the fracture fragments is observed,

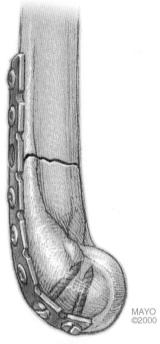

Lateral

Figure 4-11. The plate on the lateral bony column can extend distally, as the articular cartilage of the capitellum does not extend posteriorly.

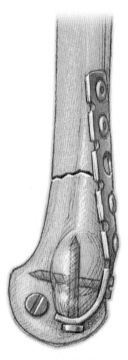

Medial

Figure 4-12. With complex "low" fractures, a plate can be constructed to bend around the medial epicondyle with screws directed into the medial epicondyle from different directions providing an "interlock" between the screws.

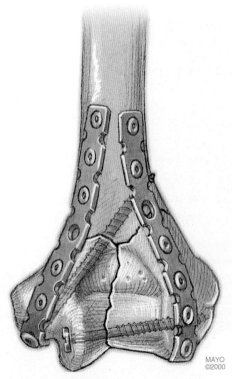

Figure 4-13. An alternative with the contoured plate bent around the medial epicondyle is to pass a screw through the plate and into the lateral column.

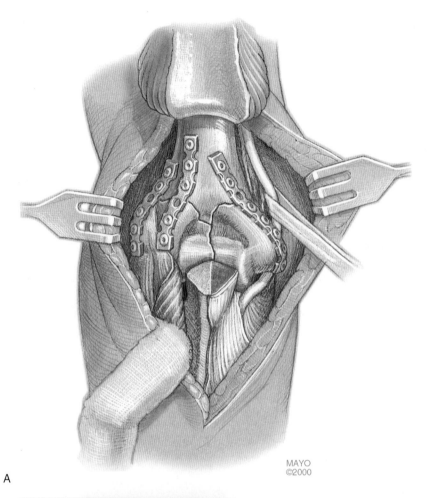

MAYO
©2000

A

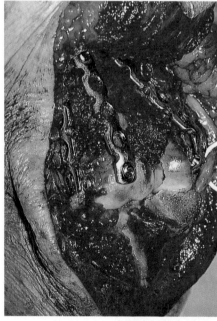

B

Figure 4-14. A,B: Another option is to place three plates with one along the lateral column, one posterior on the lateral column, and one bent around the medial epicondyle.

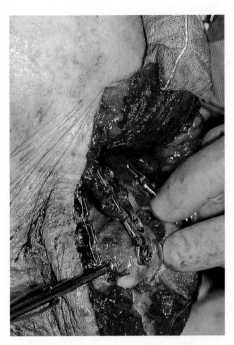

Figure 4-15. A transverse screw is placed through the lateral plate and across the trochlear fracture fragments.

it would be best to revise or alter the fixation at this point using the alternative plate application described earlier.

The olecranon osteotomy is reduced under direct vision. My preference for internal fixation continues to be tension band wires with two obliquely placed Kirschner wires providing rotational control (Fig. 4-16). Care is taken to bend the proximal ends of the Kirschner wires and seat them onto the proximal olecranon both to prevent proximal migration and to avoid the prominence of the wire interfering with full elbow motion (Fig. 4-17). At the completion of the fixation the elbow is again put through a range of motion to test the security of the internal fixation.

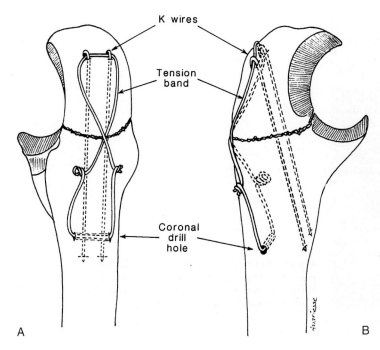

K wires

Tension band

Coronal drill hole

A

B

Figure 4-16. A,B: The olecranon osteotomy is secured with oblique Kirschner wires and a tension band wire.

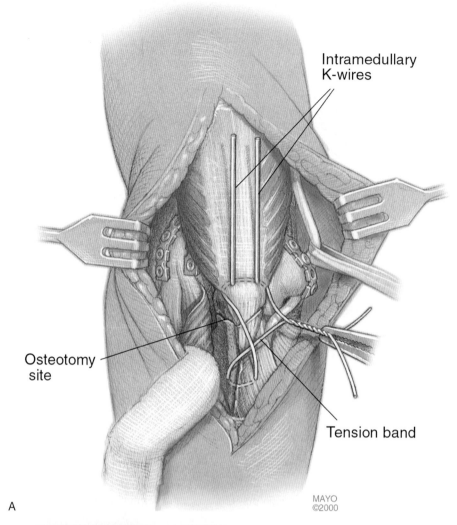

Intramedullary
K-wires

Osteotomy
site

Tension band

MAYO
©2000

A

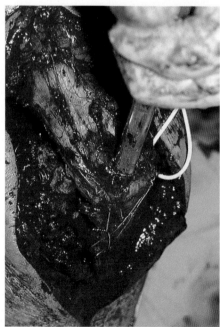

B

Figure 4-17. A,B: Attention should be paid to tapping the bent ends of the Kirschner wires into the proximal olecranon to diminish local discomfort.

The tourniquet is let down and hemostasis is carefully secured. Over a large suction drain the wound is closed in layers. A bulky dressing using Dacron batting is applied and a resting splint of plaster is applied to the elbow in full extension. A resting splint for nighttime use only with the elbow in extension helps to lessen the problem with flexion contracture.

The most common pitfalls of this type of surgery relate to the operative approach to the distal humerus: inadequate exposure, ulnar nerve mobilization, unrecognized articular comminution, fractures of the bony columns just above the articular surfaces, and stable plate fixation.

To address these pitfalls I would emphasize several specific aspects of the exposure and procedure: extensile exposure through olecranon osteotomy, wide mobilization of the ulnar nerve, careful identification and provisional fixation of the articular fragments, custom placement of plates distal on the posterior aspect of the lateral bony column and bent around the medial epicondyle, direct screws into the cortical bone of the bony columns, and careful fixation of the olecranon osteotomy. Adherence to these concepts makes the difference between a successful and an unsuccessful procedure.

In some instances, severely comminuted fractures in the elderly patient who is not active might be better treated with a primary total elbow arthroplasty (9) (see Chapter 18).

POSTOPERATIVE MANAGEMENT

Active motion is initiated on the first postoperative day. The patient is instructed to lie supine and forward-flex the involved shoulder to bring the elbow overhead. With the uninjured arm supporting the involved forearm, gravity is used to assist elbow flexion. A similar approach is used for elbow extension exercises, but in this case the patient sits upright and gently assists the forearm into extension (Fig. 4-18).

Active and patient-assisted flexion-extension exercises are continued throughout the first 3 to 4 weeks. A splint is applied only for the first few weeks and only during sleep with the elbow extended. Radiographs should be obtained frequently to assess the stability of the internal fixation. It is imperative that the surgeon monitor the patient and coordinate the rehabilitation process. A trained physical therapist can be helpful to similarly serve as a monitor, but passive activities and resisted exercises are to be avoided.

At 6 weeks postoperatively if radiographic union is progressing satisfactorily, the patient may begin light resisted exercises to restore muscle tone and strength.

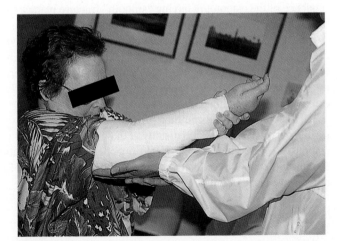

Figure 4-18. Postoperatively, active motion is begun by the patient under the guidance of a physical therapist. Gravity is used to assist elbow flexion and extension.

RESULTS

As expected, the nature of the injury has possibly the greatest influence on outcome. However, the ability to apply the principles of rigid fixation and early motion also will influence the final result. Most activities of daily living can be performed with a range of motion from 30 to 130 degrees. Loss of full extension is more easily compensated for than is loss of flexion. Typically, pronation and supination are unaffected by this fracture. With current techniques approximately 80% can attain an adequate arc of flexion even after severe fractures (1–8).

REHABILITATION

Rehabilitation following distal humerus fractures should be expected to require between 12 and 16 weeks *after* fracture union. This reality influences the editor (BFM) to favor replacement in the older patient with severe comminution. Muscle strengthening and endurance form the basis of a supervised exercise program. Typically, lack of full extension exists, and I often treat this with dynamic and/or static types of splints. Once fracture union has been assured, passive therapy modalities can be initiated.

COMPLICATIONS

Failure of fixation occurs in about 5%, and this usually results from a lack of secure fixation of the implants at the time of surgery. Clinically, fixation instability is heralded by pain and limited motion, and ultimately is confirmed by radiographic documentation of implant loosening or breakage. If suspected within the initial 6 weeks, consideration for reoperation or referral to an individual or center with extensive experience is appropriate. Cast immobilization is appealing to many but all too often results in an extremely limited range of motion.

Nonunion is being more frequently seen as the operative approach to these fractures becomes more widely accepted. Management is difficult and includes rigid fixation with two or even three plates, decompression of the ulnar nerve, and release of the anterior capsule. When this occurs in the older patient, the disability may be profound. In this patient, Morrey has reported reliable salvage with joint replacement arthroplasty (9).

Nonunion of an olecranon osteotomy occurs in about 5% of patients and has been associated with a variety of methods of techniques of internal fixation. This is in part the consequence of the osteotomy having "smooth" fracture planes, thus being intrinsically unstable. The use of a chevron-shaped osteotomy should minimize this problem.

Infection, although uncommon and more often associated with open fractures, can prove catastrophic. If infection is suspected, extensive wound debridement, lavage, and parenteral antibiotics are to be instituted immediately. If the internal fixation is stable and the infection is being actively managed, it is advisable to retain the fixation, as fracture union can take place even in the face of active infection.

Ulnar nerve palsy is a common problem that can be prevented or minimized by mobilizing the nerve proximally and distally at the time of surgery. If seen postoperatively and not responsive to rest and corticosteroid injection, early exploration can offset the profound disability that may be associated with a progressive motor deficit associated with ongoing ulnar nerve ischemia.

ILLUSTRATIVE CASE

An 85-year-old practicing attorney fell, landing on her left nondominant upper extremity. Radiographs revealed a complex, multifragmented intraarticular fracture of the distal humerus. Anteroposterior and lateral radiographs reveal a low multifragmented intraarticular fracture of the distal humerus (Fig. 4-19). Through an olecranon osteotomy the articular surface was reduced and secured back onto the bony columns of the distal humerus with three strategically placed plates. Autogenous iliac crest bone graft was used (Fig. 4-20). The comminuted extraarticular fragments were secured under the plates with attention taken to preserve soft-tissue attachments. Anteroposterior and lateral radiographs demonstrate bony union along with maintenance of the articular anatomy (Fig. 4-21). The patient was able to return to functional activities within 6 weeks following surgery (Fig. 4-22). She recovered 110 degrees of elbow flexion and lacked 40 degrees of elbow extension.

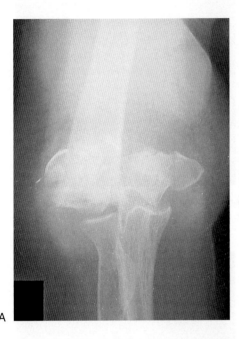

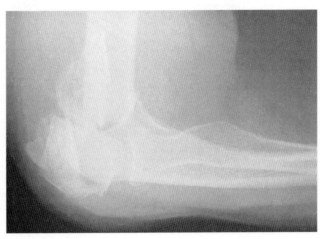

A

B

Figure 4-19. Comminuted Y condylar fracture in elderly female seen on AP (**A**) and lateral projections (**B**).

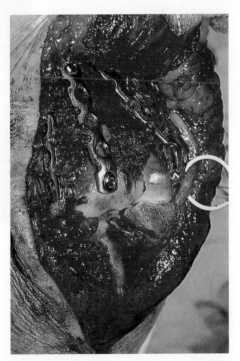

Figure 4-20. Three plates were employed to stabilize fracture distally. The comminution was treated by autogenous iliac bone graft.

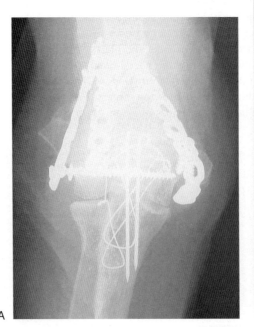
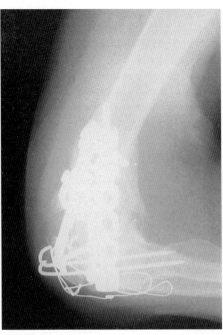

A   B

Figure 4-21. Near anatomic restoration is seen on the AP (**A**) and lateral projections (**B**).

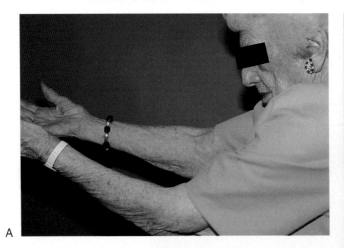
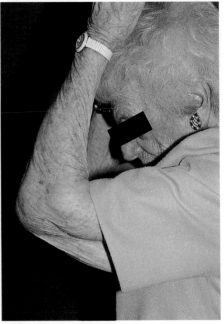

A

Figure 4-22. A useful arc of motion from 50 degrees (**A**) to 105 degrees (**B**) was obtained.

B

RECOMMENDED READINGS

1. Aitken GK, Rorabeck CH. Distal humeral fractures in the adult. *Clin Orthop Rel Res* 1986;207:191–197.
2. Gabel GT, Hanson G, Bennett JB, et al. Intraarticular fractures of the distal humerus in the adult. *Clin Orthop Rel Res* 1987;216:99–107.
3. Helfet DL, Schmerling GJ. Bicondylar intra-articular fractures of the distal humerus in adults. *Clin Orthop* 1993;292:26–36.
4. John H, Rosso R, Neff U, et al. Operative treatment of distal humeral fractures in the elderly. *J Bone Joint Surg* 1994;76B:793–796.
5. Jupiter JB, Mehne DK. Fractures of the distal humerus. *Orthopaedics* 1992;15:825–833.

6. Jupiter JB, Morrey BF. Fractures of the distal humerus. In: Morrey BF, ed. *The elbow and its disorders,* 3rd ed. Philadelphia: WB Saunders; 2000.

7. Jupiter JB, Neff U, Holzach P, et al. Intercondylar fractures of the distal humerus. *J Bone Joint Surg* 1985;67A:226–239.

8. Mehne DD, Jupiter JB. Fractures of the distal humerus. In: Browner B, ed. *Skeletal trauma.* Philadelphia: WB Saunders; 1991:1146–1176.

9. Morrey BF, Adams RA. Semiconstrained joint replacement arthroplasty for distal humeral nonunion. *J Bone Joint Surg* 1995;77B:67–72.

10. Perry CR. Transcondylar fractures of the distal humerus. *J Orthop Trauma* 1989;3:98–106.

5

Radial Head Fractures

Bernard F. Morrey

In recent years, with improved technique, the treatment of radial head fracture by internal fixation has become increasingly accepted (6). As the procedure is now well accepted, several fixation devices and strategies may be used (3,4,5,15). The major burden on the surgeon is the proper patient selection as well as meticulous technique.

Two treatment options are discussed here, osteosynthesis and prosthetic replacement.

INDICATIONS/CONTRAINDICATIONS

Three factors are considered important to define a candidate for radial head fixation after fracture:

- **Fracture type.** The best indication for open reduction and internal fixation is a Mason type II radial head fracture (4,9,11,14,15). This includes a fracture of less than 30% of the radial head, or the classic "slice fracture" that is displaced more than 3 mm.
- **Associated injury causing instability** (8,11,13,17,19). These complications include associated elbow dislocation, isolated medial collateral ligament disruption, and Essex-Lopresti injury. This topic is dealt with in detail in Chapter 7.
- **Age.** All type II radial head fractures may be considered amenable for open reduction and internal fixation in those under 50 to 55 years of age. Type II fractures with associated instability should be fixed at virtually any age (Chapter 7).

Type I radial head fracture is best treated without surgical intervention (8,10). Internal fixation should also not be used in a fracture that is too comminuted to be fixed (type III) (8,11). This problem is best suited for implant replacement. As improved radial head implants are being developed and with increased understanding of "complex instability," we include the technique for prosthetic implant replacement later in this chapter.

B.F. Morrey, M.D.: Mayo Medical School and Department of Orthopaedics, Mayo Clinic and Mayo Foundation, Rochester, Minnesota.

PREOPERATIVE PLANNING

Equipment

The AO miniset is adequate for most fractures (Fig. 5-1). The Herbert screw is available and might be used. It has the advantage of stabilizing the fracture before insertion of the screw, but it is expensive. It is not necessary to have both systems available.

If the fracture is comminuted or primarily involves the radial neck, then an AO miniplate system should be available (10).

Associated Injury

It is of paramount importance to determine if ligament injury has occurred. The effect of radial head fixation is usually adequate in most instances, so direct ligamentous repair is not necessary. If the elbow remains unstable after radial head fracture fixation, one might be prepared for the concurrent application of a distraction device (see Chapter 8).

In an Essex-Lopresti injury, the status of the wrist must be assessed. After the radial head fracture has been treated the injury at the wrist is managed either by reduction and splinting in full supination, by cross-pinning of the ulna, or by direct suture of the triangular fibrocartilage (20).

SURGERY

The patient is placed under a general anesthetic and the extremity is prepared and draped with a nonsterile tourniquet. An arm table may be used. I prefer the position described for other reconstructive procedures with the patient being in the supine position and the arm being brought across the chest.

Technique

For an isolated repair, a classic Kocher or "distal J" specific for purpose incision is made (Fig. 5-2) and the interval between the anconeus and extensor carpi ulnaris identified and entered (Figs. 5-3 and 5-4). A portion of the extensor carpi ulnaris is elevated sufficiently to allow exposure of the lateral collateral ligament complex (Fig. 5-5). If it has not been

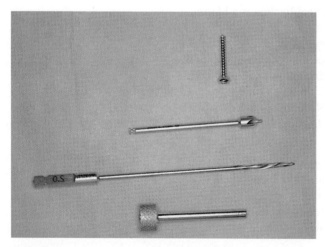

Figure 5-1. Most fractures are managed with the 2.7-mm miniscrew system, which includes a countersink to lessen the likelihood of screw head prominence.

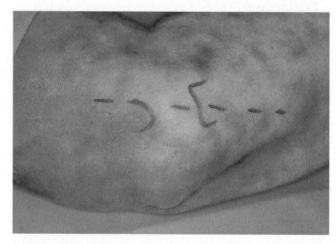

Figure 5-2. With the patient in a supine position with the arm brought across the chest, the distal portion of the Kocher incision is made over the radial head and over the lateral epicondyle.

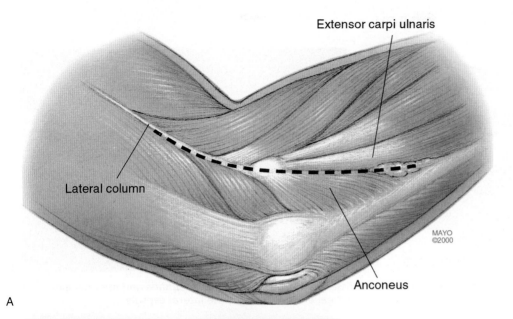

Extensor carpi ulnaris

Lateral column

Anconeus

MAYO
©2000

A

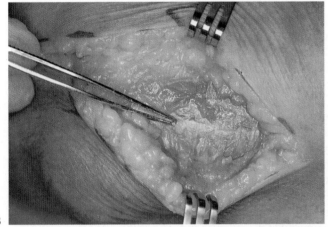

B

Figure 5-3. A,B: The interval between the anconeus and extensor carpi ulnaris is well visualized here.

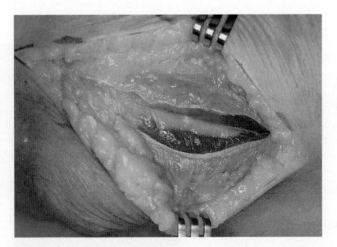

Figure 5-4. This interval is entered and the muscles are retracted.

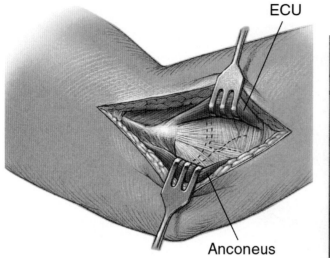

ECU

Anconeus

A

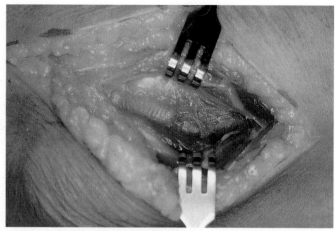

B

Figure 5-5. A,B: Sharp dissection of the extensor carpi ulnaris and minimal elevation of the anconeus by a periosteal elevator reveals the lateral capsule.

torn by the injury, an incision is made in the capsule anterior to the lateral complex that attaches to the ulna (Fig. 5-6). If the elbow is stable, sufficient reflection of the common extensor tendon is necessary to allow adequate exposure of the radial head. A band is used to reflect the common extensor tendon, and a small rake retracts the inferior posterior aspect of the capsule.

The wound is cleared of hematoma. If there are loose fragments without soft tissue, they may be removed from the wound and the surface cleansed with a water pick (Fig. 5-6). If the soft tissue remains on any of the loose fragments, great care is taken to maintain this as a source of blood supply to the fragment. If there is a single slice fracture, it is readily fixed to the remaining portion of the radial head. The articular surface is reduced anatomically and held with a tenaculum (Fig. 5-7). The cortical elements are likewise reduced anatomically. It should be noted that as with tibial plafond fractures, there may be a plastic deformation of the articular surface such that the articular surface and the cortical margins may not simultaneously appear to be anatomically reduced. In this instance, preference is, of course, given to the anatomic reduction of the articular surface. The reduced fracture frag-

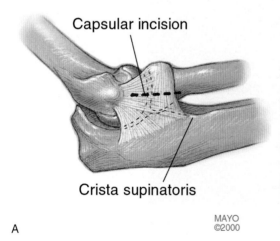

Capsular incision

Crista supinatoris

MAYO
©2000

A

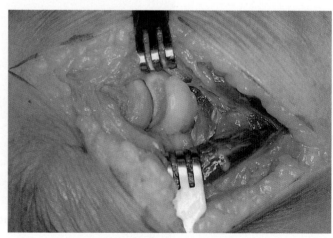

B

Figure 5-6. The lateral capsule is opened just anterior to the lateral complex, which originates at the humerus and attaches to the ulna (**A**). The fracture has been identified and the hematoma cleaned with a water pick (**B**).

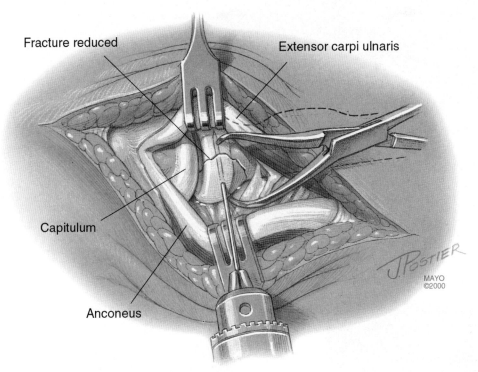

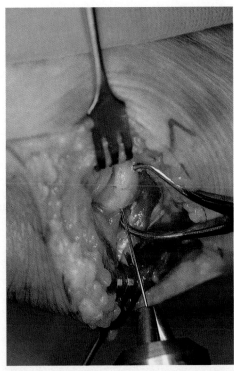

Figure 5-7. A,B: The fracture has been reduced. A K-wire is used to secure the fracture and it is placed in the anterior half of the fracture fragment.

ment is stabilized with a single 0.425 K-wire. This is placed through the anterior half of the fragment (Fig. 5-7). The forearm is then rotated to expose the remainder of the fractured segment. A 2.0-mm hole is first drilled using a tissue protector (Fig. 5-8). The precise depth of the screw hole is determined with the depth gauge, and the fracture fragment is then overdrilled with a 2.7-mm drill (Fig. 5-9). The hole is tapped (Fig. 5-10) and countersunk with a hand-held instrument (Fig. 5-11) and the appropriate-length screw is inserted (Fig. 5-12).

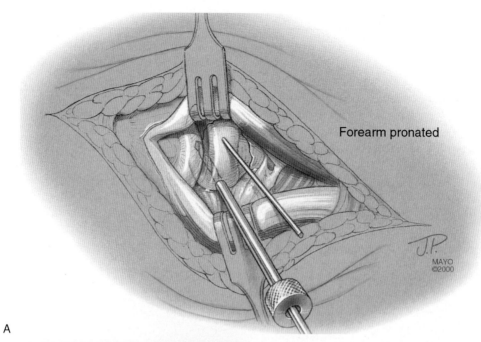

A

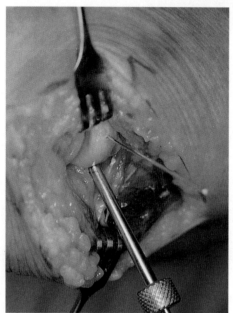

B

Figure 5-8. A,B: The forearm is slightly pronated, exposing the posterior half of the fracture fragment. A drill sleeve is used and a 2.0-mm drill bit is employed.

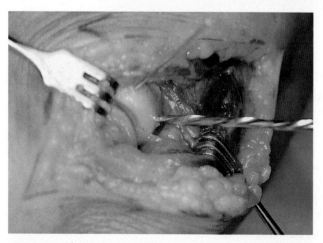

Figure 5-9. A 2.7-mm drill bit is then used to overdrill the fracture fragment to receive the 2.7-mm screw. Care should be taken not to split small slice fracture fragments with the overdrilling process.

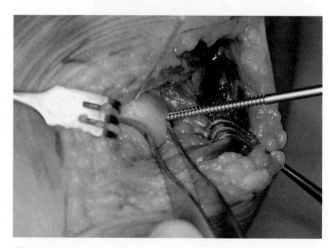

Figure 5-10. The screw hole is tapped to receive the 2.7-mm screw.

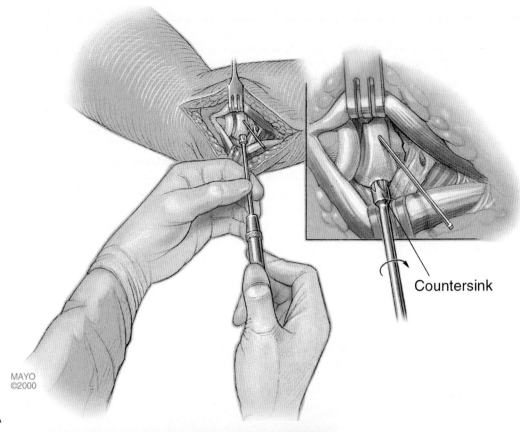

Countersink

A

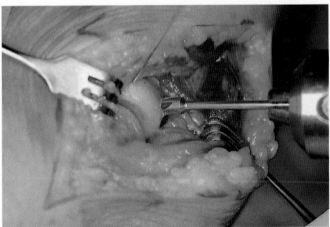

B

Figure 5-11. A,B: A hand-held countersink instrument is used so that the screw head fits flush with the surface of the fracture fragment.

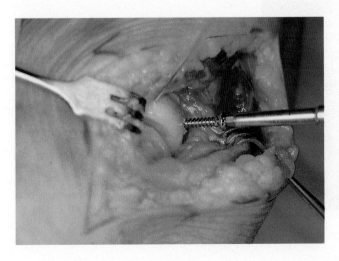

Figure 5-12. A 2.7-mm screw is then inserted across the fracture fragment, preferably perpendicular to the fracture surface. The errors in screw length should be with the screw slightly short rather than slightly long. Anticipation of the slightly increased depth of insertion after the countersink should also be taken into consideration.

MAYO
©2000

The forearm is slightly supinated, the K-wire is removed, and an identical technique is used to insert a second screw parallel to the first in the region of the K-wire.

If the fracture is comminuted, the small center fragments are first reduced and stabilized by reduction to the larger fragment. This may then be stabilized with a small K-wire or a bone-holding clamp. A sharp towel clip may also be used. The mini-AO screws are used to compress the fracture fragments to the stable column. Particular care is taken to avoid the screw extending past the cortex on the opposite side.

Special care is taken to close the rent or the incision in the lateral capsule. The lateral ulnar collateral ligament (LUCL) complex must be assessed to assure competency. Incisions anterior to the LUCL protect this structure if it was not torn at the time of radial head fracture. The final closure should not be so tight as to cause restriction of pronation and supination. This should be tested after closure of the capsule to ensure there is not excessive fric-

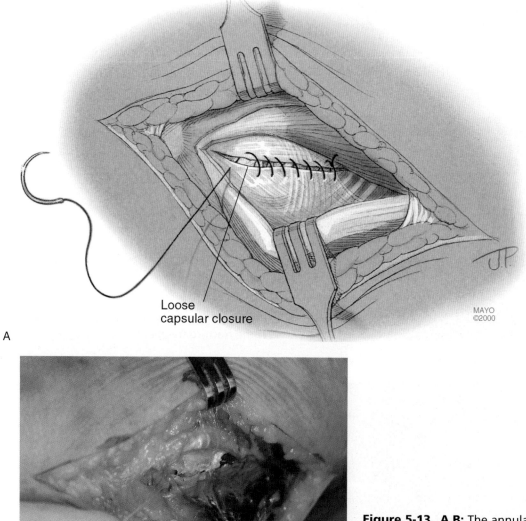

Loose capsular closure

MAYO ©2000

A

B

Figure 5-13. A,B: The annular ligament is only loosely closed. Great care should be taken not to overlap this structure, as it may be a source of irritation with subsequent pronation and supination.

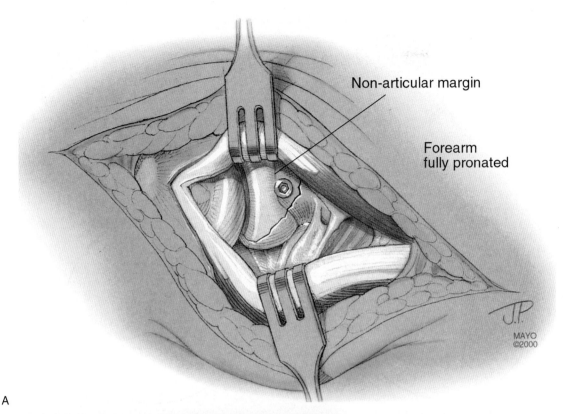

Non-articular margin

Forearm
fully pronated

A

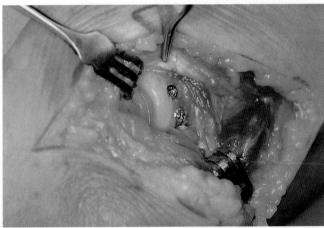

B

Figure 5-14. Note the screw going through the nonarticular portion of the margin of the radial head with the broader portion that articulates with the lesser sigmoid notch appearing below (**A**). Both screws have been inserted and are flush with the surface, and they are not a source of irritation (**B**).

tion or compression with the radial head (Fig. 5-13). An intraarticular drain is placed and absorbable sutures are used to close the Kocher's interval. Subcutaneous tissue and skin are closed in a routine fashion.

It is worth noting that the slice fracture typically occurs with the forearm partially pronated. The slice thus occurs through the part of the radial head that does not articulate with the lesser sigmoid notch. The screw heads are off the articular surface (Fig. 5-14) and do not articulate with the ulna (Fig. 5-15).

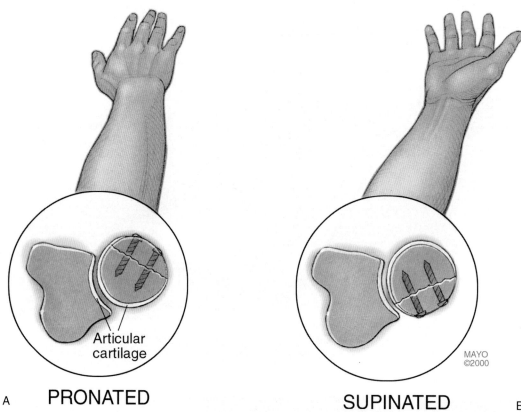

A   **PRONATED**   **SUPINATED**   B

Figure 5-15. The fixation can be applied through a margin of the radial head that does not articulate with the ulna either in full pronation (**A**) or in full supination (**B**).

POSTOPERATIVE MANAGEMENT

If absolute rigidity has been obtained with the fixation device, a posterior splint is applied for 3 days and a portable continuous passive motion (CPM) machine may be used for approximately 2 to 3 weeks. Patients are cautioned to avoid active motion, since this causes increased pressure on the radiohumeral joint. Radiographs are taken at 3 weeks. If the fracture is stable, then gentle-active and active assisted motion are allowed, and passive pronation and supination is encouraged, avoiding flexion in pronation, as this causes increased stress on the fracture (10). Radiographs are taken again at 6 weeks. It is anticipated that early osseous healing should have begun by this time. A period of 3 months is typically required for complete fracture healing. Motion recovery may be delayed for 6 to 12 months from injury.

RESULTS

There are several smaller but no large series of long-term follow-up after this procedure (4,8,9,18). For the type II fracture, approximately 90% appear to have a united fracture with a satisfactory result (14,15). The results of type III radial head fractures are less commonly reported (13). Success ranges from that comparable to the slice fracture to as low as 30% to 33%. A recent study in our laboratory demonstrated improved functional result with strength approaching normal in the uncomplicated fracture (2). The strength of the open reduction with internal fixation (ORIF) group was superior to both those having resection and those treated without surgery.

COMPLICATIONS

The most common complication of radial head fixation is failure of fixation and forearm motion loss. This is seen particularly in those fractures with comminution or with collateral ligament insufficiency causing increased stresses on or scarring to the repaired fracture fragments. The treatment for displacement is delayed radial head excision (1). Resection should not occur in the first 5 to 7 days after the initial injury, but if displacement occurs resection should be deferred for approximately 3 to 4 weeks.

If the fracture fails to unite in 8 to 12 weeks, delayed excision is preferred over additional attempts at fixation.

In some instances, particularly if fixation was not the only procedure, or fixation followed attempts at manipulation or debridement, ectopic bone may occur. Little treatment is available in the acute stage. Typically, the process must mature and then may be excised at a later date. This does complicate and compromise the ultimate result of the procedure, and prevention is far more desirable than the treatment after ectopic bone has formed.

ILLUSTRATIVE CASE

This 38-year-old patient sustained a valgus injury to the elbow, disrupting the medial collateral ligament and causing a compression fracture of the neck of the radius (Fig. 5-16). The technique described earlier was employed to insert a miniplate at the margin of the radial head after the fracture was reduced (Fig. 5-17). At 1 year the fracture has healed (Fig. 5-18) and the patient has a range of motion of 10 to 145 degrees, flexion of 70 degrees, and supination of 80 degrees. There is no pain.

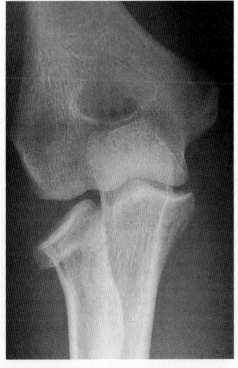

Figure 5-16. A radial/head neck fracture dislocation in a 38-year-old physician.

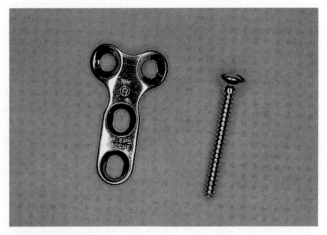

Figure 5-17. At reduction, the radial head was intact, and a miniplate was used employing the 1.0-AO cortical screws.

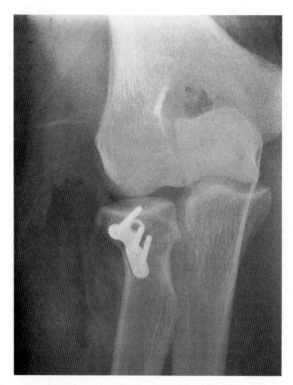

Figure 5-18. One year after treatment the patient's fracture has healed with minimal depression and the patient has a near-normal arc of motion.

RADIAL HEAD REPLACEMENT

The following are our current indications and technique for a new modular radial head replacement. Although the technique is specifically that of the rHead prosthesis by Avanta (San Diego, CA), the principles are, in general, valid for other designs (7).

INDICATIONS/CONTRAINDICATIONS

The following conditions indicate radial head replacement:

A. Acute trauma (6).
  1. Comminuted radial head fracture requiring resection associated with ligament injury.
     a. Elbow dislocation (2).
     b. Distal radioulnar joint injury (Essex-Lopresti injury) (20).
  2. Comminuted radial head fracture requiring resection with associated fracture(s).
     a. Coronoid type II or III fracture (comminuted or noncomminuted) (16).
     b. Olecranon type III fracture (displaced or comminuted and unstable) (13).
  3. After radial head excision with evidence of medial collateral ligament insufficiency (11) or ulnohumeral instability.
B. Reconstruction.
  1. With interposition arthroplasty if the radial head is excised and residual elbow instability persists (12).
  2. For stabilization of the forearm and elbow after an Essex-Lopresti injury (6,13).
  3. Failed silicone radial head implantation if required for stability.

Certain conditions contraindicate this procedure or require special consideration:

A. Acute trauma.
1. Older patient with a comminuted radial head fracture requiring radial head excision without evidence of elbow instability or other associated injury (greater than age 65).
2. Open fracture of the radial head, olecranon or associated elbow dislocation with high risk for sepsis.
3. Mason type I or II radial head fractures.
4. Mason type III radial head fracture not associated with elbow or forearm instability (2,14).
B. Reconstruction (6,14).
1. In reconstructions if the proximal radius is malaligned with the capitellum.
2. Proximal radial shaft fractures associated with comminuted radial head fracture.
3. Disease of or injury to the capitellum (e.g., osteochondrosis).

Absolute contraindications to radial head replacement include:

1. Prior sepsis or concern regarding wound contamination.
2. Known sensitivity constituents.
3. Skeletal immaturity.
4. Insufficient soft tissues to provide for lateral or medial elbow stability.
5. For reconstruction if the resected radius is malaligned with the capitellum.

SURGERY

Positioning and capsular exposure is as described earlier for internal fixation. The lateral capsule is entered slightly anteriorly to the collateral ligament, and the annular ligament and capsule are reflected anteriorly and posteriorly to expose the radial head. A portion of the lateral collateral ligament and anterior capsule can be reflected from the lateral epicondyle and anterior humerus to expose the capitellum if necessary. Efforts are made not to detach the lateral ulnohumeral ligament, but if greater exposure is required, the ligament is reflected from its humeral origin. If the ligament has been disrupted, then the exposure progresses through the site of disruption to expose the radiohumeral joint. The common extensor tendon and anterior capsule are retracted as needed for adequate exposure (Fig. 5-19).

An accurate radial neck cut requires a resection guide. The device is inserted over the capitellum with the axis alignment rod being oriented over the ulnar styloid (Fig. 5-20). This alignment replicates the anatomic axis of forearm rotation. Test forearm rotation with the axis guide in place to ensure proper alignment. The proximal flange of the axis guide is placed against the articular surface of the capitellum, and the cutting guide is then adjusted proximally or distally for the desired extent of radial head resection.

During resection of the radial head the forearm is pronated and supinated to create a resection perpendicular to the axis of rotation as defined by the resection guide (Fig. 5-21). This includes sufficient resection to allow the device to articulate with the ulna at the lesser sigmoid notch. The distal extent of resection is the minimal amount that is consistent with the restoration of function as dictated by the fracture line or previous radial head resection but still compatible with implant insertion.

Varus stress and rotation of the forearm allow exposure of the medullary canal, especially if the elbow is unstable. If the stability does not allow exposure of the proximal radius, careful reflection of the origin of the collateral ligament from the lateral epicondyle may be necessary to permit adequate exposure to the medullary canal. The canal is entered with a starter awl using a twisting motion. With the forearm in midrotation, the curved broach is introduced down the canal (Fig. 5-22).

The appropriate-sized trial stem is inserted by rotating down the canal with the tip oriented opposite of the radial tuberosity (Fig. 5-23). The appropriate-sized head is then applied (Fig. 5-24). Tracking, both in flexion and extension and in forearm rotation, should be carefully assessed. Malalignment of the radial osteotomy cut will cause abnormal tracking during flexion/extension and/or forearm pronation and supination.

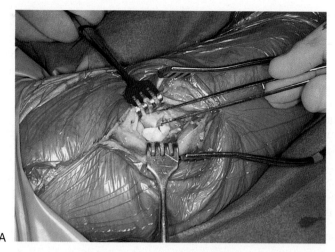

A

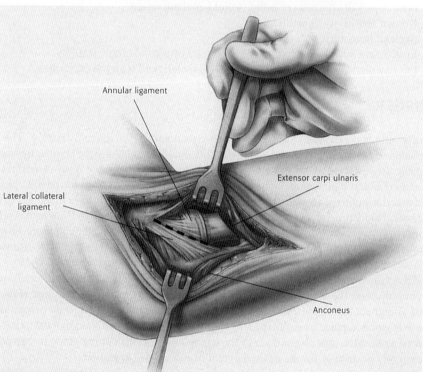

Annular ligament

Extensor carpi ulnaris

Lateral collateral ligament

Anconeus

B

Figure 5-19. A,B: After a type III radial head fracture the right elbow joint is exposed through Kocher's interval and the fracture is identified. If the collateral ligament is intact, reflection from the humeral attachment to a variable extent may be necessary to insert the implant.

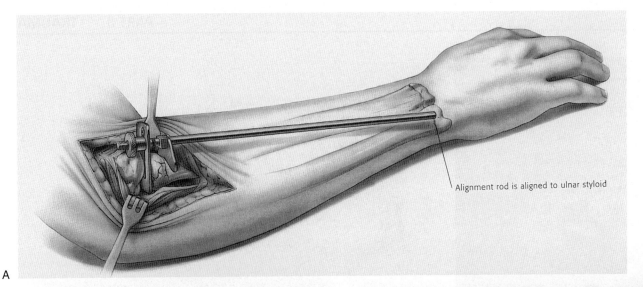

A

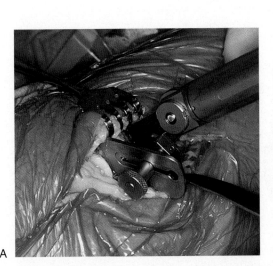

B

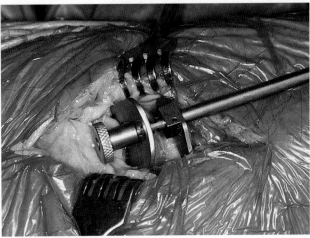

C

Figure 5-20. The alignment device is inserted in the joint. The distal portion is placed over the ulnar styloid (**A,B**) and the proximal portion rests against the capitellum (**C**).

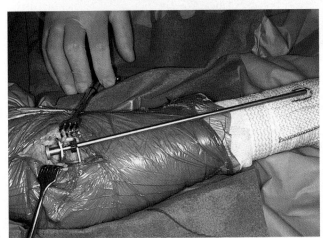

A

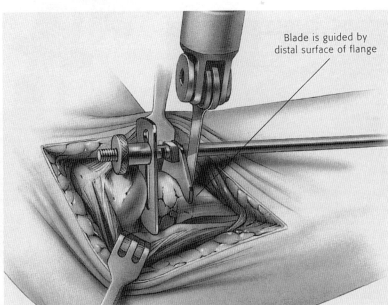

B

Figure 5-21. A,B: An oscillating saw is used to resect the neck perpendicular to the axis of rotation by using the resection guide and rotating the forearm during resection.

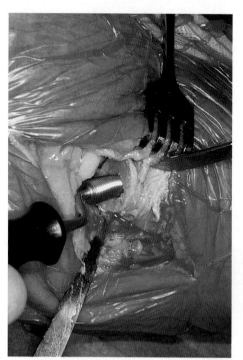

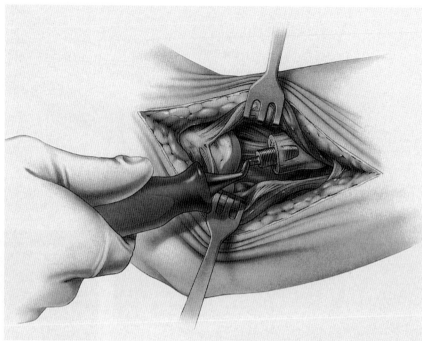

A   B

Figure 5-22. A,B: Insertion of the broach down the canal is facilitated by the curvature, which matches the stem of the implant.

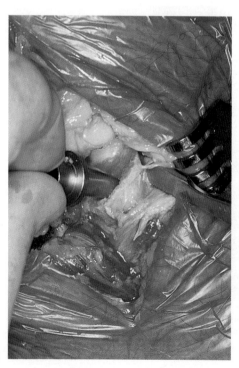

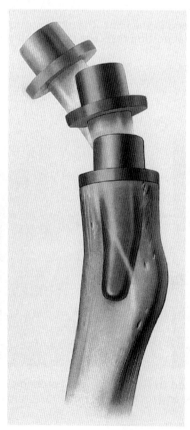

A   B

Figure 5-23. A,B: The curved trial stem of the implant is readily inserted down the canal.

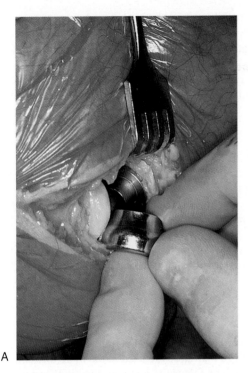

A

Figure 5-24. A,B: The appropriately sized head
is applied.

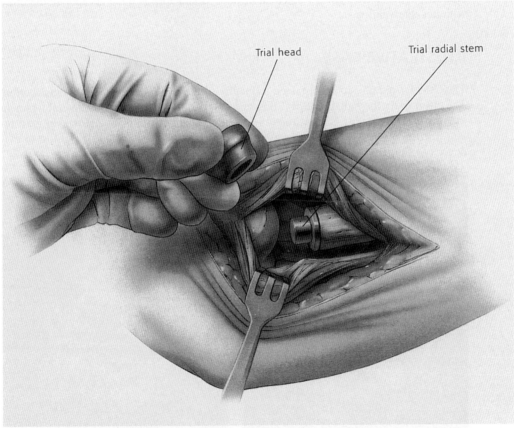

Trial head   Trial radial stem

B

   Once proper size, alignment, and positioning of the implant have been determined, the
prosthetic radial stem is inserted with a rotational motion down the medullary canal and
tapped in place with the impactor. Bone cement (PMMA) may occasionally be used if secure press-fit fixation is absent. The modular head is next placed over the taper using longitudinal distraction and/or varus stress to distract the radiocapitellar interface sufficiently

to permit the radial head to be inserted. The radial head implant is secured using the impactor. Alignment is again assessed (Fig. 5-25).

Note: Care should be taken to protect the taper from damage, including but not limited to scratches and contact with bone cement.

Closure for internal fixation is noted earlier. Once again, reconstitution of the LUCL is essential. If this appears inadequate, it should be reinforced with a No. 5 nonabsorbable Bunnell or Krachow stitch.

POSTOPERATIVE MANAGEMENT

Passive flexion and extension are allowed on the second day, assuming the elbow is considered stable. The goal of radial head replacement and soft-tissue repair is to achieve elbow stability. Both flexion/extension and pronation/supination arcs are allowed without restriction. Active motion can begin by day 5.

Long-term aftercare requires surveillance as with any prosthetic replacement. If the implant is asymptomatic and tracks well, routine removal is not necessary at this time.

RESULTS

In spite of the recent interest, there are few detailed outcomes of recent implants in the peer-reviewed literature (7). In general, it is recognized that these are used in the more difficult clinical circumstances (6). An outcome of 80% satisfactory is quite acceptable therefore with this intervention.

ILLUSTRATIVE CASE

This 30-year-old physician sustained a fracture of the radial head and elbow dislocation. The effort to fix the radial head was unsuccessful and the medial ulnar collateral ligament did not heal (Fig. 5-26). Reconstruction with the radial head implant and tendon graft reconstruction of the MCL were successful and the patient has minimal discomfort or evidence of instability (Fig. 5-27).

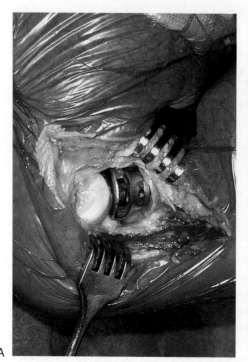
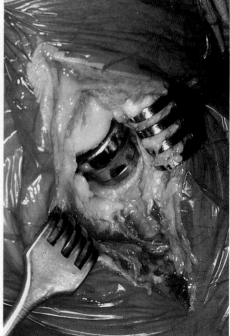

A   B

Figure 5-25. Proper tracking is assessed during flexion (**A**) and extension (**B**).

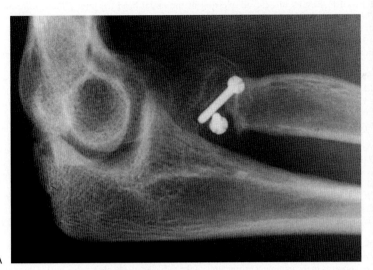

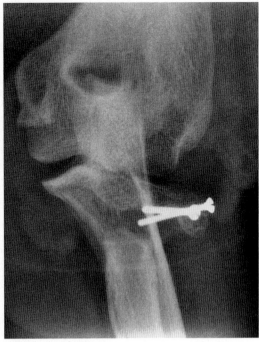

Figure 5-26. A 30-year-old physician underwent reduction and fixation of type III radial head fracture with concurrent elbow dislocation. The fracture went to a nonunion (**A**) and the medial collateral ligament failed to heal (**B**).

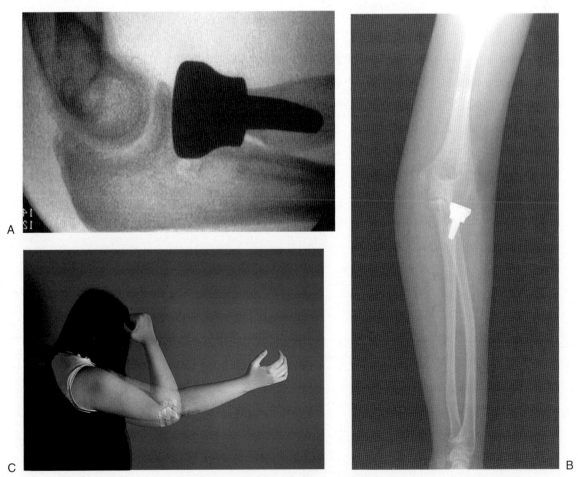

Figure 5-27. Treatment with implant and MCL reconstruction. The implant is well positioned and the elbow is stable (**A,B**). At 4 weeks the patient has excellent motion and stability (**C**).

RECOMMENDED READINGS

1. Broberg MA, Morrey BF. Results of delayed excision of the radial head fracture. *J Bone Joint Surg* 1986;68A:669–675.
2. Broberg MA, Morrey BF. Results of treatment of fracture dislocations of the elbow. *Clin Orthop* 1987;March(216):109–119.
3. Bunker TD, Newman JH. The Herbert differential pitch bone screw in displaced radial head fractures. *Injury* 1985;16:621.
4. Esser RD, David S, Taavao T. Fractures of the radial head treated by internal fixation: late results in 26 cases. *J Orthop Trauma* 1995;9:318.
5. Gupta GG, Lucas G, Hahn DL. Biomechanical and computer analysis of radial head prostheses. *J Shoulder Elbow Surg* 1997;6:37–48.
6. Hotchkiss RN. Displaced fractures of the radial head: internal fixation or excision? *J Am Acad Orthop Surg* 1997;5:1–10.
7. Judet T, Garreau de Loubresse C, Piriou P, Charnley G. A floating prosthesis for radial-head fractures. *J Bone Joint Surg* 1996;78B:244–249.
8. King GJW, Evans DC, Kellam FJ. Open reduction and internal fixation of radial head fractures. *J Orthop Trauma* 1991;5:21.
9. Konlic E, Perry CR. Indications and technique of open reduction and internal fixation of radial head fractures. *Orthopedics* 1992;15:837–842.
10. Leung KS, Tse PYT. A new method of fixing radial neck fractures. Brief report. *J Bone Joint Surg* 1989;71B:326.
11. Morrey BF, Tanaka S, An KN. Valgus stability of the elbow: a definition of primary and secondary constraints. *Clin Orthop* 1991;April(265):187–195.
12. Morrey BF. Current concepts in the treatment of fractures of the radial head, the olecranon, and the coronoid. *J Bone Joint Surg* 1995;77A:316–327.
13. Morrey BF. Complex instability of the elbow. *J Bone Joint Surg* 1997;79A:460–469.
14. Morrey BF. Radial head fracture. In: Morrey BF. *The elbow and its disorders,* 3rd ed., Philadelphia: WB Saunders; 2000.
15. Odenheimer K, Harvey JP Jr. Internal fixation of fractures of the head of the radius. *J Bone Joint Surg* 1979;61A:785.
16. Regan W, Morrey BF. Fractures of the coronoid process of the ulna. *J Bone Joint Surg* 1989;71A:1348.
17. Sanders RA, French HG. Open reduction and internal fixation of comminuted radial head fractures. *Am J Sports Med* 1986;14:130.
18. Shmueli G, Herold HZ. Compression screwing of displaced fractures of the head of the radius. *J Bone Joint Surg* 1981;63B:535.
19. Soler RR, Tarela JP, Minores JM. Internal fixation of fractures of the proximal end of the radius in adults. *Injury* 1979;10:268.
20. Trousdale RT, Amadio PC, Cooney WP, et al. Radioulnar dissociation: a review of twenty cases. *J Bone Joint Surg* 1992;74A:1486–1497.

6

Management of Olecranon Fractures and Nonunion

Ralph W. Coonrad and Bernard F. Morrey

INDICATIONS/CONTRAINDICATIONS

Since olecranon fractures involve the articular surface, two imperatives must be met if open reduction and internal fixation are to be carried out:

1. Fixation must be stable enough to permit mobilization within 5 days.
2. Anatomic or essentially normal surface reduction (within 1 mm) and normal sigmoid notch contour must be achieved.

Failure to attain either of these goals will lead to limited motion and a poorer result. Results of all elbow surgery are based on pain, motion, strength, and stability.

The management of elbow fracture indications seems to relate more appropriately to the selection of fixation than to whether or not to operate. The choice of one of several treatment options for olecranon fractures is based entirely on fracture type. Various modifications of Colton's (3) original classification of fracture types have been described. Morrey's (12) classification based on displacement, comminution, and stability has been more workable in the authors' hands (Fig. 6-1). Several treatment options are described, depending on the fracture type.

Avulsion Fractures

Avulsion fractures are essentially triceps tendon ruptures with attached large or small fragments that are best discussed in the context of triceps mechanisms insufficiency (Chapter 11).

R.W. Coonrad, M.D.: Division of Orthopedic Surgery, Duke University, Lenox Baker Childrens Hospital, Durham, North Carolina.

B.F. Morrey, M.D.: Mayo Medical School and Department of Orthopaedics, Mayo Clinic and Mayo Foundation, Rochester, Minnesota.

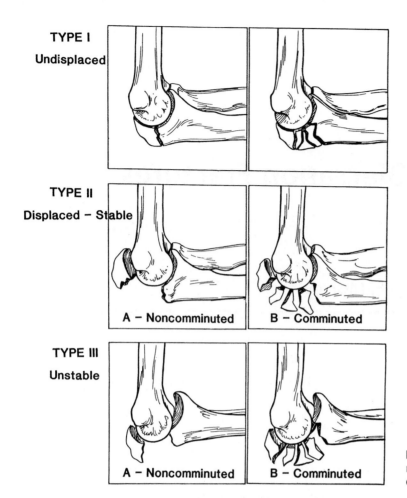

TYPE I
Undisplaced

TYPE II
Displaced – Stable

A – Noncomminuted   B – Comminuted

TYPE III
Unstable

A – Noncomminuted   B – Comminuted

Figure 6-1. The Mayo classification of olecranon fractures. (With permission, Mayo Foundation.)

Fracture Classification

We have found the basis of olecranon fracture management is predicated on variable displacement, comminution, and joint stability. These considerations are reflected in the Mayo classification of olecranon fractures (Fig. 6-1).

Type I: Nondisplaced Fractures Nondisplaced fractures that are entirely stable when tested by flexing and extending the elbow can be mobilized after 3 to 5 days of splinting for comfort (Fig. 6-2). Questionably stable fractures, particularly when comminuted or with some articular surface separation, even though less than 2 mm, may require 3 to 4

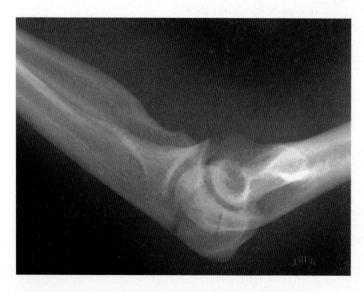

Figure 6-2. Comminuted, undisplaced, and stable olecranon fracture in a 26-year-old man treated satisfactorily in a protective splint for 3 weeks but with range of motion daily after 5 days.

weeks of immobilization in midflexion. In such instances, the authors feel immediate rigid internal fixation to permit mobilization within 5 days is preferable to accepting the loss of motion usually accompanying elbow injuries after longer immobilization.

Type II: Displaced Stable Fractures In noncomminuted stable fractures, fracture fragments that are transverse or oblique, involving less than 50% of the proximal sigmoid notch, should probably be excised in the elderly patient (5,9). All others with sufficient bone stock are treated by an intramedullary screw or Kirschner wire and tension band fixation (9,13,19). A large intramedullary screw with tension band is equal in energy to failure to tension band wiring with two Kirschner wires by the AO technique (18) and has fewer complications in our hands. The following are examples of the preceding technique and two alternate methods of fixation that are widely accepted for this type of fracture:

1. Tension band wiring with two Kirschner wires (9,13) (Fig. 6-3).
2. An obliquely placed cancellous bicortical screw or an intramedullary screw with or without tension band wiring. The former is best used with an oblique fracture (Fig. 6-4).
3. Noncomminuted stable fractures involving more than 50% of the sigmoid notch are best treated, in the authors' hands, with a contoured plate, described later (9,13) (Fig. 6-5).
4. Comminuted stable fractures of the olecranon often involve central fragmentation. All fragments are salvaged if at all possible and stabilized with an AO 3.5-mm DC, one-third tubular, or reconstruction contoured plate (6,9,13), using bone grafts from the iliac crest to fill or buttress defects along with additional interfragmentary screw fixation. Comminuted fractures involving less than 50% of the sigmoid notch can be safely excised if ligamentous integrity is assured and is the treatment of choice in the elderly patient (1,5,11).

Type III: Unstable Displaced Fractures Unstable displaced fractures of the olecranon are uncommon, often comminuted, and unstable because of injury to the collateral ligament that inserts at the medial aspect of the coronoid process (16). Roentgenographic recognition of Regan-Morrey types II and III displaced coronoid fractures (15) is sometimes difficult; however, the importance of restoring displaced coronoid fractures both for the anterior buttress effect on the joint and for the stabilizing effect of the anterior oblique ligament insertion cannot be overstressed. With unstable elbow injuries, fragment excision is contraindicated. Bone defects are buttressed with iliac bone grafts.

In the authors' hands, a contoured AO plate (6,13) with interfragmentary screw fixation has proven to be the stable construct (Fig. 6-6). With a more distal fracture involving the ulnar shaft, a longer plate is used (2). Alternatively, the combination of a dorsally applied AO plate and tension band with K-wires or intramedullary screw may be used.

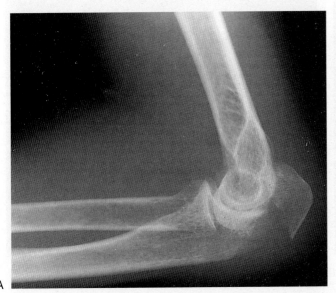
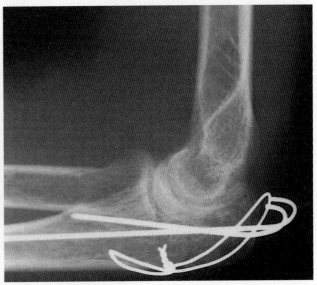

A   B

Figure 6-3. Pre- (**A**) and postoperative (**B**) radiographs of a displaced, stable, Morrey type IIA olecranon fracture treated with Kirschner wires and tension band wire by the AO technique and mobilization at 5 days with satisfactory result; healing by 3 months.

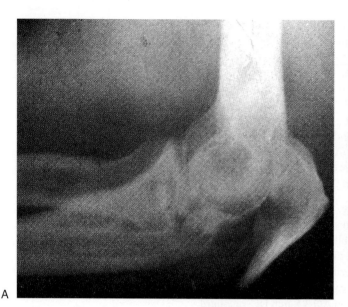
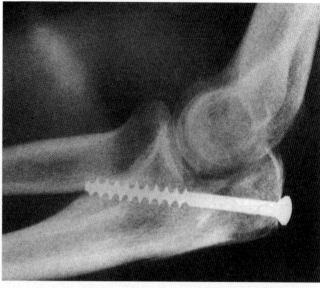

Figure 6-4. Pre- (**A**) and postoperative (**B**) radiographs of a displaced, stable, Morrey type IIA comminuted olecranon fracture treated with bicortical oblique screw fixation with a range of motion result limited by only 5 degrees. (From Wadsworth TG. Adult trauma. In: Wadsworth TG, ed. *The elbow.* New York: Churchill Livingstone; 1982.)

When fixation of unstable fractures is at all questionable, as with severe comminution, an external fixator or distraction device should be applied to compensate for the potential instability and still permit early motion. The reader is referred to Chapter 8 for details of application and use of the distraction device. With severe comminution and instability in the elderly patient, resection of bone is likely to be disabling, and consideration may need to be given to primary total elbow implant arthroplasty.

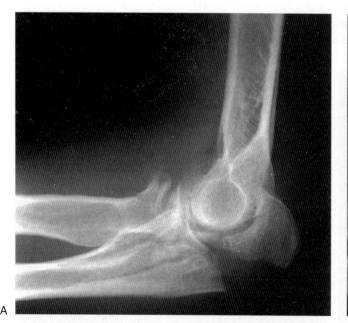
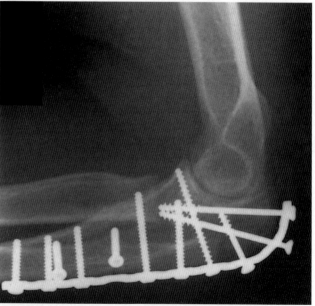

Figure 6-5. Pre- (**A**) and postoperative (**B**) radiographs of a displaced, stable, Morrey type IIA olecranon fracture in a 46-year-old man treated with reconstruction plate and interfragmentary screws with excision of the comminuted radial head. Motion regained was from 10 to 135 degrees with full rotation.

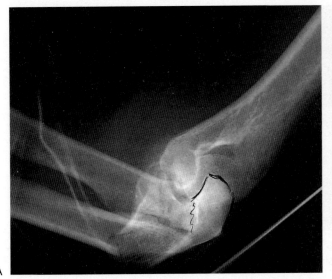
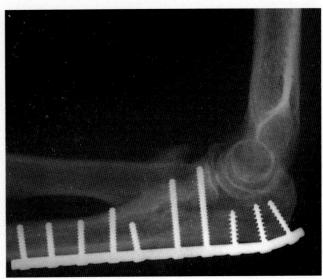

A   B

Figure 6-6. Preoperative radiograph (**A**) of an open unstable, displaced, and comminuted olecranon fracture (type IIIB) in a 42-year-old woman treated with a plate and recovered 25 to 135 degrees of painless anteroposterior (AP) motion and 90 degrees of pronation with 75 degrees supination (**B**).

PREOPERATIVE PLANNING

Resection rather than internal fixation may be a consideration and is preferable in the elderly or osteopenic patient with a noncomminuted or comminuted stable fracture involving 50% or less of the proximal olecranon (1,5,10,11). In all other instance, internal fixation should be used, with the choice being determined by the type of fracture as classified earlier. If instability is present the injury is considered one of complex instability and managed as described in Chapter 7.

SURGERY

Perioperative antibiotics are administered, with the initial dose given at the time of the surgical procedure. A tourniquet to 100 mm Hg above systolic pressure is checked before, during, and at the end of the operative procedure. (Tourniquet calibration is checked with each use.) Exsanguination before tourniquet inflation is by total elevation of the extremity for 60 seconds, rather than with an Esmarch bandage, to make visualization of the vascular structures easier.

A 10 × 10 (3M) drape is applied to isolate the tourniquet from seepage of prep solution beneath the tourniquet (burns have been reported). Skin preparation is carried out with betadine solution after a 5-minute scrub.

The patient is supine or turned one-third away from the side of the involvement with the arm across the chest (authors' choice) or prone with the arm over a padded table. The arm can be extended from either position away from the table for C-arm fluoroscopic use.

Type I: Nondisplaced Fractures

If internal fixation is felt advisable to avoid more than 5 to 7 days of immobilization, treatment is the same as for type II displaced stable fractures, described later.

Type II: Displaced Stable Fractures

Displaced noncomminuted stable fractures with 50% or less involvement of the sigmoid notch are treated with one of the three following methods, listed in order of the authors'

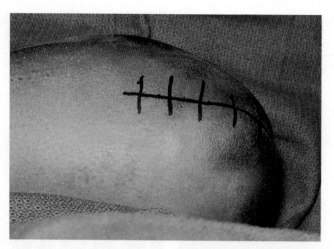

Figure 6-7. Approach to the proximal ulna and radial head through a posterior incision.

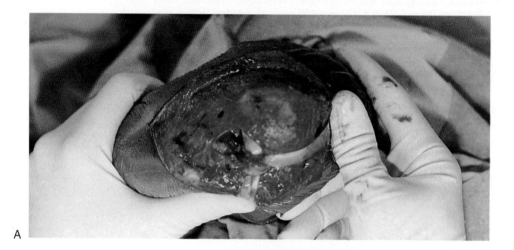

A

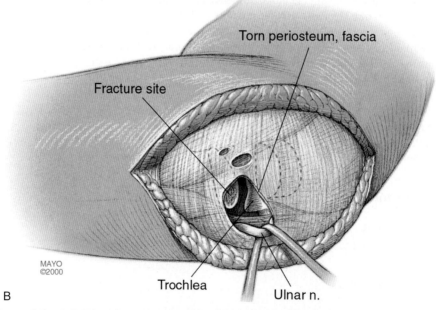

Torn periosteum, fascia

Fracture site

Trochlea   Ulnar n.

MAYO
©2000

B

Figure 6-8. A,B: The ulnar nerve is routinely identified but transferred only if necessary. It is protected with a Penrose drain.

preference: intramedullary screw, with wire technique; tension band technique; bicortical screw fixation.

Intramedullary Screw, Tension Band Technique The skin incision is midline over the olecranon (Fig. 6-7) and extended proximally and distally if necessary, incising the superficial fascia and elevating the anconeus from the lateral aspect of the ulna (17). By reflecting the proximal fragment, sufficient visualization is available to perform anatomic reduction of the fragment (Fig. 6-8). Care is taken to preserve and/or repair the radial ulnar collateral ligament. Alternatively, if the radial head, anterior capsule, and coronoid are to be visualized, the Kocher approach is used, developing the interval between the anconeus and extensor carpi ulnaris as described in Chapter 1.

The ulnar nerve is routinely identified and protected with a 1/4-inch Penrose drain (wet and untied) around it, transferring the nerve subcutaneously if necessary (Fig. 6-8).

A 5-mm tongue of distal periosteum is taken with the proximal olecranon major fragment after identifying that the fracture line is not already separated, and the soft tissue attached to the major fragments is disturbed as little as possible (Fig. 6-9). Laterally and me-

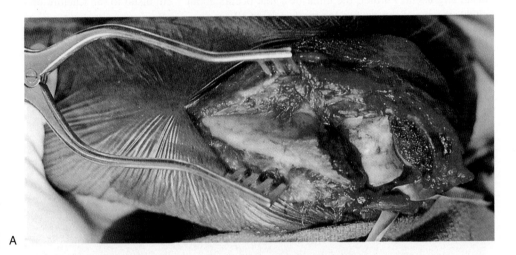

A

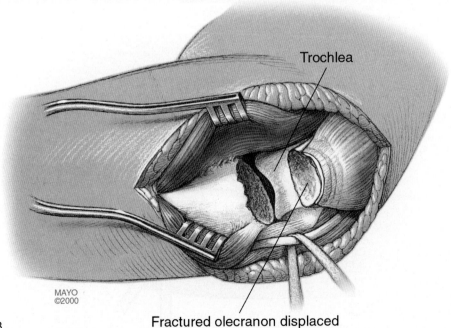

B

Figure 6-9. A,B: The fractured fragment is retracted by dissecting it free of the periosteum, which has usually been ruptured from the fracture.

dially, the triceps retinaculum and the periosteum are incised and the fracture(s) are identified and cleaned of hematoma; the fragments are temporarily reduced and held in place with a ratcheted towel clip or K-wire (Fig. 6-10). Accurate approximation of the fracture surfaces dorsally, laterally, and at the sigmoid notch level is achieved, and any defect of buttressing of a central fragment is accomplished with bone graft from the ilium.

A 3.2-mm drill bit is used as a guide for the intramedullary screw, and a drill hole at the level of and in line with the medullary canal is made in the proximal fragment (Fig. 6-11). The hole in the proximal fragment is enlarged by a 4.5-mm drill bit, and a 6.5-mm tap is used in the cortex of the proximal fragment and taken distally into the medullary canal of the distal segment for a distance of 7 to 10 cm. Exposure for the tap, and subsequently for screw placement, is made with a 1- to 2-cm longitudinal incision in the triceps tendon in the midline over the posterior olecranon (Fig. 6-12). I also use fluoroscopic verification of the position of the fracture and fixation.

Note: If the insertion in the proximal fragment is not proper to ensure anatomic reduction, it may be enlarged to allow the proximal position of the screw to accommodate the distal alignment. Further, the ulnar bow that occurs about 7 cm distal to the fracture precludes the use of screws any longer than 10 to 12 cm.

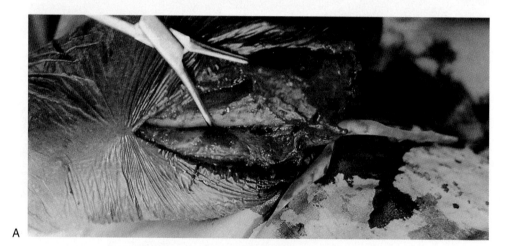

A

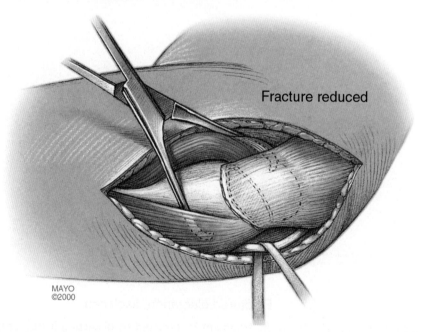

Fracture reduced

MAYO
©2000

B

Figure 6-10. A,B: The fracture is reduced and stabilized with a bone holding forceps.

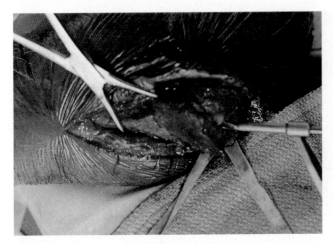

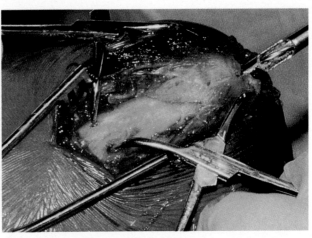

Figure 6-11. The proximal drill hole is very carefully made to ensure anatomic alignment of the fracture and correct orientation with the distal shaft fragment.

Figure 6-12. Intramedullary fixation should extend distally for approximately 7 cm; the proximal fragment is prepared with a 6.5-mm tap.

Depending on the ulnar bow, a 6.5-mm, 10- to 12-cm AO screw (Fig. 6-13) (unthreaded proximally and with 32-mm distal threads) is then inserted over the washer and across the reduced fracture site, but incompletely tightened (Fig. 6-14). The screw threads must achieve firm cortical fixation in the intramedullary canal. C-arm fluoroscopic verification is made.

A 2-mm drill hole (for the tension band wire) is then made transversely through the distal fragment 3 mm anterior to the dorsal cortex and 3 to 4 cm distal to the fracture, or more than equal distance from the proximal tip of the olecranon to the fracture site (Fig. 6-15). A 15-gauge tension band wire is passed beneath the triceps tendon and under the washer and screw. This may be facilitated by a large-bore intracatheter needle (Fig. 6-16), twisted in a figure-eight fashion dorsally over the periosteal sleeve of the olecranon, and threaded through the transverse hole in the distal fragment. It is then twisted in a loop on each side by the AO method. This will permit more uniform compression as the wire is tightened.

The intramedullary screw is tightened to a compression level while observing the sigmoid notch, with care taken to avoid any collapse of its normal semicircular contour (Fig. 6-17).

The tension band wires are then tightened with a wire twister on each side (Fig. 6-18). They are cut to a 4-mm length and reflected volarward and toward the ulna (Fig. 6-19). Fluoroscopic C-arm verification is made.

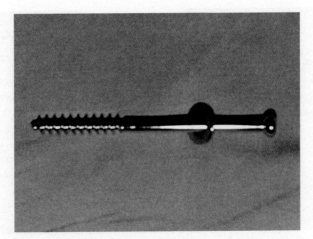

Figure 6-13. A 6.5-mm cancellous screw 10 to 12 cm in length is introduced down the canal. This should cross the fracture site at least 7 cm.

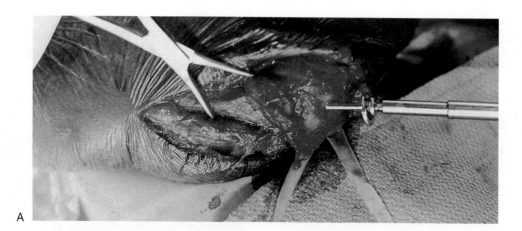

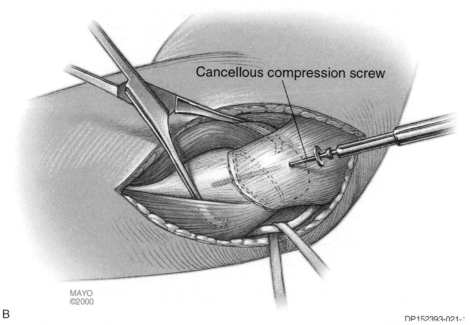

Cancellous compression screw

MAYO
©2000

B

DP152393-021-1

Figure 6-14. A,B: Exposure to insert the drill and screw is most readily obtained by a simple triceps splitting incision over the insertion at the posterior olecranon.

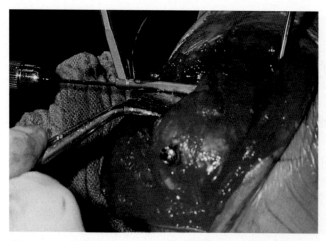

Figure 6-15. A transverse drill hole is made about 3 mm anterior to the dorsal cortex 3 or 4 cm distal to the fracture.

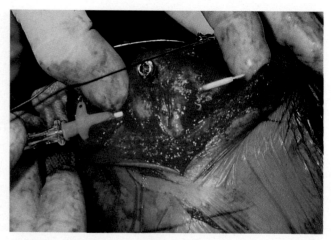

Figure 6-16. A tension band is passed beneath the triceps tendon. This is facilitated by a large-bore needle to serve as a cannula.

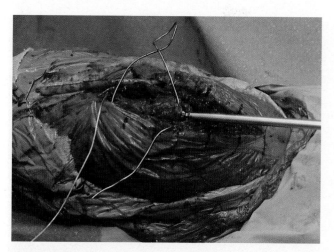

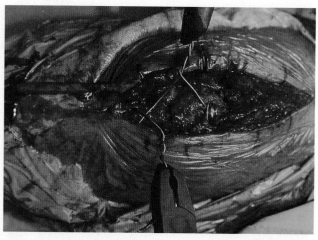

Figure 6-17. The distance between the coronoid and the tip of the olecranon is directly observed as the screw is being tightened. This distance must not be narrowed.

Figure 6-18. Medial and lateral tightening of the tension band system is performed to apply uniform compression across the fracture site.

The periosteum, triceps aponeurosis, and deep fascia on each side are repaired with 0 Vicryl interrupted sutures; the subcutaneous tissue is closed with interrupted 2-0 Vicryl, and skin is closed with 4-0 continuous Vicryl subcuticular suture. After using Steri-strips for skin approximation, a dry dressing and skin adhesive are applied and followed by six- to eight-thickness equally and snugly applied sheet cotton beneath a light cast (two rolls of fiberglass casting material) with the elbow in full extension.

Sensation and neurologic function are recorded in the operating and recovery room, and the patient is sent to the recovery room with the extremity at 60 degrees of elevation, maintained with pillows.

Case Presentation This technique was useful to fix the Mayo type I fracture in a 45-year-old active male (Fig. 6-20). The patient attained normal motion and strength.

Tension Band Technique With the tension band technique, incision and exposure are identical to the intramedullary screw and band technique described earlier.

After accurate visualization and fracture reduction medially, laterally, and dorsally, and with any central sigmoid notch impaction reduced and buttressed with autogenous bone from the ileum or lateral epicondyle, two 2-mm parallel Kirschner wires, to resist torque and displacement forces, are inserted under C-arm fluoroscopic control so that they extend from the posterior dorsal aspect of the olecranon, traverse the fracture site obliquely, and

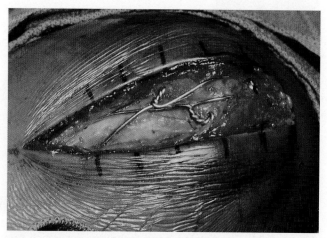

Figure 6-19. The wires are cut and bent to avoid irritation.

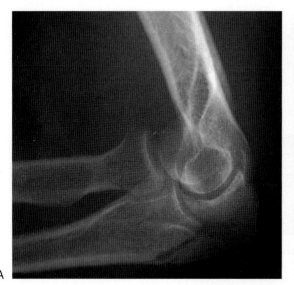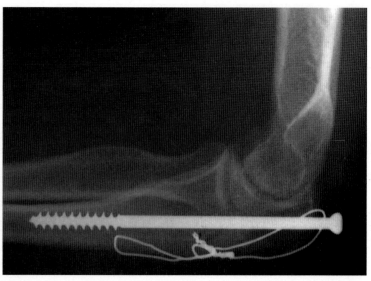

A   B

Figure 6-20. A,B: Figure 6-20. Intramedullary screw and tension band technique for a Morrey type IA fracture.

extend just through the anterior ulnar cortex distal to the coronoid process (Fig. 6-21). The wires are cut and bent toward the ulna.

An 18-gauge wire for a tension band is passed beneath the triceps tension and looped around the two bent Kirschner wires by the AO technique directly over bone and brought out distally in a figure-eight fashion and threaded transversely through a 2-mm drill hole through the ulna as described earlier. The tension band attachments to bone and K-wires are inserted dorsal to the midaxis of the ulna, and with the elbow flexed serve to further compress the fracture site. Radiographic verification of the construct and reduction is made.

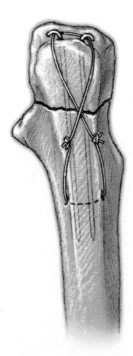

Pins oblique, cortex engaged

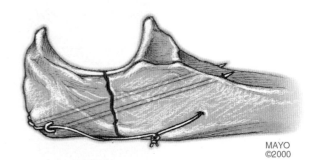

MAYO
©2000

Figure 6-21. The tension band technique for which two pins are inserted down the midaxis of the ulna or obliquely to engage the anterior cortex. Radiographic verification is required to be sure the pins have not violated the sigmoid notch.

Note: The oblique orientation of the K-wires penetrating the anterior cortex has largely eliminated the problem of K-wire back-out, requiring removal. Further, although somewhat controversial, we are not convinced the cables offer any advantages over simple 18-gauge wire (8).

Bicortical Screw Fixation   When using bicortical screw fixation, incision and exposure are identical with those described earlier.

With the fracture temporarily held reduced with a K-wire or ratcheted towel clip, the 3.2-mm drill bit used as a guide is removed and the hole is enlarged to 4.5 mm in the proximal fragment. A 6.5-mm tap is inserted through the ulnar cortex distal to the coronoid and a 6.5-mm AO screw over a washer and of proper length to achieve bicortical compression is inserted and tightened. Radiographic verification of fixation and reduction is made. A tension band is ordinarily unnecessary with oblique bicortical fixation.

Types IIB and III

Displaced, stable comminuted fractures (type IIB) and displaced, unstable noncomminuted and comminuted fractures (type IIIA, B) are treated by contoured plate technique if possible. The distractor is applied if necessary (Chapter 7).

Contoured Plate Technique   Incision and exposure are identical to those described earlier.

With exposure of the major fragments under direct vision, and using C-arm fluoroscopic control, reduction is achieved and maintained with temporary Kirschner wires and interfragmentary screw fixation. The fracture reduction is visualized on each of the sigmoid notch and dorsally.

A 3.5-mm low-contour dynamic compression (LCDC) eight-hole AO plate (authors' choice), a 3.5-mm DC, or a reconstruction plate is contoured to permit 90-degree insertion of one screw at the proximal end down the center of the olecranon, with the plate on the dorsal surface (Fig. 6-22A). Contouring of the plate is achieved with bending irons and the bending press. The next two screws, if possible, are inserted in a divergent pattern and pointing anteriorly within the proximal fragment. Subsequent screws are placed in a compression mode, and any fracture of the coronoid process is reduced and fixed with one of the screws. Visualization of the coronoid can usually be made through the fracture site of the separated olecranon fragments before reduction. Bicortical screw fixation is used to ensure direction and length of the screws. The advantage of the LCDC plate is that the screw heads are flush with the plate and are not often prominent enough to require later removal. A compression device is not typically necessary, as the plate is reserved for comminuted fractures. If an intramedullary 6.5-mm or larger-caliber screw is to be used with the con-

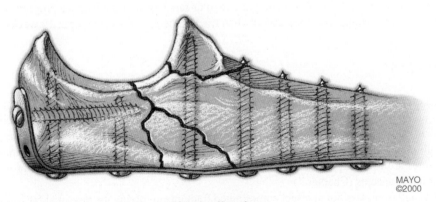

Neutralization

Figure 6-22. Contoured eight-hole 3.5-mm LCDC AO plate with three screws in the proximal larger fragment with bicortical screw fixation where possible, distal to the sigmoid notch.

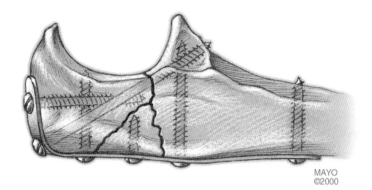

MAYO
©2000

Figure 6-23. Contoured eight-hole reconstruction plate with bicortical screw fixation. Maintenance of the contour and width of the greater sigmoid notch is essential.

struct, the proximal hole in the 3.5-mm LCDC plate must be enlarged preoperatively or a 4.5-mm reconstruction plate must be used. The LCDC plate is less likely to fracture than a tubular or reconstruction plate. Meticulous care is taken to maintain the normal contour of the sigmoid notch (Fig. 6-23).

Valgus instability of the elbow, present on stress testing after stabilization of the olecranon fracture, indicates the need for medial or lateral collateral ligament repair (described in Chapter 14) and, if medial, is followed by an application of a distractor device for 4 weeks to prevent subluxation and permit active motion (described in Chapter 8).

POSTOPERATIVE MANAGEMENT

The extremity is immobilized in a well-padded fiberglass splint in full extension for 5 days.

The upper extremity is maintained at 60 degrees total elevation for 2 to 3 days with pillow support and with the hand kept 1 foot above head height 100% of the time, whether recumbent, in a recliner chair, or standing.

The splint is removed at 5 days. Similar elevation overhead is encouraged for another week. Because edema and swelling are usually quite minimal at this time, the elbow can be taken through a range of active assistive motion. Motion is increased by additional sessions and by greater range each day thereafter.

At 2 weeks, Steri-strips are removed, a dressing is usually unnecessary, and active assistive motion is carried out through a full range at least four to six times daily.

Anteroposterior (AP) and lateral radiographs are repeated at 3 days, 1 week, and 4 weeks postoperatively.

Physical therapy rehabilitation is not necessary and is even considered contraindicated by the authors. Carrying of weights is also contraindicated.

The patient is encouraged to maintain a regular range of motion exercise program with specific strengthening exercises added when fracture healing is evident or at 12 weeks.

RESULTS

Most olecranon fractures treated by open reduction do well (4,7), with an overall satisfactory rating of at least 90% (12). Satisfactory results in undisplaced fractures are obtained in 95% of cases. In displaced stable noncomminuted and comminuted fractures satisfactory results occur in 90% of patients. Poorer results in the unstable displaced and comminuted fractures are to be expected, but the outcomes are improving with current and improving treatment concepts (Chapter 7).

The author prefers not to resect comminuted fractures involving the proximal 50% of the sigmoid notch except in the elderly, where excision is preferable. In most instances, a contoured plate with screw fixation will adequately stabilize most comminuted fractures of the olecranon, and fragment retention is important in the authors' opinion, since even the proximal olecranon offers significant architectural stability to the joint.

COMPLICATIONS

Complications are not uncommon with comminuted fractures involving more than 60% of the sigmoid notch, with fractures of the coronoid process, and with instability. This problem is discussed in detail in Chapter 7. Problems include motion loss, nonunion, ulnar neuropathy, malunion, and posttraumatic arthrosis. Some motion loss occurred in 75% of fractures in a Mayo Clinic series, with 50% having a loss of 20 to 60 degrees and 20% having a loss of more than 60 degrees. If rigid fixation is achieved, motion loss is almost directly proportional to the period of immobilization and edema or swelling about the joint. With adherence to a postoperative regimen of immobilization limited to 5 days with the elbow in full extension and the strict elevation of the elbow above shoulder height for 2 weeks, motion loss from swelling and edema can be significantly minimized. Ulnar neuropathy has been reported from 3% to 10% and can be minimized or avoided with careful protection and handling of the nerve, utilizing subcutaneous transposition if necessary. Nonunion is most commonly a result of inadequate primary fixation and has been reported in up to 5% of patients. Loss of blood supply to the major fragments and excessive soft-tissue stripping often play an important role in the incidence of nonunion. Malunion is uncommon following open reduction but may occur with the more severely comminuted open injuries delaying or excluding adequate reduction. Posttraumatic arthrosis is more likely to develop in the unstable comminuted fracture with coronoid and radial head fractures or with failure of internal fixation requiring reoperation (10). Because of the significant impact of nonunion, we discuss this problem in detail.

NONUNION

Even with careful attention to the principles described earlier, nonunion may occur with a reported incidence of up to 5%. There are two types of olecranon nonunions with significant difference in management: undisplaced and displaced. The treatment of nonunion follows principles of primary fracture treatment and therefore depends entirely on the type as classified earlier. Although the blood supply and vascularity of the cancellous olecranon are felt to be sufficient without bone grafting when reconstruction for nonunion is carried out, the authors use routine iliac inlay or onlay grafting.

The following factors determine the treatment options for olecranon nonunion:

1. When nonunion occurs in the proximal 50% of the olecranon, excision is an acceptable alternative and is the treatment of choice in the elderly or osteoporotic patient.
2. If there is no gross deformity the inlay bone plug technique is used.
3. For gross deformity, rigid low-profile dynamic compression plating (LDCP) plate fixation with or without an intramedullary screw but always with an onlay corticocancellous "bone plate" is the preferred strategy (14).

Undisplaced, Symptomatic Nonunion

Lateral Inlay Plug Bone Graft For minimally displaced nonunion this technique has worked well. Incision and exposure are identical to those used for the acute fracture, with the exception of the patient being positioned in the prone posture with the arm over a padded armrest to permit use of a fluoroscopic C-arm. This position is chosen to permit ease of obtaining a better corticocancellous graft from the posterior rather than the anterior iliac crest. Care should also be taken to carefully identify and protect the ulnar nerve (Fig. 6-24). Any previously placed metal is removed and the area of pseudarthrosis is identified through the periosteum.

The pseudarthrosis is debrided of fibrous tissue to viable bone with a rongeur, curette, and motorized bur, avoiding the removal of any vascularized bone (Fig. 25).

Using a 7/16-inch Cloward circular plug cutter, corticocancellous plugs of bone (additional in case of loss) are taken from the posterior iliac crest (Fig. 6-26), and an additional

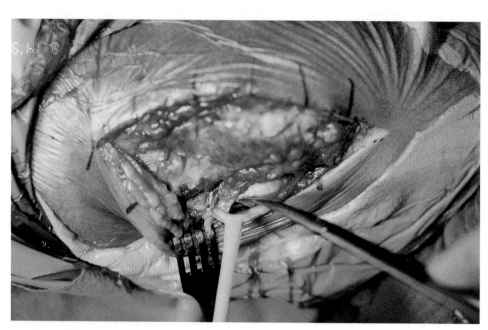

Figure 6-24. Because exposing nonunions is typically more difficult, particular care should be made to identify the ulnar nerve to avoid injury.

piece of cancellous bone is cut to fit the pseudarthrosis defect in the olecranon at the site of nonunion.

Large AO 6.5-mm intramedullary screw and tension band wire fixation is carried out as described earlier. Particular care is taken to avoid any change in the normal contour of the sigmoid notch as compression is accomplished with the compression screw.

A corresponding 7/16-inch Cloward circular cutting drill is then used to make a hole at

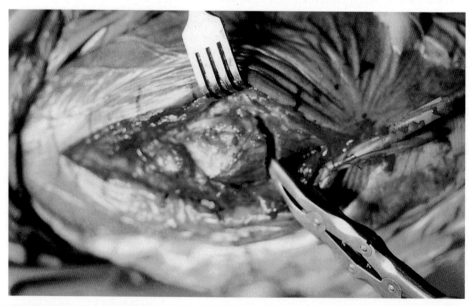

Figure 6-25. The pseudarthrosis is debrided of fibrous tissue. If reasonable stability is present, the nonunion is not completely taken down. If it is grossly unstable, then both surfaces must be refashioned.

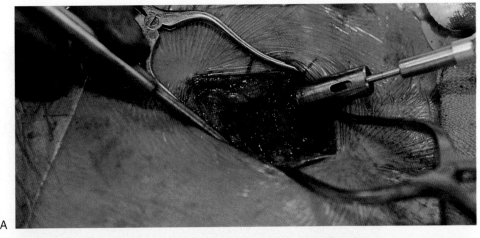

A

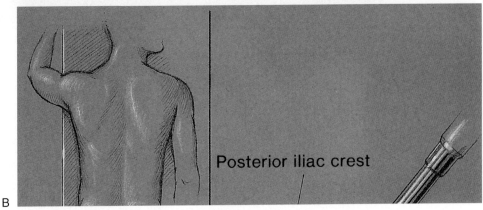

Posterior iliac crest

B

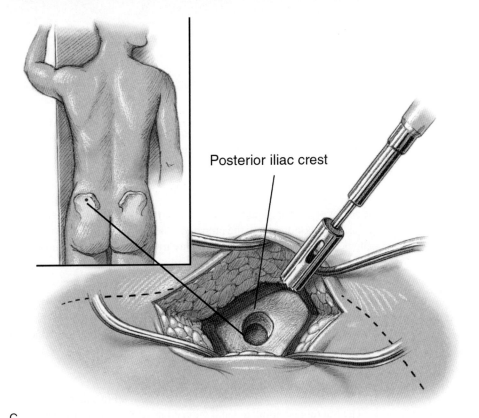

Posterior iliac crest

C

Figure 6-26. A,B: A trephine (Cloward) is used to remove bone plugs from the posterior iliac crest. This can be done with a percutaneous technique. **C:** Several plugs may be removed.

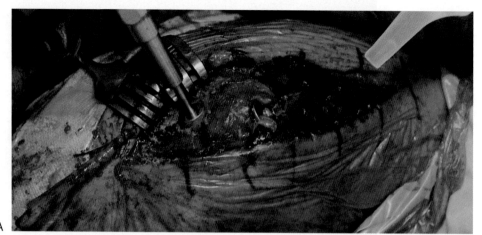

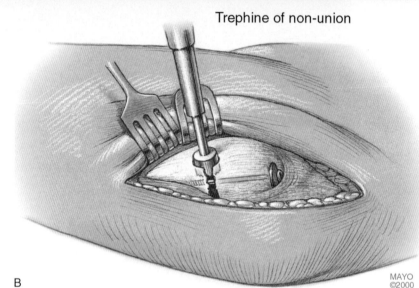

Trephine of non-union

MAYO
©2000

Figure 6-27. A,B: A circular trephine (Cloward) then is used to remove a plug of bone at the site of the pseudarthrosis allowing an effective bone graft site in the presence of an intramedullary fixation device.

the site of olecranon pseudarthrosis laterally (Fig. 6-27), and the previously harvested plug of iliac graft is tapped into the prepared hole (Fig. 6-28). Additional small fragments of cancellous bone graft may be placed in any irregularity in the pseudarthrosis site.

The wires and the intramedullary screw are tightened.

Displaced Fractures

If not essential for stability, resect. If restored ulnohumeral articulation is required for joint function, then mobilize, reduce, and fix.

Technique

1. The ulnar nerve is identified and protected in all instances.
2. The fracture is mobilized and reduced in such a way as to restore ulnohumeral function according to the principles described in Chapter 7.
3. For bone grafting, one of us (BFM) always employs structural differential cortical cancellous "bone plate" harvested from the posterior iliac crest (Fig. 6-29). This may be ap-

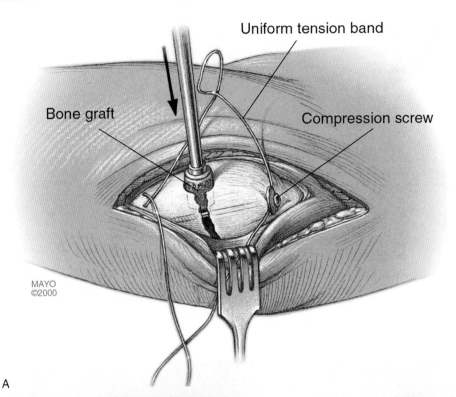

Uniform tension band

Bone graft

Compression screw

MAYO
©2000

A

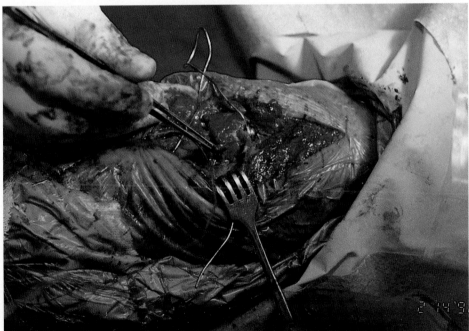

B

Figure 6-28. A,B: The bone plugs are impacted into the circular defect created at the site of the pseudarthrosis.

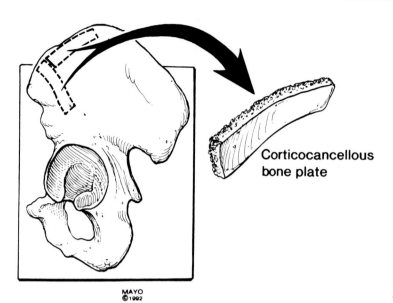

Corticocancellous
bone plate

MAYO
©1992

Figure 6-29. In all instances of displaced nonunion a 4- to 5-cm × 1.5-cm graft is harvested from the posterior iliac crest.

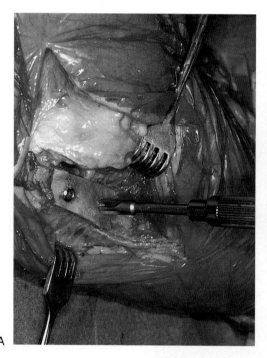

A

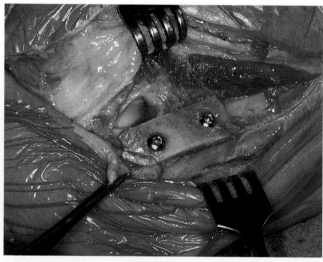

B

Figure 6-30. The plate of bone is secured with bone screws with the heads countersunk (**A**). At least one screw is placed on either side of the nonunion (**B**).

plied to the medial or lateral face of the ulna. The plate is secured with bone screws and the heads are countersunk to avoid irritation (Fig. 6-30).

4. Fixation.
   a. Compression. If adequate stock is present, we prefer axillary fixation with a threaded AO cancellous screw (Fig. 6-31).
   b. Neutralization. If the fracture does not allow compression, an LDCP plate is applied either medially or laterally, depending on the position of greatest rigidity. In all instances, the essential component is the harvest and application of a cortical/cancellous onlay "plate" 4.5 cm × 1.5 cm attached by screws to the opposite ulnar cortex (Fig. 6-32) (14).

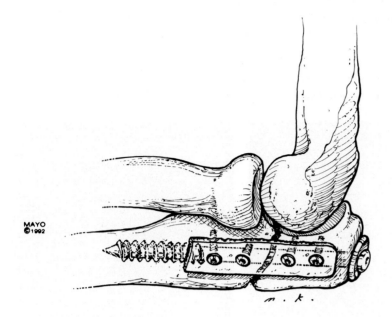

MAYO
©1992

Figure 6-31. With adequate bone surface present, intramedullary fixation is effective treatment for olecranon nonunion supplemented by a cortical cancellous "bone plate" applied by screw fixation.

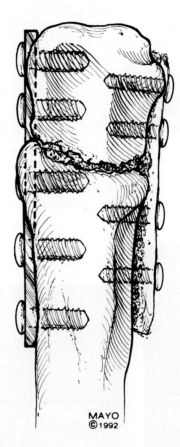

MAYO
©1992

Figure 6-32. With osseous deficiency, neutralization plate fixation is applied with the cortical cancellous "bone plate" applied to the opposite cortex.

ILLUSTRATIVE CASES

Case 1

An olecranon osteotomy was used to expose a distal humeral fracture. After 9 months a nonunion was evident and established (Fig. 6-33A). The bone plug and compression

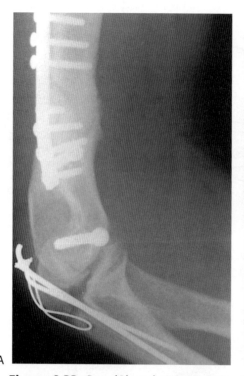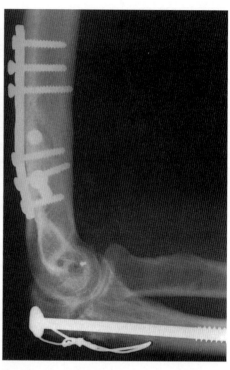

Figure 6-33. Pre- (**A**) and postoperative (**B**) views of an olecranon nonunion at 9 months following a surgical osteotomy to repair a lower humeral fracture, and treated by bilateral iliac corticocancellous plug bone grafts with excision of the pseudarthrosis, cancellous grafting of the defect, and fixation with a 6.5-mm intramedullary bone screw and tension band wiring. Union was painless and solid at 9 months with 35 to 120 degrees of motion.

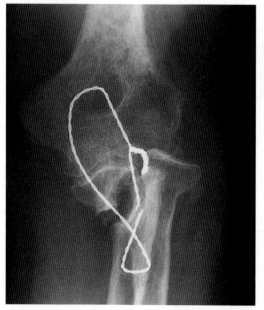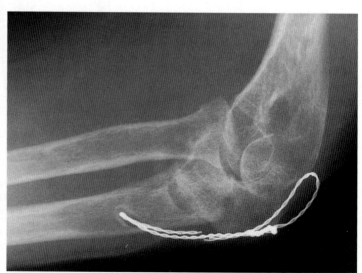

Figure 6-34. A,B: Established nonunion of olecranon with instability of the articulation.

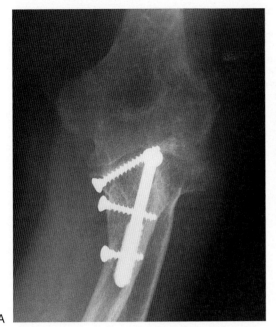
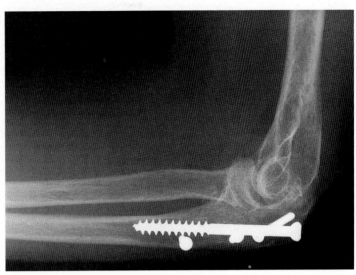

A   B

Figure 6-35. A,B: Excellent result with axial stability from AO cancellous screw and "bone plate" applied with three screws.

screw technique was successful in obtaining union (Fig. 6-33B) and a functional arc from 35 to 120 degrees.

Case 2

Tension wiring failed and the forearm was unstable (Fig. 6-34). Displaced olecranon nonunion 2 years after injury in a 45-year-old female. Mobilization of the fragment and rigid fixation with an intramedullary screw and a "bone plate" graft resulted in healing at 6 months with an arc of 35 to 130 degrees flexion and minimal pain (Fig. 6-35).

RECOMMENDED READINGS

1. Adler S, Fay GD, MacAusland WR Jr. Treatment of olecranon fractures: indications for excision of the ole-cranon fragment and repair of the triceps tendon. *J Trauma* 1962;2:597.
2. Beck C, Dabezies EJ. Monteggia fracture dislocation. *Orthopedics* 1984;7:329.
3. Colton CL. Fractures of the olecranon in adults: classification and management. *Injury* 1973;5:121.
4. Eriksson E, Sahlen O, Sandohl U. Late results of conservative and surgical treatment of fractures of the ole-cranon. *Acta Chir Scand* 1957;113:153.
5. Gartsman GM, Sculco TP, Otis JC. Operative treatment of olecranon fractures. *J Bone Joint Surg* 1981;63A:718.
6. Heim U, Pfeiffer KM. *Internal fixation of small fractures,* 3rd ed. Berlin: Springer-Verlag; 1988.
7. Kiviluoto O, Santavirta, S. Fractures of the olecranon: an analysis of 37 consecutive cases. *Acta Orthop Scand* 1978;49:28.
8. Kozin SH, Berglund LJ, Cooney WP, et al. Biomechanical analysis of tension band fixation for olecranon fracture treatment. *J Shoulder Elbow Surg* 1996;5:442–448.
9. MacAusland WR Jr, Wyman ET. Fractures of the adult elbow. *Instr Course Lect* 1975;24:169–181.
10. Maeko D, Szabo RM. Complications of tension-band wiring of olecranon fractures. *J Bone Joint Surg* 1985;67A:1396–1401.
11. McKeever FM, Buck RN. Fracture of the olecranon process of the ulna: treatment by excision of fragment and repair of triceps. *J Am Med Assoc* 1947;135:1.
12. Morrey BF. Current concepts in the treatment of fractures of the radial head, the olecranon, and the coronoid. *J Bone Joint Surg* 1995;77A:316–327.
13. Muller ME, Allgower M, Schneider R, et al. *Manual of internal fixation: techniques recommended by the AO Group,* 2nd ed. New York: Springer-Verlag; 1979.
14. Papagelopoulos PJ, Morrey BF. Treatment of olecranon fracture nonunions. *J Bone Joint Surg* 1994;76B:627–635.
15. Regan WM, Morrey BF. Fractures of the coronoid process of the ulna. *J Bone Joint Surg* 1989;71A:1348.

16. Schwab GH, et al. Biomechanics of elbow instability: the role of the medial collateral ligament. *Clin Orthop* 1980;146:42.
17. Taylor TKF, Scham SM. A posteromedial approach to the proximal end of the ulna for internal fixation of olecranon fractures. *J Trauma* 1969;9:594.
18. Wadsworth TG. Screw fixation of the olecranon after fracture or osteotomy. *Clin Orthop* 1976;119:197–201.
19. Murphy DF, Greene WB, Gilbert JA, et al. Displaced olecranon fractures in adults. Biomechanical analysis of fixation methods. *Clin Ortho Related Research* 1987;224:210–214.

7

Fractures of the Coronoid and Complex Instability of the Elbow

Bernard F. Morrey and Shawn W. O'Driscoll

Complex instability of the elbow is defined as an injury that destabilizes the elbow because of interarticular fracture and disruption to the ligamentous structures (2). Others add soft-tissue involvement, including neural and vascular injuries, as essential for the diagnosis of complex injury, but these associated problems are uncommon (8).

In general terms, the collateral ligaments provide approximately 50% of the varus/valgus stability of the joint, and the articular surfaces provide an additional 50% (4). The anterior band of the medial collateral ligament and the ulnar part of the lateral collateral ligament are the primary constraints to valgus and posterolateral rotatory instability, respectively. Both the ulnar and radial parts of the lateral collateral ligament resist varus.

The significance of a coronoid fracture is becoming somewhat clearer. Treatment of a fractured coronoid is an essential element of managing complex elbow instability. The amount of the coronoid required for stability depends on the ligamentous integrity and that of the radial head but is always at least 50% (Fig. 7-1). This becomes important in preoperative planning and surgical approach, which are necessary for effective restoration and fixation of coronoid fractures.

The radial head has been shown to be, and hence defined as, a secondary stabilizer of the elbow (5). When the medial and lateral ligaments are intact, it is not required for stability. If the medial collateral ligament or coronoid are damaged, it emerges as an important secondary stabilizer. Hence the value of either fixing the fracture, if possible, or replacing the head with a prosthesis is clear in the face of these specific associated injuries. Procedures to address fractures of the radial head and olecranon are discussed in detail in Chapters 5 and 6.

The basic principle of management in fracture of the proximal ulna is restoration of the ulnohumeral joint. This principle cannot be overstated (3,6).

B.F. Morrey, M.D.: Mayo Medical School and Department of Orthopaedics, Mayo Clinic and Mayo Foundation, Rochester, Minnesota.

S.W. O'Driscoll, M.D., PH.D.: Orthopedic Surgery, Mayo Medical School, Mayo Foundation, Rochester, Minnesota.

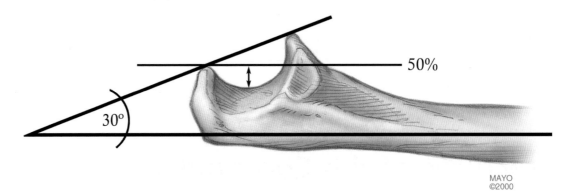

Figure 7-1. Coronoid 50% rule. A line from the tip of the olecranon and parallel to the shaft passes through 50% of the coronoid.

The specific contribution of the olecranon in resisting various loading configurations is proportional to the amount of olecranon articulation present. The critical amount necessary for maintenance of stability is at least 50%. In some instances the elbow is unstable, with less than 50% of the olecranon fractured because of a concomitant fracture of the coronoid. For this reason each elbow is individually assessed for instability.

CLASSIFICATION

Regan and Morrey (7) have described three fracture types, depending on the extent of the fracture (Fig. 7-2). As more experience is gained with these fractures, it is now recognized

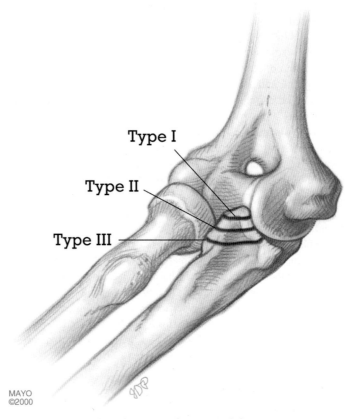

Figure 7-2. Regan-Morrey classification of coronoid fractures. Some type II and all type III are unstable.

that a varus moment applied to the elbow in an extended position may create a sagittal coronoid fracture. This fracture usually includes the attachment of the ulnar collateral ligament on the sublime tubercle (Fig. 7-3) and might be termed a type IV or anterior medial fracture.

Type I Fracture

Type I fractures represent small shear fractures of the tip of the coronoid and serve mainly as an indicator that the elbow has dislocated or at least displaced sufficiently to have sustained an injury of the collateral ligaments (7).

Type II Fracture

In type II fractures, as much as 50% of the coronoid is involved and the elbow is considered unstable unless proven otherwise. If posterior displacement occurs with less than 40 to 45 degrees of flexion, the residual articulation is considered inadequate and the ulnohumeral joint must be stabilized. If the fracture fragment is large enough for fixation, osteosynthesis through the anterior capsule is performed. If the fragment is too small for fixation, then a heavy number 5 suture is placed over the fragment (or fragments), which is brought to its anatomic location and tied through drill holes placed in the ulna. A threaded 0.045 or 0.062 Steinmann pin can be placed through the ulna into the fragment to buttress it as well. In the latter situation, or even if osteosynthesis has been carried out but there is concern about stability and the rigidity of fixation, the system is neutralized by the application of a hinged external fixator. The external fixator eliminates or neutralizes the posteriorly directed forces that are applied to the fracture site by the muscles that flex and extend the elbow joint (Fig. 7-4). The device allows motion of the ulnohumeral joint while placing a distal distraction force on the ulna, thus protecting the articulation. The distraction de-

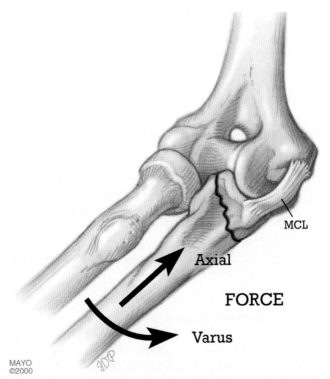

MAYO
©2000

Figure 7-3. A sagittal fracture occurs from varus axial load with or without comminution and usually involves attachment of the anterior medial collateral ligament.

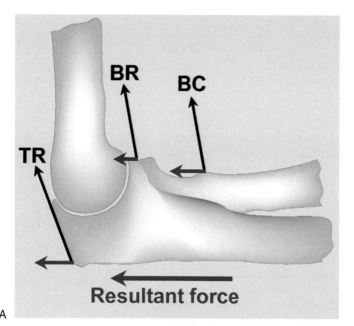
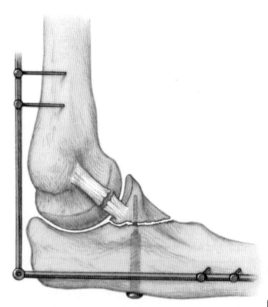

A
B

Figure 7-4. Complex instability of the elbow. Posterior directed forces occur from the posteriorly directed pull of the biceps, brachialis, and triceps (**A**). If fixation is inadequate, neutralization of coronoid fixation is carried out with an external fixator (**B**).

vice is maintained for 3 to 6 weeks, depending upon the nature of the injury (1) (see Chapter 8).

Type III Fracture

Type III fractures are the most difficult to treat since, by definition, the ulnohumeral joint is grossly unstable. If the coronoid is a large fragment and has not been comminuted, it may be fixed with a screw or plate, and screws and the joint will be stable.

INDICATIONS/CONTRAINDICATIONS

Indications for Fracture Fixation (2,3,6)

1. Type II fractures with an intact radial head and in which the elbow is grossly unstable when flexed less than 50 or 60 degrees.
2. Type II coronoid fractures in which the radial head has been fractured and the elbow has been dislocated ("terrible triad" injury).
3. All type III fractures.
4. Isolated anteromedial coronoid fractures, because of their propensity for slight articular incongruity and subluxation.

Relative Contraindications

For fear of ectopic bone formation avoid surgical exposure of the coronoid if greater than 5 to 6 days after injury, but only if the ulnohumeral joint is reduced. A persistently unstable joint with articular incongruity is less successfully treated later than is an elbow with heterotopic ossification.

PREOPERATIVE PLANNING

Assess the extent of fracture. If less than 50% of the coronoid is involved, a line from the tip of the olecranon through the base of the fracture is parallel to or intersects the line of axis of the ulna posterior to the olecranon. If greater than 50% has been fractured, this line intersects the long axis distally.

Preparation for surgery includes several considerations. The posterior skin incision affords medial or lateral deep exposure. If a radial head fracture requires removal, a deep lateral approach may be adequate. If the radial head is intact or the ulnar nerve is symptomatic, the deep medial approach is used. Usually, the lateral collateral ligament (LCL) is disrupted, so this is carefully repaired along with the coronoid fixation.

Finally, if the fixation is tenuous, an external fixator is applied (see Chapter 8).

SURGERY

Exposure: Medial Column

Position The patient is supine, an elbow table is applied, and the arm is draped free with a nonsterile technique.

Incision

With the arm initially across the chest, we prefer a posterior incision to allow medial exposure of the fracture as well as lateral exposure of the lateral collateral ligament should this be necessary. A 12-cm posterior incision is made just medial to the tip of the olecranon (Fig. 7-5). A subcutaneous flap is elevated medially, exposing the ulnar nerve posterior to the intermuscular septum. The intermuscular septum is identified and preserved or released from the medial epicondyle if ulnar nerve transposition is anticipated (Fig. 7-6). The soft

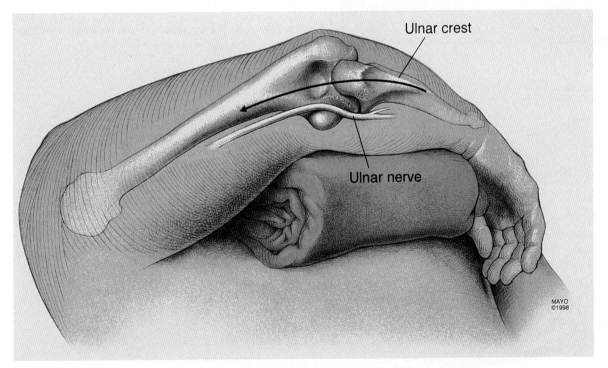

Figure 7-5. A posterior incision is preferred to expose the coronoid from the medial column.

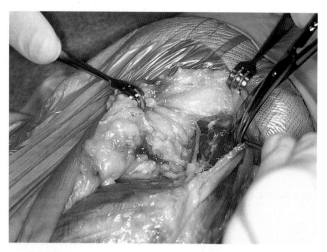

Figure 7-6. The intramuscular septum is identified. In this instance the ulnar nerve is identified and protected.

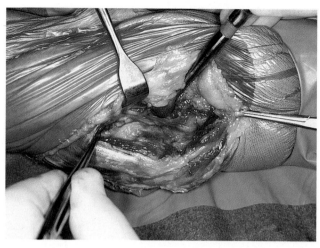

Figure 7-7. The brachialis and pronator teres muscles have been elevated from the anterior capsule.

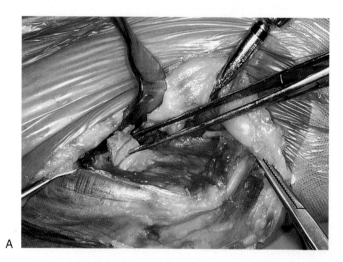

A

Figure 7-8. A,B: The anterior capsule is exposed and entered revealing a type II coronoid fracture.

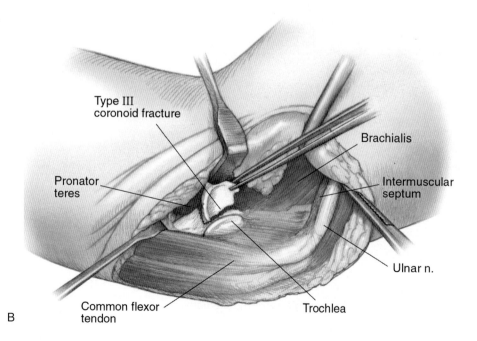

B

Type III
coronoid fracture

Brachialis

Pronator
teres

Intermuscular
septum

Common flexor
tendon

Trochlea

Ulnar n.

tissues are elevated from the anterior aspect of the septum and a periosteal elevator elevates the brachialis from the anterior cortex of the distal humerus. The pronator is elevated, leaving a portion of the flexor carpi ulnaris (FCU) as a cuff for reattachment at closure. Take care to preserve the medial collateral ligament. The muscle flap is elevated from the capsule (Fig. 7-7). The fibers of the brachialis are swept from the anterior capsule, which is divided for exposure of the joint surface with a longitudinal incision. The fracture is identified (Fig. 7-8)and reduced with a sharp tenaculum. A 0.045 or 0.062 K-wire stabilizes the fracture (Fig. 7-9). For some fractures (type II) fixation with a 2.7-mm screw is adequate (Figs. 7-10 and 7-11). With type II or type III comminuted fractures not amenable to screw or suture fixation, a carefully contoured plate may be used to buttress the fixation construct. Exercise caution putting screws through the fragments, as they may fragment.

Suture Technique

If the fracture is relatively small or comminuted, one or two no. 2 or no. 5 suture is passed over the fragment or through drill holes if possible and through the capsule that is attached to it. If possible, a Krachow suture is placed in the brachialis tendon at its insertion (Fig.

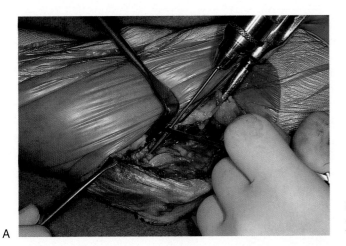

A

Figure 7-9. A,B: The fracture is stabilized with a K-wire, and a 2.0 drill bit is used to drill coronoid fragment. The fragment is often too small to allow overdrilling.

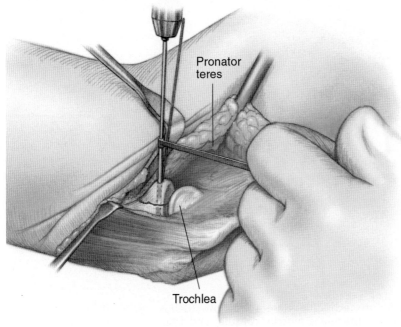

Pronator teres

Trochlea

B

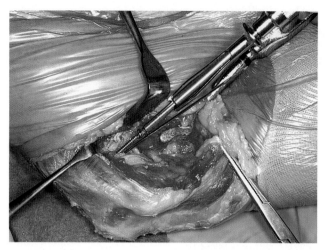

Figure 7-10. The fracture is secured with a 2.7-mm screw.

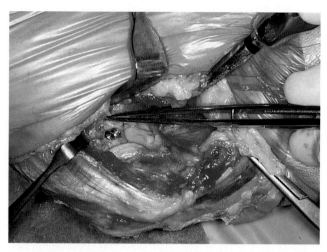

Figure 7-11. If a large enough fragment exists, two screws are preferable.

7-12). Two or three drill holes are placed retrograde from the subcutaneous border of the ulna into the base of the fracture and close to the articular surface (Fig. 7-13). Care is taken to ensure that the fragments are pulled into place in a fashion that places the bone fragment(s) close to the joint surface. The sutures are then passed through the holes with a suture passer. The fragment is reduced and the sutures are tied (Fig. 7-14).

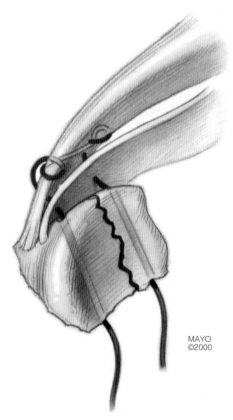

MAYO
©2000

Figure 7-12. Suture technique. Here a Krachow stitch is used to secure the brachialis muscle, capsule, and fractured fragments.

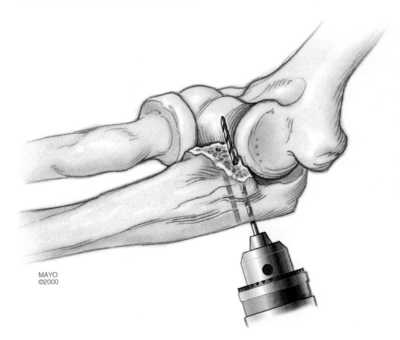

Figure 7-13. The drill is directed retrograde from the dorsal aspect of the ulna into the bed of the fractured coronoid.

Lateral Ulnar Collateral Ligament Repair

Note: In all instances fractures of the coronoid are closed by repair of the disrupted ligaments. Application of a hinged external fixator may be indicated as well as needed (see Chapter 8).

A coronoid fracture almost always involves disruption of the lateral collateral ligament and may involve an medial collateral ligament (MCL) injury as well. Most have associated radial head fractures. The combination of elbow dislocation and fractures of the coronoid and radial head has been termed the *terrible triad.* With this injury we proceed with treatment of the coronoid, radial head and a careful ligamentous repair as described in Chapter 5.

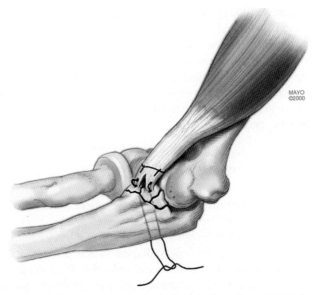

Figure 7-14. The suture is tied with the elbow in 90-degree flexion.

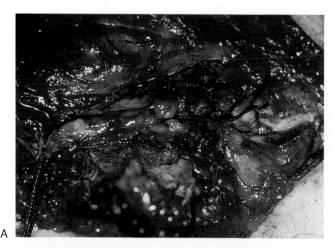

A

Figure 7-15. A,B: A disrupted lateral ulnar collateral ligament is stabilized with a running locked stitch (Krachow) that is secured to the humerus through drill holes.

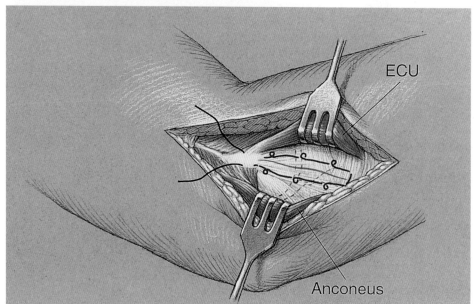

B

In the terrible triad special attention is paid to the lateral collateral ligament complex. A heavy nonabsorbable suture is passed through a drill hole exiting at the anatomic origin of the LUCL at the humerus (Fig. 7-15). Using a Krachow stitch, the suture passes along the length of the ligament, including the ulnar insertion of the ligament at the tubercle of the supinator crest. The stitch proceeds proximally and again passes through the humeral origin and is tied with the elbow reduced, the forearm is in neutral rotation, and the elbow is flexed 45 to 90 degrees. Medially, the same technique is used if the medial collateral ligament has been torn.

POSTOPERATIVE MANAGEMENT

If the fracture fragments are stable, the patient is instructed in passive range-of-motion exercises with gravitational varus stress eliminated (i.e., in vertical plane, which can also be performed overhead while lying supine). The senior author prefers a continuous passive motion (CPM) for this injury. Repeat radiographs are taken after 7 to 10 days and at 6 weeks to ensure the maintenance of reduction. If a contracture of 30 or more degrees is present at 6 weeks, a static adjustable splint program is commenced (see Chapter 9). If the external fixator is applied, full motion is immediately allowed and encouraged using a CPM machine for 21 hours a day for 3 to 4 weeks. Active motion is allowed as tolerated when out of the CPM and while the fixator is in place. The device is removed at 4 to 6 weeks.

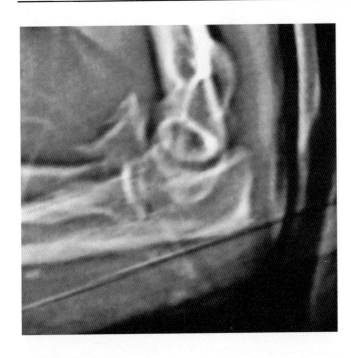

Figure 7-16. This 40-year-old thoracic surgeon sustained a type II coronoid fracture after a fall from a bike.

ILLUSTRATIVE CASE

A 48-year-old surgeon fell from a bicycle and sustained a fracture dislocation of the left elbow. A type III coronoid fracture was observed (Fig. 7-16). This was reduced and fixed with two 3.0-mm AO screws applied with the lag technique. A DJD II external fixator was applied (Fig. 7-17). At 8 weeks he has an arc of 40 to 130 degrees (Fig. 7-18). He returned to surgery at 10 weeks.

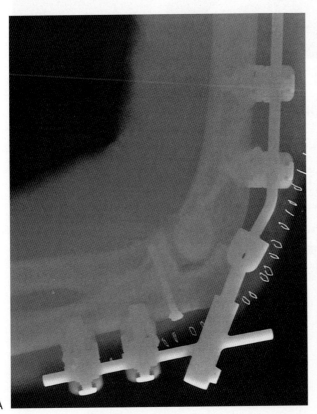
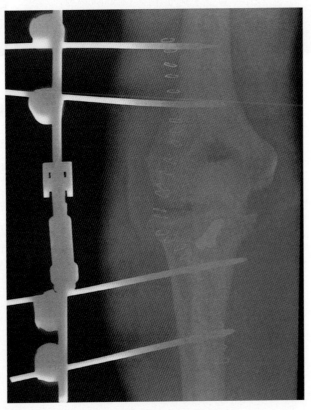

A   B

Figure 7-17. A,B: The fracture was fixed with two screws and stabilized with the half-pin configuration of the DJD II.

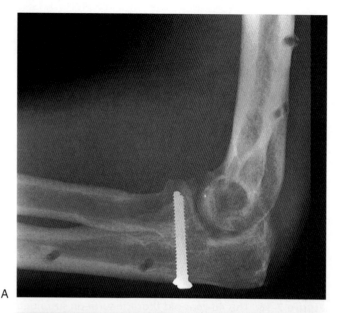

A

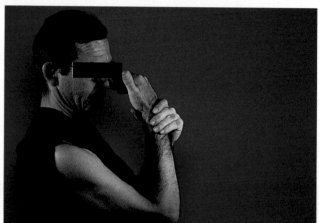

Figure 7-18. A-C: Excellent function was restored by 10 weeks.

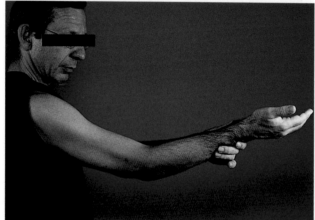

B

C

RECOMMENDED READINGS

1. Cobb TK, Morrey BF. Use of distraction arthroplasty in unstable fracture dislocations of the elbow. *Clin Orthop* 1995;312:201–210.
2. Morrey BF. Complex instability of the elbow. *J Bone Joint Surg* 1997;79A:460.
3. Morrey BF. Current concepts in the treatment of fractures of the radial head, the olecranon, and the coronoid. *J Bone Joint Surg* 1995;77A:316–327.
4. Morrey BF. Fracture of the radial head. In: Morrey BF, ed. *The elbow and its disorders,* 2nd ed. Philadelphia: WB Saunders; 1993:383–404.
5. Morrey BF, Tanaka S, An K-N. Valgus stability of the elbow: a definition of primary and secondary constraints. *Clin Orthop* 1991;265:187–195.
6. O'Driscoll SW, Jupiter JB, King GJW, et al. The unstable elbow. *J Bone Joint Surg* 2000;82A:724–738.
7. Regan W, Morrey BF. Fracture of the coronoid process of the ulna. *J Bone Joint Surg* 1989;71-A:1348–1354.
8. Regel G, Seekamp A, Blauth M, et al. Complex injury of the elbow joint. *Unfallchirurg* 1996;99:92–99.

8

Articulated External Fixators

Bernard F. Morrey and Robert N. Hotchkiss

Two principal goals are simultaneously sought with use of the articulated external fixator: (a) to allow active or passive motion, (b) to protect the articular surface and the collateral ligaments.

INDICATIONS/CONTRAINDICATIONS

Protection of the articular surface is required in the following situations:

1. Coronoid fracture with or without fixation.
2. Olecranon fracture with tenuous fixation.
3. Distal humeral articular fractures.
4. Unstable ulnohumeral joint after acute collateral ligament disruption.
5. Combination of instability with any of the preceding fractures (complex instability).

Reconstruction

As an adjunct for individuals undergoing release for a stiff elbow.

This is the most common in the posttraumatic condition but occasionally is used with inflammatory stiffness. The use of distraction is generally indicated in these circumstances.

1. There has been a significant amount of dissection, suggesting that maintaining the intraoperative motion will be difficult.
2. If the pathology has modified the joint contour, requiring refashioning of the joint surface, with or without an interposition membrane.
3. When an interposition procedure is performed.

B.F. Morrey, M.D.: Mayo Medical School and Department of Orthopaedics, Mayo Clinic and Mayo Foundation, Rochester, Minnesota.

R.N. Hotchkiss, M.D.: Hand Service, Hospital for Special Surgery; and Clinical Surgery (Orthopaedics), Weill Medical College, New York, New York.

4. If the collateral ligament has been reconstructed or repaired in association with the release.

For the most part the following conditions are relative contraindications.

1. Inexperience with the use of external fixation devices is considered a relative contraindication. Application of this device is technically demanding and requires accurate placement of the skeletal pins.
2. If uncertainty exists with regard to the anatomic location of the neurovascular structures due to posttraumatic destruction of the joint, the distraction device should be used only with extreme caution. (The pins, under these circumstances, may be inserted under direct vision.)
3. Local sepsis is a relative contraindication to the application of this device.
4. The presence of some fracture fixation devices in the distal humerus or proximal ulna.
5. Preemptive medical condition (e.g., severe osteoporosis).

Preoperative Planning

Reliable identification of the axis of rotation and rigid skeletal fixation can be obtained by use of an articular device that replicates the axis of rotation.

Skeletal fixation on the ulna with the Dynamic Joint Distractor (DJD) II allows protection or neutralization of the articular surface for a variety of clinical circumstances.

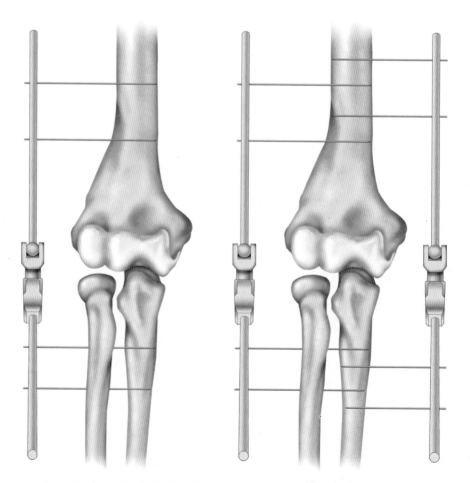

Figure 8-1. Half- and full-pin fixation with uni- or bilateral frame application offers significant application flexibility and clinical uses for the DJD II.

Motion in flexion/extension is allowed without encumbrance, particularly in both the articular surface and the collateral ligaments.

Options: The DJD II may be used in either a monolateral or a bilateral configuration. This allows a great deal of flexibility of use and indications (Fig. 8-1).

SURGERY

The patient is placed supine with a sandbag under the scapula. The arm is draped free with a nonsterile tourniquet and is brought across the chest (Fig. 8-2). The elbow is exposed according to the pathology present. Regardless of the exposure or pathology, the essential landmarks for axis pin placement are critical.

On the lateral aspect of the capitellum, a tubercle is present at the site of the origin of the lateral collateral ligament. This tubercle also represents the geometric center of curvature of the capitellum, which is the site of the flexion axis of the elbow and is the point through which a 3-mm Apex humeral reference pin will pass (Fig. 8-3).

On the medial aspect of the distal humerus, the axis of rotation lies just anterior and inferior to the medial epicondyle. The axis pin is placed in this region or slightly anterior and proximal to this location (Fig. 8-3). This represents a safe zone relative to the ulnar nerve.

Hence these two loci are used to position the humeral (axis) reference pin guide (Fig. 8-3). For a lateral frame application a 3-mm Apex humeral reference pin is drilled or tapped 10 to 20 mm into the distal humerus. If there is gross distortion, the center of the trochlea is the desired location for the pin, since the ulna rotates on the humerus and rotation on the capitellum is a secondary feature. If a medial frame is to be applied, the ulnar nerve is identified and protected at the time of insertion of the 3-mm Apex humeral reference pin.

Articular Fracture The articular fracture is approached according to surgeon preference, the specific pathology, and the treatment goals (see Chapter 1). Olecranon fractures are easily exposed and the fixator is readily applied (Chapter 6). Fractures involving the coronoid require more extensive exposures, as described later for the release of the stiff elbow (Chapter 7). Distal humeral fractures may be treated by exposure with olecranon os-

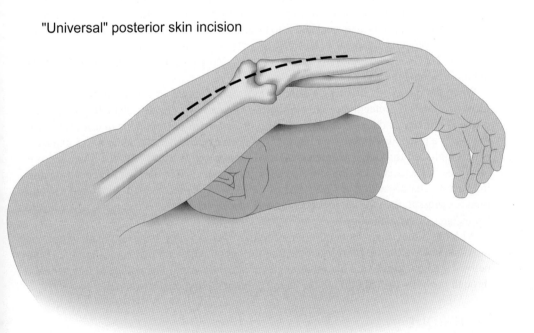

Figure 8-2. The patient is supine, the arm is brought across the chest, and most commonly a posterior skin incision is employed.

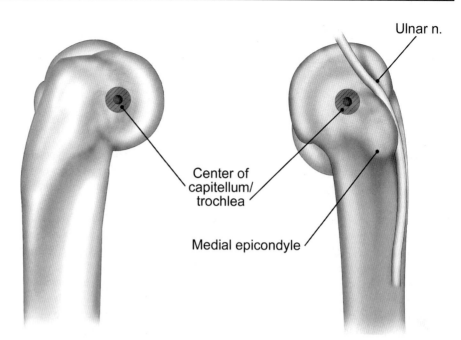

Figure 8-3. The axis landmark on the distal humerus laterally is the axis of the projected center of the capitellum. Medially, the axis is at the anterior inferior aspect of the medial epicondyle.

teotomy or a triceps reflection technique (Chapters 1 and 4). If the fracture fixation device(s) or collateral ligament reattachment precludes the introduction of a 3-mm axis pin, a small Kirschner wire is inserted in a manner to replicate the axis of rotation.

The Stiff Elbow If the elbow is being treated for stiffness, the previous incision is entered, and an extensile lateral Kocher-type joint release is used.

Typically, the triceps is reflected from the tip of the olecranon (Mayo Modified Kocher). However, in some instances, such as when elbow flexion is normal, the triceps may be left intact. The capsule is exposed by releasing the common extensor tendon. If the pathology is extrinsic to the joint, the anterior capsule is excised but the lateral collateral ligament is preserved. If the joint is abnormal and is to be altered, as with an interposition arthroplasty, the lateral collateral ligament is elevated as a flap of tissue from its origin at the lateral condyle. This is tagged and reflected distally, providing an extensive exposure (Fig. 8-4), but must be repaired and reattached at closure.

When the pathology involves a joint surface that requires an extensive dissection, the identification and protection of the ulnar nerve is necessary. Ideally, a single posterior incision is utilized, and a subcutaneous dissection is carried out to the medial aspect of the triceps. If a previous Kocher skin incision has been placed laterally, ulnar nerve exposure is accomplished through a supplemental medial incision. In any event, the ulnar nerve is identified but is usually not translocated anteriorly. Instead, it is simply protected, first during the capsular dissection and later at the time of axis pin placement. If ulnar nerve symptoms are present, then the nerve is decompressed with definitive management, according to the dictates of the pathology.

With the 3-mm Apex humeral reference pin in place, 2-mm holes are made distal and proximal to the axis site for reattachment of the lateral collateral ligament (Fig. 8-5). Bunnell or Krachow sutures are placed through the radial (lateral) ulnar collateral ligament and through the holes drilled through the lateral column around the flexion pin.

TECHNIQUE

To construct the frame, follow these steps:

1. *Axis of rotation.* Determine the axis of rotation external landmarks and place the humeral (axis) reference pin guide in line with the axis of rotation. The tip of the guide

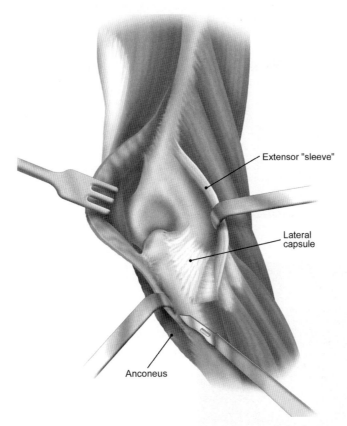

Figure 8-4. An extensile surgical exposure typically involves elevating the sleeve of extensor muscles and releasing the lateral collateral ligament.

is usually placed on the medial side while the pin guide on the lateral side as the axis pin enters laterally (Fig. 8-6).

2. *Reference pin that acts as a guide during frame construction.* Insert laterally the 3-mm-diameter self-drilling/self-tapping Apex pin through the humeral (axis) reference pin guide in the axis of rotation. For monolateral frame construction insert the pin to a depth of 15 to 20 mm. For bilateral frames it is recommended to replace the 3-mm Apex humeral reference pin by a 3-mm smooth transfixing Apex pin that is inserted across the distal humerus (see "Bilateral Frame Option").

Note: The 3-mm pin is a reference pin and is the essential reference required to ac-

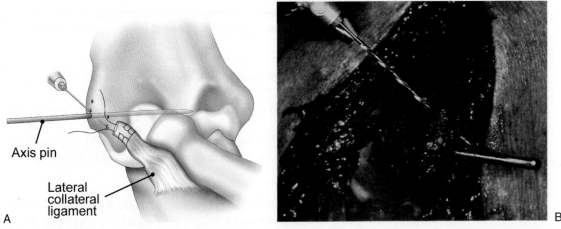

Figure 8-5. A,B: Holes that are placed around the axis of rotation allow the ligament to be reattached with an osseous attachment.

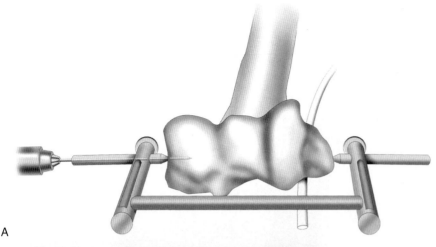

A

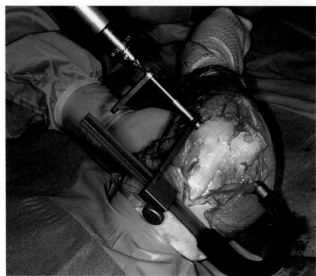

B

Figure 8-6. A,B: The C-guide with the sharp tip placed medially under direct vision allows accurate orientation of the axis reference pin even if placed only partially across the joint.

curately assemble the DJD II frame and to properly insert the humeral and ulnar pins. It will be removed after frame construction.

3. *Remove the humeral (axis) reference pin guide.*
4. *Placement of the DJD II frame on the reference pin.* The hollow-bored hinge of the DJD II is placed over the reference pin so that its hinge is exactly in the same axis of rotation as the natural axis of rotation of the elbow. Verify that the distraction device is fully compressed before frame construction.
5. *Pin insertion.* At this stage, depending on surgeon preference or features of the case, one may insert either the humeral or the ulnar pins. Humeral pin insertion is the author's choice.
6. *Humeral pin insertions.*
   a. Apply the 3-mm or 4-mm drill guide over the humeral rod so that pin guide is aligned with the lateral humerus (Fig. 8-7).
      Note: The 5-mm humeral rod is aligned to the anterior cortex of the humerus (INSERT).
   b. The proximal humeral self-drilling/self-tapping Apex 4-mm (or 3-mm) pin is inserted into the lateral cortex of the humerus through the pin guide and engages the opposite cortex.
   c. The pin guide is then removed.
   d. The proximal pin is fixed to the humeral rod with a Hoffmann II Compact pin-to-rod coupling that is then tightened using a Hoffmann II Compact wrench (Fig. 8-8).

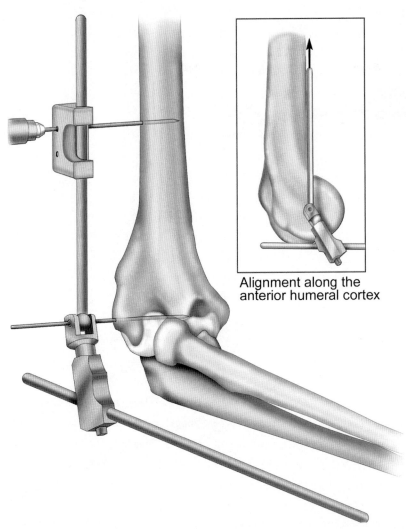

Alignment along the
anterior humeral cortex

Figure 8-7. The fixator is placed over the reference pin, and using the alignment guide a proximal half-pin is placed through the lateral and medial humeral cortices. The humeral arm of the fixator aligns with the anterior cortex of the humerus (INSERT).

Note: Hoffmann II Compact pin-to-rod couplings accept pins of both 3 and 4 mm in diameter.

e. Place the pin guide over the humeral rod more distally (closer to the hinge).

f. The second self-drilling/self-tapping Apex 4-mm (or 3-mm) pin is now inserted more distally through the pin guide (Fig. 8-9).

Note: The pins need not necessarily be parallel. If a different pin insertion angulation is required to access a more desirable area on the humerus, slightly (5 degrees) rotate the pin guide over the humeral rod until such a pin insertion area can be reached. By ensuring proper pin/rod distance, the system allows independent pin placement that is not coplanar (INSERT).

g. The pin guide is then removed from the humeral rod.

h. The distal pin is fixed to the humeral rod with a Hoffmann II Compact pin-to-rod coupling that is then tightened using a Hoffmann II Compact wrench.

7. *Ulnar pin insertions.*

a. According to the pin diameter (3 or 4 mm), place the appropriate pin guide over the ulnar rod to access the lateral aspect of the ulna.

Note: Three-millimeter pins are usually preferred, as the ulna diameter is smaller.

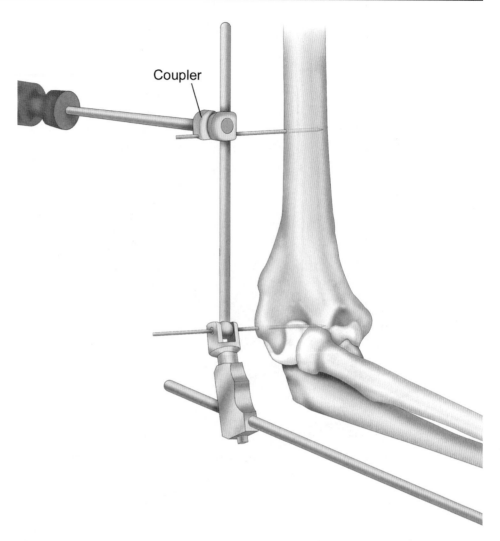

Coupler

Figure 8-8. The proximal pin is fixed to the humeral rod with the H2C coupling mechanism.

b. The distal ulnar self-drilling/self-tapping Apex 3-mm (or 4-mm) pin is inserted into the lateral cortex through the pin guide and pierces the medial ulnar cortex (Fig. 8-10).

c. The pin guide is then removed.

d. The distal pin is fixed to the ulnar rod with a Hoffmann II Compact pin-to-rod coupling, which is then tightened using a Hoffmann Compact wrench.

e. Place the pin guide over the ulnar rod more proximally (i.e., between the distraction mechanism and the distal pin).

f. The proximal self-drilling/self-tapping Apex pin can now be inserted through the pin guide (Fig. 8-11).

Note: As at the humerus, the pins are not necessarily parallel. If a different pin insertion angulation is required to reach a more adequate pin insertion area, slightly rotate the pin guide over the ulnar rod until such a pin insertion area can be reached. The system allows an independent pin placement (Fig. 8-9).

g. The ulnar pin guide is then removed.

h. The proximal pin is fixed to the ulnar rod with a Hoffmann II Compact pin-to-rod coupling, which is then tightened using a Hoffmann II Compact wrench.

i. If the indication requires the use of the proximal ulnar pin in the olecranon, it can be

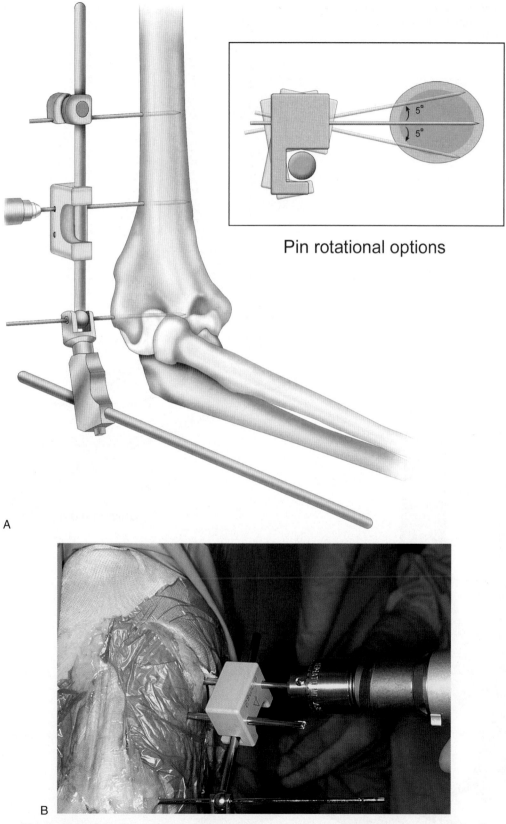

Pin rotational options

Figure 8-9. A,B: Using the pin guide, a second half-pin is placed across the proximal humerus distal to the first. If needed, a plus/minus 5 degrees of out-of-plane rotation may be introduced to provide better target as well as avoid soft-tissue injury (INSERT).

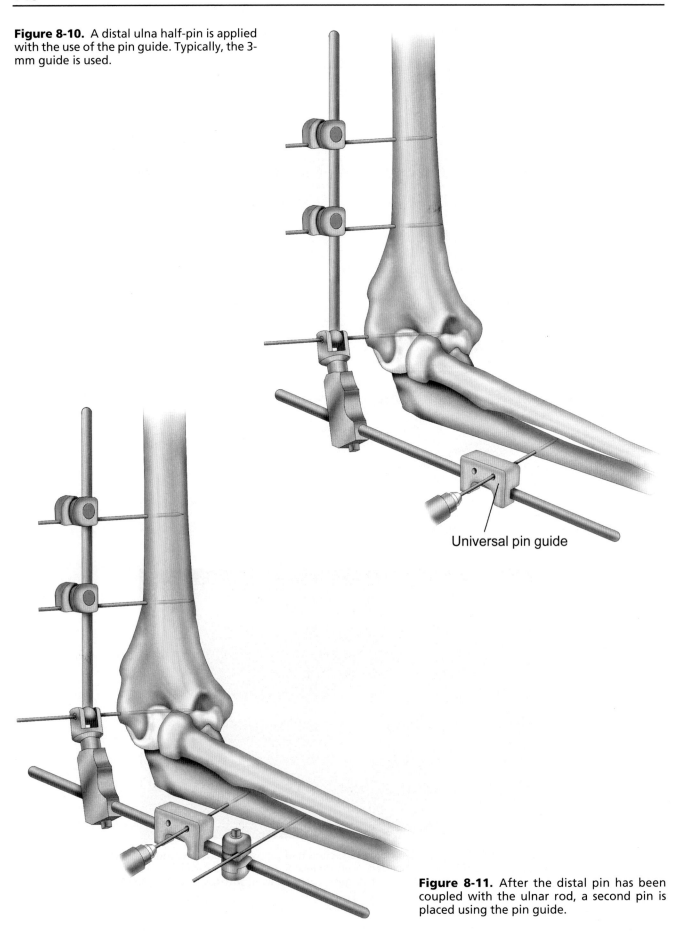

Figure 8-10. A distal ulna half-pin is applied with the use of the pin guide. Typically, the 3-mm guide is used.

Universal pin guide

Figure 8-11. After the distal pin has been coupled with the ulnar rod, a second pin is placed using the pin guide.

inserted through the pin guide. This pin will be once again attached to the ulnar rod with a Hoffmann II Compact pin-to-rod coupling, which is then tightened.

8. *Reference pin removal.* The 3-mm Apex humeral reference pin is then removed (Fig. 8-12).

9. *Distraction.* The ulna is separated from the humerus by turning the distraction screw using a Hoffmann II Compact wrench. Most commonly, 2- to 3-mm distraction is sufficient to accomplish the goals of the procedure (Fig. 8-13). Skin closure is usually deferred until the distraction is applied.

Bilateral Frame Option

If greater stability of the external fixator is desired, a second half frame is applied over the smooth transfixing Apex pin on the medial aspect. Independent half-pins are then applied on both the humerus and the ulna as described in steps 6 and 7 (Fig. 8-1).

Medial Application

Exposure of the Joint—Stiff, Ankylosed, or Posttraumatic Joint A "medial column" exposure of the elbow is most commonly used, especially if ulnar nerve symptoms are present. The medial aspect of the triceps is identified along with the ulnar nerve. The nerve is not necessarily transposed unless appropriate for the case. The intermuscular septum is identified proximal to the epicondyle and followed anteriorly to the humerus. The soft tissues are elevated from the distal humerus, and the pronator attachment is released

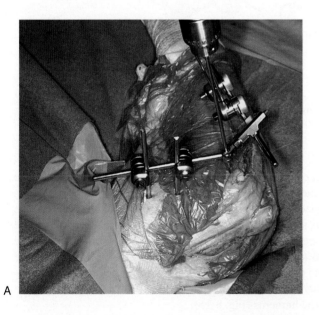

A

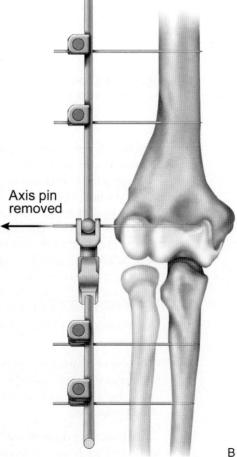

Axis pin removed

B

Figure 8-12. A,B: The reference (axis) pin is removed, leaving no interarticular fixative device.

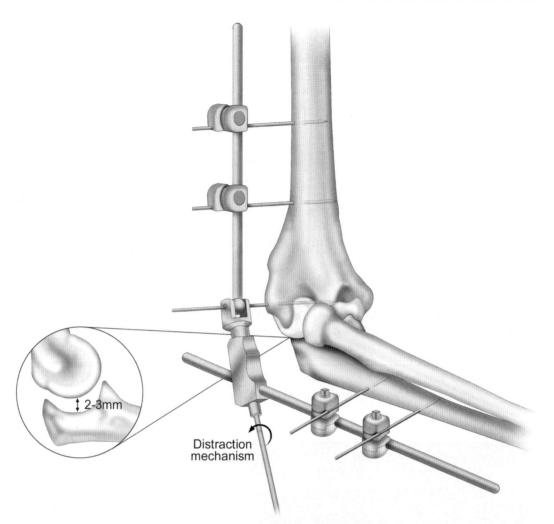

Figure 8-13. Using the hand wrench the distraction device is advanced 2 to 3 mm or until the flexion arc occurs without evidence of articular contact.

from the anterior superior aspect of the medial epicondyle. Elevating the soft-tissue sleeve allows exposure of the anterior medial capsule (Fig. 8-14).

To apply the DJD II fixator, place the humeral (axis) reference pin guide in line with the axis of rotation. The guide stylus is placed medially, and the point is placed laterally at the axis site located at the lateral tubercle. Insert medially the 3-mm Apex humeral reference pin (Fig. 8-15). The application proceeds as with the lateral description. However, care must be exercised to observe and protect the ulnar nerve and anterior neuromuscular bundle at the time of humeral pin insertion. This is best done by directly observing the entrance site of the percutaneous pins at the humerus (Fig. 8-16).

For some acute or subacute fractures in which the elbow is unstable, there is a tendency for the ulna to sublux posteriorly. In these cases, the DJD II may be applied to neutralize this tendency. The typical features of the application under these circumstances include the following:

- The use of fluoroscopy, so that the pins may be inserted percutaneously.
- Insertion of the pins distal to the coronoid to avoid any fracture fixation that may be present, but also to apply the correct distal displacement vector to help accomplish elbow joint reduction.

The patient's extremity is draped free, and a C-arm fluoroscopic unit is also draped in a sterile fashion. It may be difficult to palpate the lateral epicondyle if there is a significant

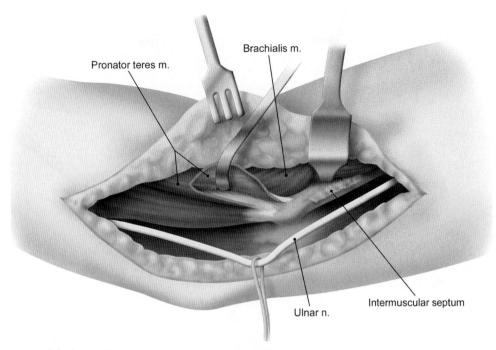

Figure 8-14. After identification of the medial intermuscular septum the pronator origin and brachialis are swept from the anterior aspect of the distal humerus.

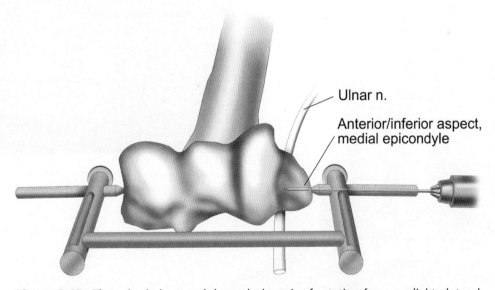

Figure 8-15. The axis pin is passed through the axis of rotation from medial to lateral using the alignment guide and medial axis target area past the inferior aspect of the medial epicondyle.

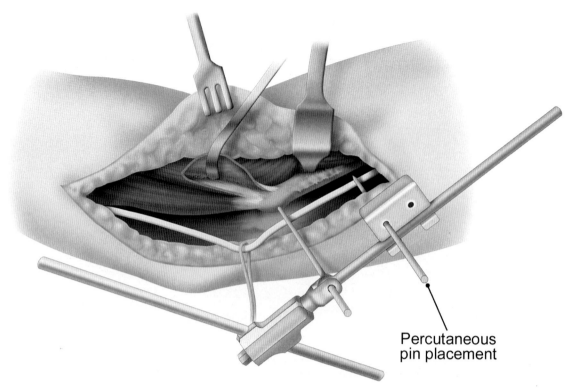

Figure 8-16. The humeral pins medially are most safely placed percutaneously under direct vision.

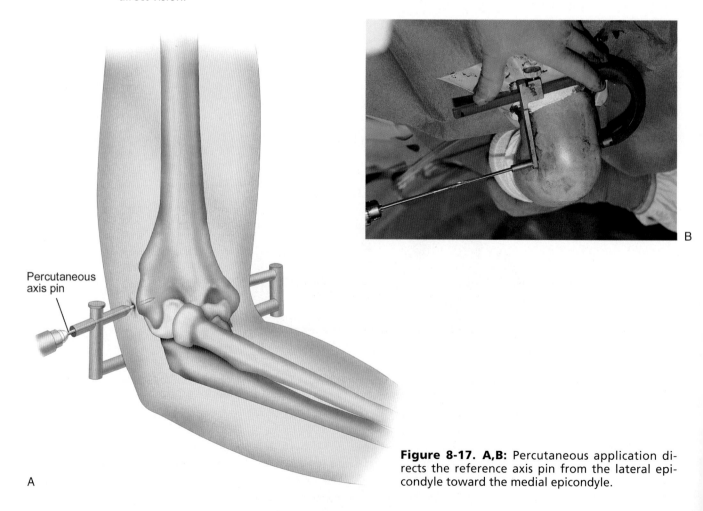

Figure 8-17. A,B: Percutaneous application directs the reference axis pin from the lateral epicondyle toward the medial epicondyle.

amount of swelling. Thus the location in the midpoint of the lateral epicondyle is identified by AP and lateral projections, using a hypodermic needle or Steinmann pin to identify the point of insertion.

A 3-mm Apex pin used as the reference pin is placed laterally and directed toward the point identified at the medial epicondyle (Fig. 8-17). The DJD II is then applied over the reference pin, and the humeral half-pins are inserted percutaneously using the appropriate pin guide (see the preceding step 6) (Fig. 8-18). Hoffmann II Compact pin-to-rod couplings are used to attach the humeral pins to the humeral rod of the DJD II. The joint is reduced as able and the ulnar pins are then applied with the appropriate pin guide. Ulnar pins are then attached to the ulnar rod with Hoffmann II Compact pin-to-rod couplings.

Note: The joint is reduced before the frame is secured; however, small adjustments to alignment can be made by advancing the distraction mechanism (Fig. 8-19).

Compass Hinge

To use the Compass hinge, the frame is first assembled. In most instances, the 150-mm ring size is the best. The geared component is always medial; the knob is always posterior (Fig. 8-20).

When the frame has been placed and appropriately assembled and adjusted, it will slide along the axis pin without significant impingement or resistance (Fig. 8-21). The clinician should make sure to allow for swelling in the postoperative period, allowing at least 2 cm of clearance from the skin to the hinge block at the time of surgery.

For release of contracture and removal of heterotopic bone, the patient is placed in the supine position with the arm on a radiolucent hand table. If the patient first requires a more

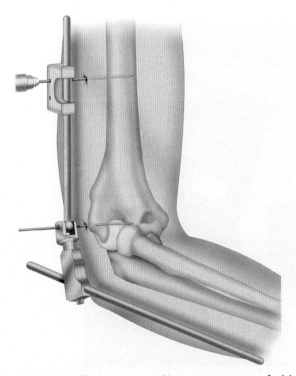

Figure 8-18. The proximal half-pin is inserted in a percutaneous fashion (of right arm). Fluoroscopy is recommended for assistance as necessary.

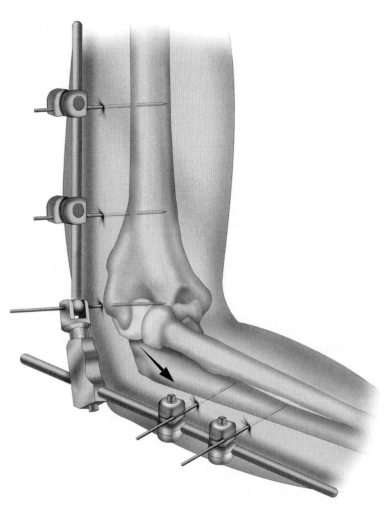

Figure 8-19. After application of the apparatus, the joint is distracted according to the needs of the pathology.

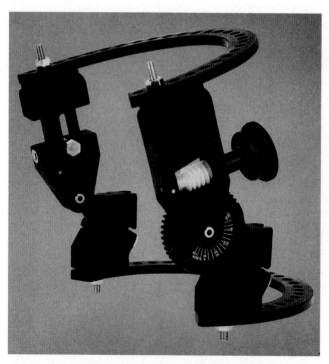

Figure 8-20. The Compass hinge employs hemi-rings and a gear mechanism that allows free motion on applied force across the mechanism.

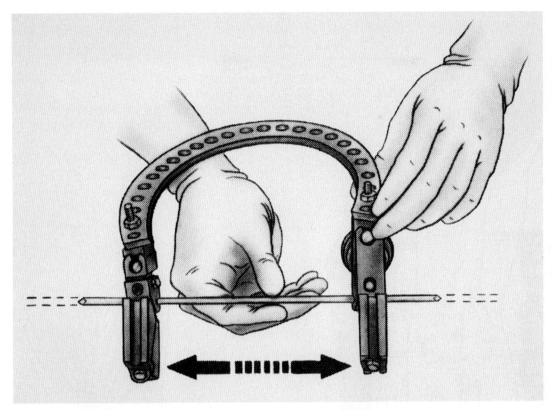

Figure 8-21. The preconstructed frame allows free slide of the axis pin.

extensive exposure of the distal humerus for fracture or reconstructive procedure, it may be useful to begin the operation with the arm over the chest, using one of the more standard posterior approaches to the elbow, either olecranon ostectomy or triceps-sparing exposure if Bryan/Morrey or a Mayo Modified Kocher release (see Chapter 1). In cases of gross instability, the prone position can be used; however, exposure of the coronoid is quite difficult in this position.

As with the DJD, a single temporary axis pin can be placed across the joint, or two half-pins can be inserted, one from the medial and the other from the lateral aspect of the joint. The alignment of the axis is crucial. It is important to take the time necessary to achieve perfect placement of this pin for alignment of the Compass hinge at the elbow. Anteroposterior and lateral radiographs ensure adequate placement. Once the two pins are coincident, the frame should still be easy to slide from medial to lateral, back and forth, before securing the axis pin from the medial side (Fig. 8-22).

The principle in placing the humeral pin is to secure the humerus in two planes, without impaling any of the major muscle/tendon units or jeopardizing any neurovascular structures. It is helpful to be familiar with half-pin systems. If internal fixation is present, the pin placement can be adjusted to avoid the plates by customizing the frame. In general, two 5-mm half-pins, medial and lateral, are required. In larger elbows or in cases in which internal fixation precludes use of the described sites, a third humeral pin may be used, usually placed laterally, superior to the spiral groove.

The medial pin is usually placed first through a two-hole Rancho cube on the undersurface of the upper ring. Both cortices should be engaged.

The lateral pin is usually placed using a two-hole post and a single-hole Rancho cube (Fig. 8-23). The lateral flare of the humerus is used for placement. The drill guide rests on

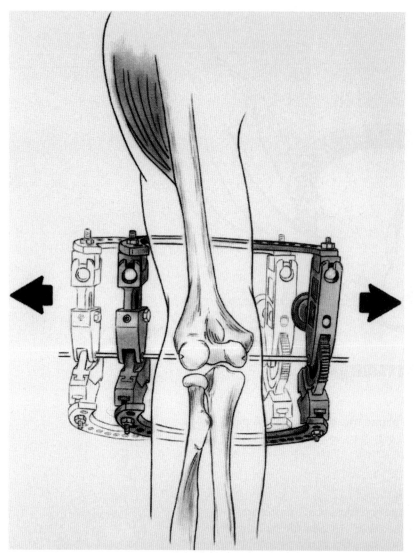

Figure 8-22. Once applied, the frame must freely slide from medial to lateral.

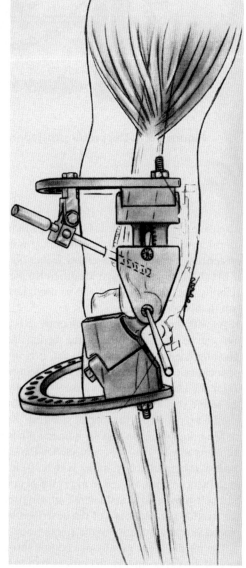

Figure 8-23. The initial fixation is with a lateral half-pin commonly deviated medially at the lateral humeral flare.

the lateral supracondylar ridge, directed anterior and distally. The radial nerve, at this level, is anterior to the pin. Humeral fixation and alignment of the axis of the hinge must be achieved before fixation of the ulna.

One 5-mm and one or two 4-mm pins are used in the ulna. The more proximal pin (5-mm) provides optimal control of the joint and is placed form the dorsal surface through the coronoid (Fig. 8-24). The smaller (4-mm) pins are used more distally in the ulna, again from the dorsal surface. If the elbow is grossly unstable, it is quite important to reduce the elbow by placing it in approximately 90 degrees of flexion when applying the ulnar fixation. Once the joint is reduced and held in position, the first two proximal ulnar pins can be placed. Once the first two pins are in place, ranging through flexion and extension and ensuring reduction of the joint is important. If there is a tendency for the elbow to subluxate, then alignment has not been achieved and the bolts must be loosened and reduction achieved.

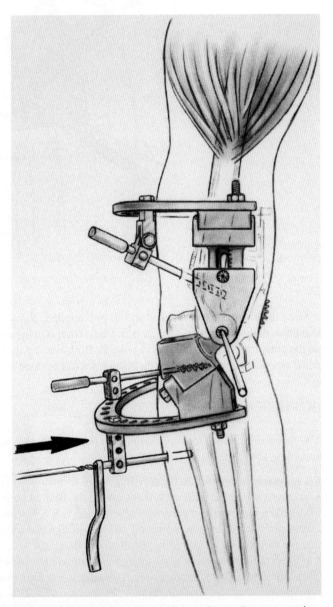

Figure 8-24. Proximal and distal ulnar pins are used to stabilize the frame to the ulna.

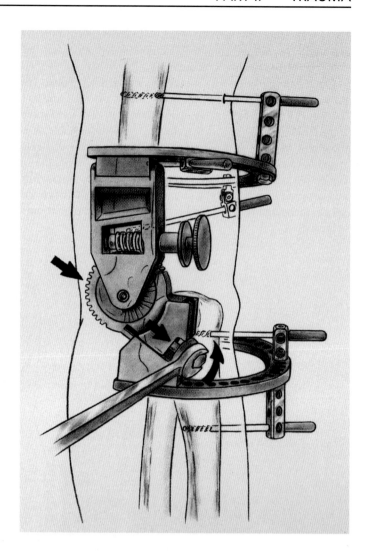

Figure 8-25. Distraction is accomplished by rotating the bolts near the ulnar ring fixation blocks.

Once the joint has been reduced and all pins applied, distraction can be applied to the system through the distraction mechanism. Distraction is achieved by turning the bolts located on the ulnar ring fixation blocks (Fig. 8-25). Both sides of the hinge should be distracted an equal amount. Use and extent of distraction should be done at the discretion of the surgeon.

POSTOPERATIVE MANAGEMENT

The following general steps are employed postoperatively, but this plan is individualized according to the specific needs of the case.

- The patient is assessed in the recovery room to ensure neurovascular competence.
- To avoid unwanted joint movement during the first 24 hours, the external fixator can be locked by the specific mechanism of either device. A Hoffmann II Compact rod is placed between the proximal humeral rod and the distal ulnar rod of the DJD II. The Compass hinge can also be locked at the distraction if desired.
- If the procedure requires early motion and complete relief of pain, appropriate analgesia should be provided to attain this goal. We often employ a brachial plexus catheter for this purpose.
- The patient is encouraged to begin passive range of motion during the first 24 to 48 hours.
- A careful inspection of the elbow is made to assess for swelling and to ensure that the device is not exerting pressure on the skin.
- Proper pin site care is necessary to reduce the risk of pin tract infection.

TABLE 8-1.

Post-op management	Time period
Axillary block	Recovery room to 48 hours
CPM	Day 1–4: Hospital—then
	Day 4–21: Stiffness
	Day 4–42: Fracture
Removal of distractor	3 weeks, soft tissue
	6 weeks, fracture
Flexion and extension splints program	12 weeks
	21 hr/d, 3 weeks
	18 hr/d, 3 weeks
	15 hr/d, 6 weeks
Long-term splints	Maintenance (night)
	3 months
	(longer as needed)

- If there is no evidence of infection and there has been adequate progress, the patient is dismissed upon surgeon's discretion with active or passive range-of-motion instructions.
- Approximately 3 weeks after the operative procedure for stiffness and 6 weeks after treatment of fracture, before the fixator is completely removed, the elbow is examined for stability. Care is taken not to forcefully manipulate the elbow. If the elbow is found to be unstable with the DJD II, the ulnar rod is reattached to the ulnar pins. If the elbow is stable, the fixator may be removed as well as the ulnar and humeral pins.

An anteroposterior and lateral radiograph is taken to ensure that the elbow is adequately reduced and stable. The patient is then treated with flexion and extension splints according to the merits of the case (Table 8-1).

ILLUSTRATIVE CASE

A 28-year-old male sustained a fracture/dislocation with a type III radial head fracture. The subluxation persisted for 3 weeks before treatment (Fig. 8-26A). The fracture was managed

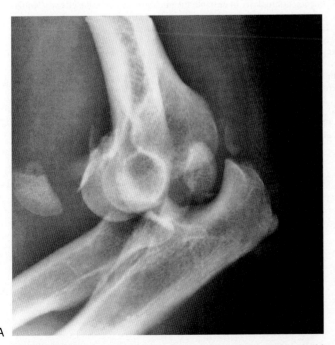
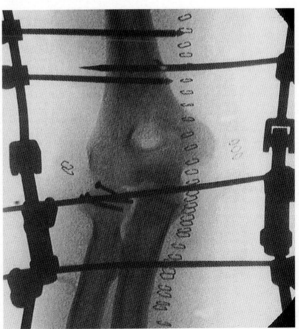

Figure 8-26. Complex dislocation with a Mason III radial head fracture dislocation (**A**). The fracture is fixed with intrafragment compression osteosynthesis and the construct is stabilized by the DJD II external fixator (**B**). *(continued)*

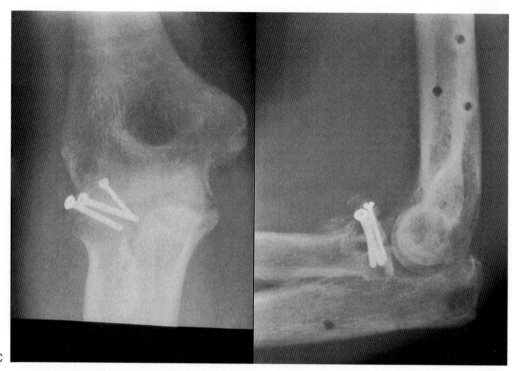

Figure 8-26. *Continued.* The fracture healed with an arc of 20 to 140 degrees of flexion and no pain (**C**).

with osteosynthesis (Fig. 8-26B). The construct was protected or "neutralized" by the DJD II (Fig. 8-26C).

RECOMMENDED READINGS

1. Cobb TK, Morrey BF. Use of distraction arthroplasty in unstable fracture dislocations of the elbow. *Clin Orthop* 1995;312:201.
2. Kasparayan NG, Hotchkiss RN. Dynamic skeletal fixation in the upper extremity. *Hand Clin* 1997;13:643.
3. Morrey BF. Distraction arthroplasty: clinical applications. *Clin Orthop* 1993;293:46.
4. Morrey BF. Post-traumatic contracture of the elbow: operative treatment including distraction arthroplasty. *J Bone Joint Surg* 1990;72A:601.
5. Morrey BF, Chao EY. Passive motion of the elbow joint. *J Bone Joint Surg* 1976;58A:501.
6. Morrey BF, Hotchkiss RN. External fixators of the elbow. In: Morrey BF, ed. *The elbow and its disorders,* 3rd ed. Philadelphia: WB Saunders; 2000.
7. Shiba R, Sorbie C, Siu DW, et al. Geometry of the humeroulnar joint. *J Orthop* 1988;6:897–906.
8. Tomaino MM, Sotereanos DG, Plakseychuk A. Technique for ensuring ulnohumeral reduction during application of the Richards compass elbow hinge. *Am J Orthop* 1997;26:646.

9

Postoperative Treatment Adjuncts

Bernard F. Morrey and Shawn W. O'Driscoll

Because the elbow is so prone to posttraumatic and postsurgical stiffness, continuous passive motion (CPM) is useful in maintaining motion and preventing stiffness.

Based on an understanding that stiffness develops from bleeding and edema occurring within minutes after surgery or trauma, and since motion has been shown to negate these changes (4,9), this treatment should commence as soon as possible following surgery, ideally in the recovery room (2,4). However, this is not always practical.

INDICATIONS/CONTRAINDICATIONS

CPM is indicated to prevent stiffness and to maintain motion obtained at the time of surgery following intraarticular fracture fixation, contracture release, synovectomy, and excision of heterotopic ossification. It may also be useful following the replacement of arthritic joints that were stiff preoperatively or in any setting in which swelling and motion restriction are anticipated.

The use of CPM is relatively contraindicated in the presence of ligamentous insufficiency if the elbow is unstable or if fracture fixation is not rigid or is tenuous. The most common contraindication is poor-quality soft tissue and concern about wound dehiscence.

PREOPERATIVE PLANNING

Effective use requires that several considerations be satisfied.

1. Access to an effectively designed device for inpatient and outpatient use (Figs. 9-1 and 9-2).

B.F. Morrey, M.D.: Mayo Medical School and Department of Orthopaedics, Mayo Clinic and Mayo Foundation, Rochester, Minnesota.

S.W. O'Driscoll, M.D., PH.D.: Orthopedic Surgery, Mayo Medical School, Mayo Foundation, Rochester, Minnesota.

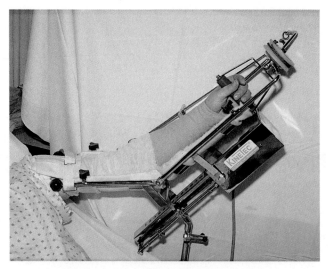

Figure 9-1. Bedside-based CPM machine.

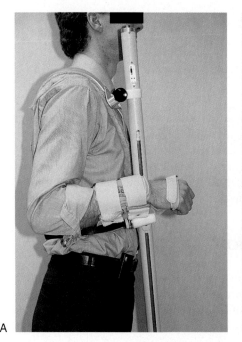

A

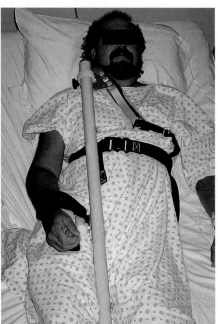

B

Figure 9-2. A,B: Portable CPM unit.

2. A nursing staff knowledgeable in the applications of CPM.
3. A compliant patient.
4. Physician understanding and commitment and communication with patient and nursing staff.

SURGERY

1. Until motion is started, it is preferable to elevate the limb with the elbow in full extension and wrapped in a compressive Jones dressing to minimize swelling.
2. A drain is usually useful to prevent periarticular accumulation of blood.
3. Before starting CPM, all circumferential wrapping (Jones, cling, etc.) should be removed and replaced with a single elastic sleeve.

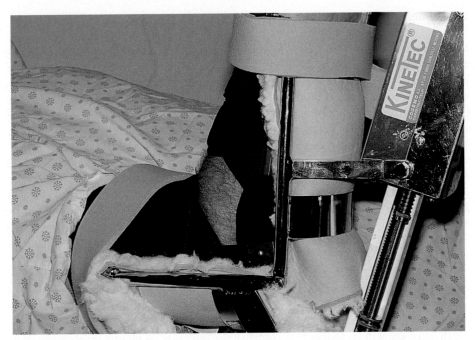

Figure 9-3. Proper position with elbow and device flexion axis coincident. In this instance the elbow is also protected in a brace.

4. The arm is carefully positioned in the CPM device and the elbow flexion axis, or brace hinge aligned with the flexion axis of the device (Fig. 9-3).
5. The hand and forearm are secured with well-padded supports (Fig. 9-4), especially if a brachial plexus block is being used.
6. The wound is examined to ensure that its integrity is not compromised during elbow flexion.

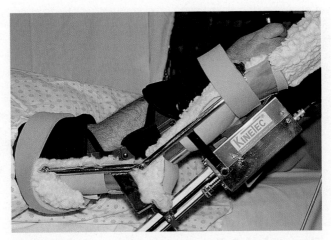

Figure 9-4. The hand and forearm are secured and carefully padded if sensory changes exist due to the brachial plexus block.

Device Selection and Adjustment

Most commonly, a stationary unit is utilized in the postoperative period. Once CPM is started, it is necessary that the full range of motion be utilized (Fig. 9-5). The tissues are being "squeezed" alternately in flexion and extension, as CPM causes a sinusoidal oscillation in intraarticular pressure. This not only rids the joint and tissue of excess blood and fluid, but prevents further edema from accumulating (4). In the first 24 hours, swelling can develop in minutes (as a result of bleeding), so CPM should be applied early and be continuous. Only bathroom privileges are allowed.

Note: This treatment requires close supervision by someone skilled with its use, so it is mandatory that the patient and family be involved and educated from the beginning regarding the principles of use and how to monitor the limb. Frequent checking and slight adjustments of position prevent pressure-related problems. The arm tends to slip out of the machine, so it must frequently be readjusted. If the full flexion arc cannot be immediately attained, the physician must increase the adjustments as rapidly as tolerated by the soft tissue.

As the number of days following surgery increases, the amount of time required for swelling to develop increases also, so that longer periods out of the machine are permitted.

As noted earlier, portable units are available, though not as effective (Fig. 9-2). CPM treatment at home should be used long enough to get the patient through the period during which he or she will be unable to accomplish the full range of motion independent of assistance. This can be several days to several weeks, usually a month.

Pain Control

In the early stages following surgery, an indwelling catheter for continuous brachial plexus block anesthesia is used (5). This permits a range from analgesia to anesthesia by varying the dose of bupivocaine, a long-acting local anesthetic. In many cases, the dose employed initially is sufficient to cause a complete or nearly complete motor and sensory block. Motor blockade requires splinting of the wrist to protect it. Moderate or complete anesthesia, as opposed to analgesia with minimal anesthesia, requires careful attention to the status of the limb overall, as the patient's protective pain response is no longer present and impending complications such as compartment syndrome can be missed.

The catheter is usually left in place for 3 days in the hospital, then removed. At that time the patient is generally able to maintain the same range of motion with oral analgesics. The

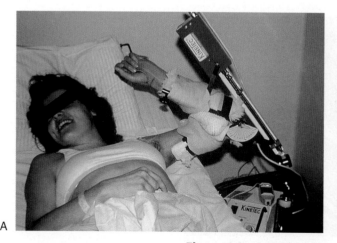
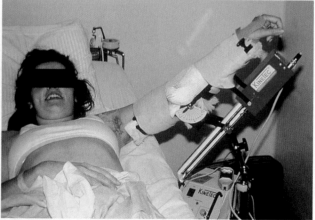

Figure 9-5. A,B: The range of motion on CPM should be full. This permits the tissues to be squeezed alternately in flexion and extension.

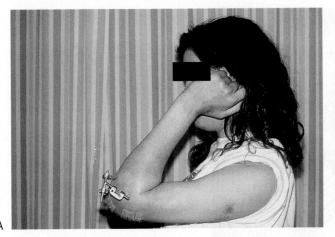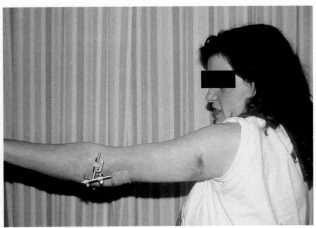

Figure 9-6. A,B: Typical range of motion seen at 3 weeks following a distraction interposition arthroplasty treated postoperatively using continuous passive motion.

goal is to have the patient leave the hospital capable of moving the elbow from about 10 to 135 degrees of motion actively.

A PCA (patient-controlled analgesia) pump with morphine has also been used effectively if a brachial plexus block is contraindicated, unsuccessful, or unavailable.

COMPLICATIONS

Bleeding may be increased, but rarely sufficiently to require a transfusion. Excessive wound or incision pressure at full flexion is the greatest concern. The incision must be visible to the surgeon in the early stages of CPM treatment. If wound compromise occurs, CPM is discontinued. Excessive pressure from an improperly applied or padded device is particularly possible in limbs rendered arthritic by the brachial block. Hematomas are drained surgically.

RESULTS

Despite widespread use of knee CPM and the scientific basis for its utility, there is little clinical evidence that clearly documents its effectiveness compared with a control population (3). Nonetheless, it is the authors' opinion, shared by others, that this is a valuable modality in selected patients (1) (Fig. 9-6).

SPLINTS

The most common complication of elbow injury and some arthritic conditions is stiffness. The accepted principle to avoid this after a fracture is rigid fixation. Early motion has also been used to decrease this sequelae after fractures and injury at the elbow (see the preceding section, "Continuous Passive Motion"). In spite of these measures, because of limitations imposed by the injury or in executing the ideal treatment, and due to the inherent biology and response to injury, stiffness of the elbow is a common problem (7). Unfortunately, aggressive physical therapy to address posttraumatic stiffness is not always successful and, in fact, may contribute to making the contracture worse.

Ankylosis develops from contracting scar tissue as a response to insult. The goal of splint treatment is to stretch the soft tissues, thus maintaining the length of the capsule and liga-

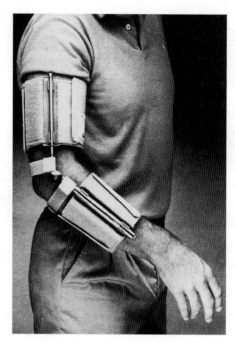

Figure 9-7. Commercially available dynamic splint. The tension and excursion may be adjusted by the patient.

ments. The question then arises as to the best method of providing a force to stretch the periarticular soft tissues: dynamic or static adjustable splinting. The selection of one program over the other is dependent on one's philosophy and interpretation of the concepts and goals of splint usage (8–10).

Dynamic Splinting

Dynamic splinting is probably the most popular means of treating impending or developing stiffness, probably because dynamic splints are readily available (Fig. 9-7). The rationale of dynamic splinting is based on considering the elbow capsule as a viscoelastic tissue. The response of such a tissue to a constant force is shown in Fig. 9-8. The response in

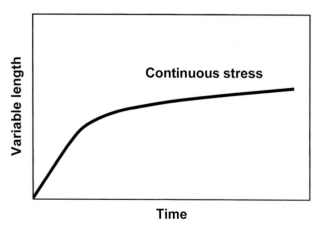

Figure 9-8. Viscoelastic tissue response to a constant force resulting in gradual stretching of the tissue. However, the potential for inflammation is not demonstrated by this curve but is possible if the force is constantly present, which is the case in dynamic loading.

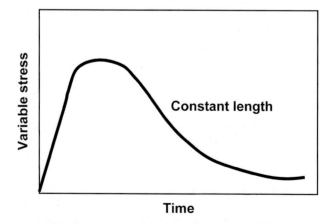

Figure 9-9. Tissue response to a single discrete force results in stress relaxation of the viscoelastic tissue over time.

the soft tissue to a persistent force is a deformation, which is called creep (10). However, the constant force may cause irritation of the soft tissue; hence inflammation is commonly associated with dynamic splinting. Nonetheless this type splinting remains a commonly employed option for many (8).

Static Adjustable Splinting

With static adjustable splinting, a specific force is applied to the elbow, which results in a discrete stress being imparted to the tissue. However, since the splint position is not further altered, the soft tissue is allowed to undergo a process called stress relaxation that occurs over a period of time in response to the fixed position (Fig. 9-9). It is felt that stress relaxation lessens the likelihood of tissue irritation and of inflammation. Thus the elbow is more amenable to this type of load application and splint philosophy, since it is inflammation that breeds additional swelling and scarring.

INDICATIONS/CONTRAINDICATIONS

The indication for elbow splint therapy is the presence of a flexion or extension contracture that is amenable to stretch deformation. Experimental data (6) and clinical experience suggest tissue is amenable to this type of therapy in three stages as follows (9): I, onset to 3 months from injury, highly effective; II, 3 to 6 months, moderately successful; III, 6 to 12 months, variably effective. A stable articulation and articular surface is a prerequisite for splint therapy to be effective in any of these stages.

Contraindications include poor-quality skin that does not tolerate the constant forces from the splint. Excessive or increasing swelling can also cause the development of neural symptoms that require splint discontinuance or program alteration as follows: sensory—alter the pressure points; motor—alter basic program or discontinue.

Static Adjustable Splints

At the present time a single brace is used to attain full extension and flexion up to 100 degrees (Figs. 9-10 and 9-11). For flexion beyond 100 degrees a second "hyperflexion" brace is used to attempt to gain further flexion (Fig. 9-12). With traditional humeral-based support, the soft tissue tends to "bunch up" in the brace in flexion, and this tendency limits further flexion. The hyperflexion brace is stabilized at the shoulder, and the elbow is flexed through a mechanism applied to the wrist with an adjustable strap.

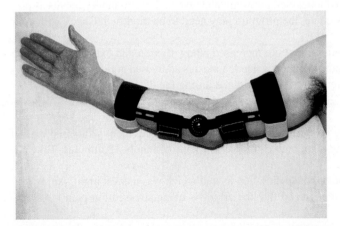

Figure 9-10. A static adjustable splint currently used by the author in which the force is directly applied to the axis of rotation.

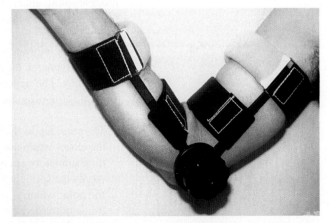

Figure 9-11. The same splint shown in Fig. 9-10 but reversed and being used in the flexion mode. Hence the splint is called the universal splint in our practice.

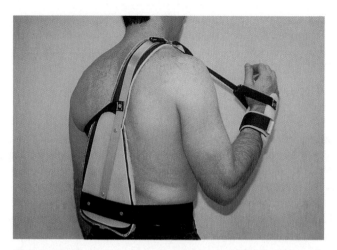

Figure 9-12. To avoid soft-tissue impingement associated with straps supporting braces about the elbow, a hyperflexion splint that frees the elbow of any encumbrance is based at the shoulder and flexion across the elbow by way of the wrist.

The extension brace is applied with the hinge aligned to the elbow flexion axis. The brace should have broad surfaces for force application at the wrist and forearm, and the support at the brachium should not cause soft-tissue constriction. The precise use is described later in a format designed to be individualized and given to the patient.

In all instances the patient assumes responsibility for the use of the brace.

General Instructions for the Use of Static Adjustable Splint(s)

The following general guidelines for the use of the static adjustable splint may be modified, depending on individual needs and progress.

1. *General goals.* To attain improved motion of the elbow, inflammation must be avoided. This is done with the use of the anti-inflammatory agents, heat and ice and education of the patient to the signs of inflammation.
2. *Cardinal signs of inflammation.* Increased soreness, increased discomfort with use, swelling or, commonly, a progressive loss of motion rather than improvement from day to day.
3. *Treatment of inflammation.* Avoid the causative factor. Be less vigorous with static adjustable splint, adhere to the heat/ice program, and take antiinflammatory agents as prescribed. If it seems inadequate, the program may need to be modified. Check with your doctor.
4. *Direction of improvement.* Often both increased elbow flexion and extension are being sought. In general, the motion which is needed most is addressed at night as well as during the day. The opposite motion is encouraged during the day.
5. Typical splint program (20-hour program, 0 to 3 weeks from injury or surgery) (Fig. 9-13).
   a. *Morning.* Upon rising in the morning the splint is removed. Gently flex and extend the elbow while taking a hot bath or shower for approximately 15 minutes. Take antiinflammatory agent.
   b. Apply the splint in the opposite direction as that which was used at night. Apply it to the point where it is recognized that the elbow is being stressed but pain is not extreme or intolerable.
   c. *Noon.* The splint may be removed for 1 hour in the morning, 1 hour in the afternoon, and 1 hour in the evening. Reapply the splint in the opposite direction after these rest periods.

IV	**I**		**II**		**III**		**IV**	
Sleep	**Breakfast**	**8 - noon**	**Lunch**	**1 - 6 pm**	**Dinner**	**6 - 10 pm**	**Nite**	**Sleep**
Flex*	Out:	Flex	Out:	Extend	Out:	Flex	Out:	Flex
Extend	1 hr#	Extend	1 hr	Extend	1 hr	Extend	1 hr	Extend

Figure 9-13. Flexion and extention visual splint (20 hours and 3 weeks). The hours are changed for the Phase II/6 hour program. *Circle direction of splinting: extension or flexion; write in duration out of splint. A sample of the "20-hour" daily program given to the patient at the time of splint prescription. A visual prescription of the splint usage program is provided to those undergoing splint therapy.

  d. *Evening.* Use the elbow when out of the splint as able during these periods and in the evening. While out of the splint if the elbow is sore or seems inflamed, apply ice for 15 minutes before bedtime. If not inflamed but stiff, apply heat for 15 minutes, gently working the joint in flexion and extension.
  e. *Night.* Before going to bed at night apply the splint in the direction needed most. Application should be sufficient to be aware that the elbow is being stressed and a person should be able to sleep comfortably for about 6 hours without being awakened by elbow pain.

If the use of the splint causes numbness and tingling that disappears when the splint is removed, it is acceptable to continue the program but to alter it to minimize nerve symptoms. If the numbness does not resolve or motor symptoms develop, discontinue the splint and call your doctor.

After reading these instructions, contact your physician if you have any specific questions.

POSTOPERATIVE MANAGEMENT

The patient is reassessed at 3 weeks and the program modified as needed. The typical phase II program follows.

Phase II: The 12- to 14-Hour Program

The duration of phase II from 3–6 weeks to 6–10 weeks.

  1. Sleep in direction needed most.
  2. In the morning, do a 15-minute warm-up. Take antiinflammatory; use extremity as tolerated for 2 hours. Then apply splint in opposite direction to that used during sleep.
  3. At noon, remove the splint for 2 hours. Reapply same splint used at night.
  4. At dinnertime, remove the splint for 2 hours. Reapply in the evening in opposite direction to that used at night.
  5. At night, apply ice if sore and inflamed. Apply heat if stiff. Remove splint 1 hour before bedtime, then apply it in the direction in which motion is needed most.
  6. Reassess after 3 weeks. Alter the program further as needed.

RESULTS

Over the period 1984 through 1997 we have prescribed approximately 360 braces for patients with various expressions of stiff elbow. We estimate an overall success rate of the splinting program as about 80%. That is, the splint was considered a beneficial adjunct. It is not a panacea. It is this experience that has resulted in the program that is currently employed. These splints are now commercially available (Prosthetic Laboratories of Rochester, Inc.; 201 1st Ave. S.W.; Rochester, MN 55902). This experience has also led to the further development of effective splints by Air Cast and other commercial vendors.

A great deal of time is spent with the patient explaining the rationale of brace management and specifically discussing the program based on the specific goals of treatment.

RECOMMENDED READINGS

1. Breen TF, Gelberman RH, Ackerman GN. Elbow flexion contractures: treatment by anterior release and continuous passive motion. *J Hand Surg* 1988;13B:286–287.
2. O'Driscoll SW, Kumar A, Salter RB. The effect of continuous passive motion on the clearance of a hemarthrosis from a synovial joint: an experimental investigation in the rabbit. *Clin Orthop* 1983;176:305–311.
3. Pop RO, Corcoran S, McCaul K, et al. Continuous passive motion after primary total knee arthroplasty. *J Bone Joint Surg* 1997;79B:914.
4. Salter RB. Motion vs. rest. Why immobilize joints? *J Bone Joint Surg* 1982;64B:251–254.
5. Stinson LJ, Lennon R, Adams R, et al. The technique and efficacy of axillary catheter analgesia as an adjunct to distraction elbow arthroplasty: a prospective study. *J Shoulder Elbow Surg* 1993;2:182–189.
6. Billingham RE, Russell PS. Studies on wound healing, with special reference to the phenomenon of contracture in experimental wounds in rabbits' skin. *Ann Surg* 1956;144:961–981.
7. Broberg MA, Morrey BF. Results of treatment of fracture dislocations of the elbow. *Clin Orthop* 1987;March(216):109–119.
8. Kottke FJ, Pauley DL, Ptak RA. The rationale for prolonged stretching for correction of shortening of connective tissue. *Arch Phys Med Rehabil* 1966;47:345–352.
9. Morrey BF. The use of splints with the stiff elbow. In: Heckman JD, ed. *Perspectives in orthopedic surgery,* Vol. I, No. 1. St. Louis: Quality Medical Publishing; 1990:141–144.
10. Richard R, Shanesy CP, Miller SF. Dynamic versus static splints: a prospective case for sustained stress. *J Burn Care Rehabil* 1995;16:284–287.

PART III

Soft-Tissue Injury

10

Distal Biceps Tendon Rupture

Bernard F. Morrey

Although once thought to be an uncommon injury, most surgeons now see distal biceps tendon rupture with increasing frequency. Since the first edition, increased concern about ectopic bone and a growing interest in suture anchors has emerged. An early diagnosis is important, since the prognosis with early reattachment is excellent.

INDICATIONS/CONTRAINDICATIONS

Indications

There is little question that acute rupture of the distal biceps tendon should be reattached to the radial tuberosity as soon as possible (1,2,11–13). The average age of patients is approximately 55, and virtually every report in the literature has been of a male. In our practice at Mayo we have treated two females from among 70 with this diagnosis, both with partial ruptures. Usually the patient is involved with heavy labor or activity, which further emphasizes the need of early definitive treatment.

The tendon almost always fails by complete avulsion of its insertion from the radial tuberosity (12). Surgical procedures have been described using a modified Henry approach (6,11) or through a two-incision approach described by Boyd and Anderson (4). The advantage of the anterior Henry approach is that it is less likely to create ectopic bone. The disadvantage is that it puts the radial nerve at jeopardy (6,11,13).

However, it must be emphasized that the two-incision approach currently used is *not* that described by Boyd and Anderson. The advantage of the two-incision technique is that it lessens and virtually eliminates the likelihood of injury to the radial nerve (12). The original Boyd-Anderson approach exposes the ulna, and hence can be associated with ectopic bone (7). Through the years we have employed the Mayo modification of the Boyd-Anderson approach, which does *not* expose the ulna and hence is associated with very little ectopic bone (9).

B.F. Morrey, M.D.: Mayo Medical School and Department of Orthopaedics, Mayo Clinic and Foundation, Rochester, Minnesota.

Delayed reattachment is difficult because the tendon retracts. If this has occurred, reattachment or embedding the biceps tendon into the brachialis is easy but rarely acceptable today.

Contraindications

Reattachment is contraindicated in patients who do not have significant functional impairment. This might be seen in a sedentary patient, but rarely does such an individual sustain this injury. An attempt to reattach this tendon if there has been a delay of more than 3 weeks requires careful thought, as the tendon typically is retracted into the biceps muscle and is not of adequate length to reach the radial tuberosity (12). Furthermore, the tract of the tendon to the tuberosity will have scarred and become obliterated, making the surgery much more difficult.

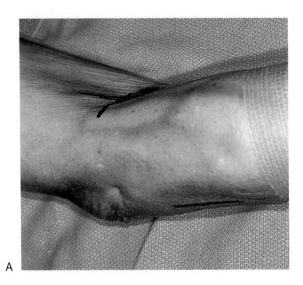

A

Figure 10-1. A,B: The two-incision technique employs a simple 4-cm transverse incision in the antecubital space and a 5- to 7-cm incision over the posterior aspect of the proximal forearm.

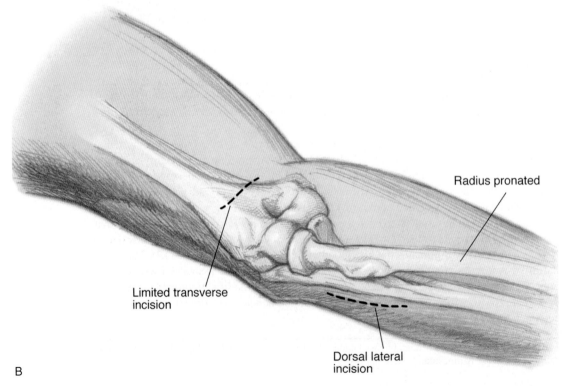

Radius pronated

Limited transverse incision

Dorsal lateral incision

B

Delayed reconstruction is a difficult surgical procedure (8) and typically is referred to those with experience with this procedure. The author prefers the achilles allograft for this procedure as described herein.

PREOPERATIVE PLANNING

If more than 4 weeks has passed since the injury occurred, be prepared to perform a more detailed dissection in the antecubital space. If the tendon has retracted, restoration of length with an achilles allograft is preferred. The patient must be prepared for these eventualities.

SURGERY

Immediate Reattachment

Incision The arm is prepped and draped with the patient supine. A sandbag may be placed under the shoulder to allow the arm to be brought across the chest comfortably. Under a general anesthesia, a single 4-cm transverse incision in the antecubital crease is employed (Fig. 10-1).

Tendon Preparation By digital palpation or limited dissection, the tendon is identified, dissected free of soft tissue, and delivered from the wound (Fig. 10-2). The end of the tendon tends to be bulbous and is trimmed to allow it to fit well into the tuberosity. After the tendon has been trimmed, two No. 5 Mersilene sutures are placed through the torn portion entering the end of the tendon. A crisscrossed (Bunnell) suture or locking stitch (Krakow) is employed (Fig. 10-3). A curved clamp is then introduced into the tunnel previously occupied by the biceps tendon (Fig. 10-4). It is directed by palpation to and then past the tuberosity between the radius and ulna. Rotation of the forearm confirms proper position of the instrument on the ulnar side of the radius. The curved hemostat is advanced until it punctures the muscle and subcutaneous tissues of the dorsal aspect of the forearm (Fig. 10-4). An incision is then made over the site of prominence splitting the common extensor and supinator muscles (Fig. 10-5). With full forearm pronation the tuberosity is identified and cleaned of soft tissue.

Reattachment Preparation A high-speed bur is used to excavate the cancellous bone from the midportion of the tuberosity (Fig. 10-6). After an adequate orifice 10 to 12 mm × 7 to 8 mm has been made to receive the tendon, three drill holes are placed on the radial side of the tuberosity (Fig. 10-7). This is simplified by allowing the forearm to supinate slightly to bring this margin of the radial tuberosity into better alignment. The

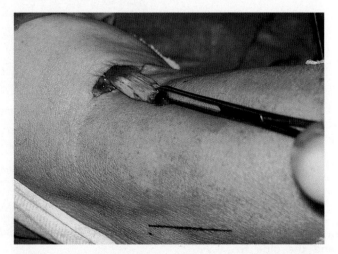

Figure 10-2. The tendon is identified by digital palpation and delivered through the skin incision, revealing a bulbous degenerative process at the site of disruption.

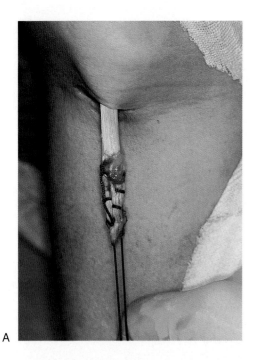

A

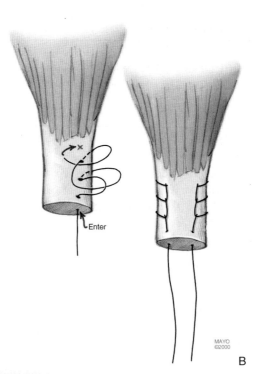

B

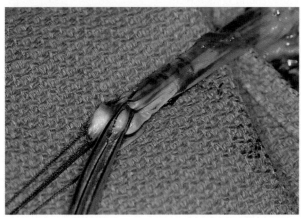

C

Figure 10-3. A–C: Two No. 5 nonabsorbable sutures are inserted by the crisscross Bunnell or Krachow locking technique.

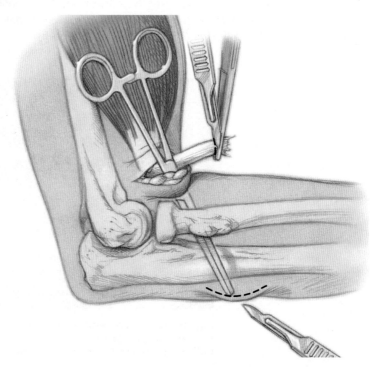

Figure 10-4. The curved hemostat is passed between the radial tuberosity and the ulna to emerge through the common extensor muscle mass and tent the skin on the proximal posterolateral aspect of the forearm.

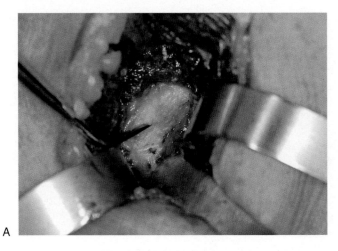

A

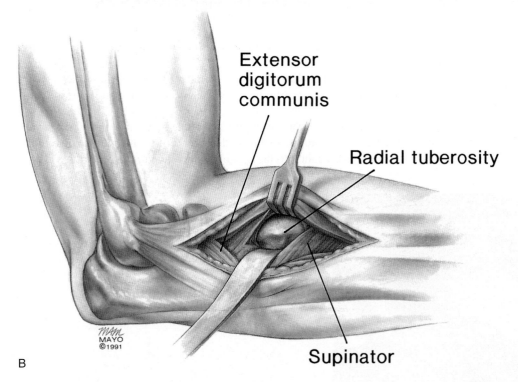

Extensor
digitorum
communis

Radial tuberosity

Supinator

B

Figure 10-5. A,B: An incision is made over this prominence, the muscle is split, the forearm is fully pronated, and the tuberosity is exposed.

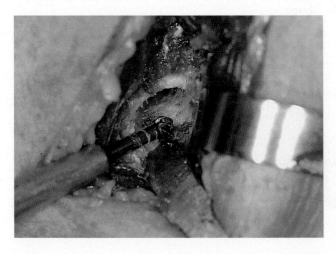

Figure 10-6. The greater tuberosity is excavated with a high-speed bur in such a way as to receive the distal biceps tendon.

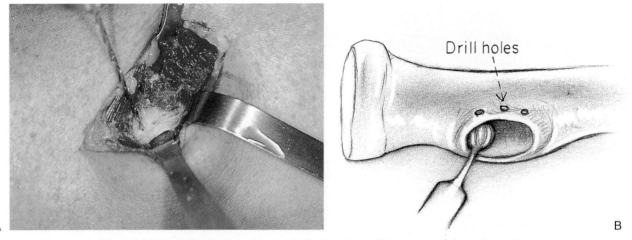

A   B

Figure 10-7. A,B: Three holes are drilled in the radial aspect of the tuberosity.

holes should be placed in such a way as to leave sufficient bone to avoid osseous rupture or pullout of the sutures (Fig. 10-8).

Reattachment of the Tendon The biceps tendon is retrieved from the antecubital incision and the sutures are grasped by the curved hemostat. The instrument is again directed through the tunnel and out the second incision (Fig. 10-9). The tendon is then brought through the tunnel from the antecubital space and drawn past the ulnar side of the tuberosity (Fig. 10-10). The sutures are threaded into each of the holes at the margin of the tuberosity. One suture is brought into the proximal and one into the center hole. The sec-

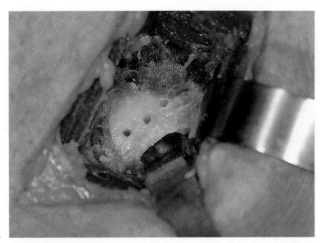

Figure 10-8. A,B: Care is taken to provide sufficient space between the holes to provide secure fixation in bone.

A

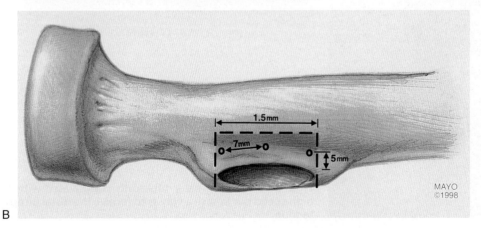

B

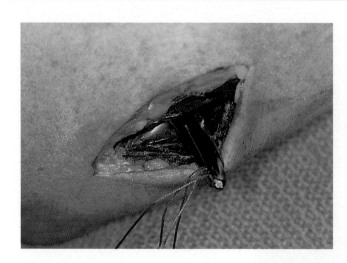

Figure 10-9. The sutures are grasped again with a curved hemostat and introduced through the tunnel of the biceps tendon to emerge through the forearm incision.

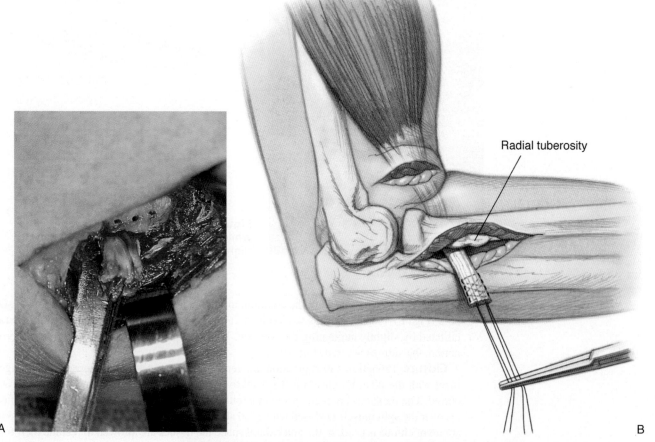

Radial tuberosity

A

B

Figure 10-10. A,B: The tendon is then pulled through the forearm wound.

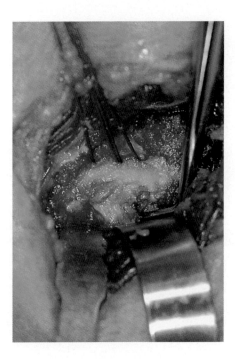

Figure 10-11. The distal aspect of the biceps tendon is threaded into the excavated portion of the radial tuberosity. The sutures are brought through the three holes, with the center hole used for one arm of each of the sutures.

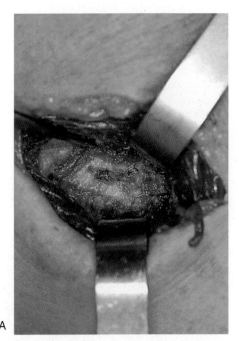

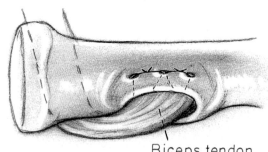

Biceps tendon   B

A

Figure 10-12. A,B: The sutures are tied while the forearm is allowed to supinate slightly to facilitate this process.

ond suture is brought through the common middle hole and its other end through the distal hole (Fig. 10-11). The biceps tendon is threaded into the tuberosity; once again this is facilitated by slightly supinating the forearm. With the arm remaining in less than full pronation, the sutures are tied (Fig. 10-12).

Closure Pronation and supination are gently tested to ensure that there is no impingement with the ulna. Extension is assessed to ensure that excessive shortening has not occurred. The incisions are then closed in a routine fashion. At the proximal forearm the fascia over the split muscle is closed with a 2-0 absorbable suture, and a subcutaneous and skin suture of choice is used. In the antecubital space the tissues are allowed to resume their former position, a drain is left in the antecubital space, and the remainder of the wound is closed in layers as desired.

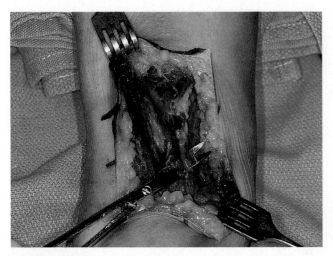

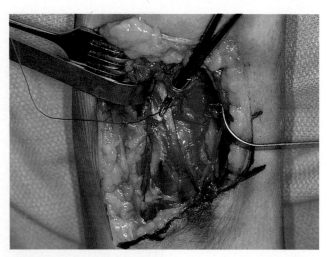

Figure 10-13. A Henry anterior exposure identifies the tendon and lacertus fibrosis.

Figure 10-14. The radial nerve is identified emerging from the interval between the brachial radialis and lateral aspect of the biceps (above retractor). The recurrent radial artery is identified and ligated.

ANTERIOR APPROACH/SUTURE ANCHORS

Technique: Suture Anchors

Suture anchors employ a Henry or modified Henry skin incision (Fig. 10-13). The radial nerve is identified at the lateral margin of the biceps muscle and followed distally to the supinator muscles (Fig. 10-14). The fascia is split and the recurrent radial artery is ligated, allowing exposure of the tuberosity (Fig. 10-15).

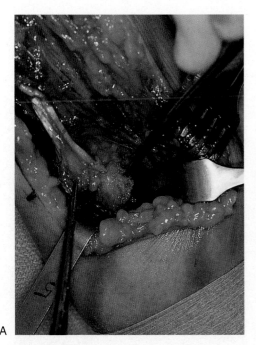

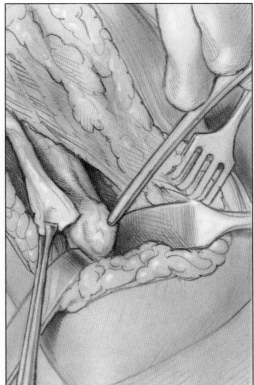

Figure 10-15. A,B: The tuberosity is exposed.

MAYO
©2000   B

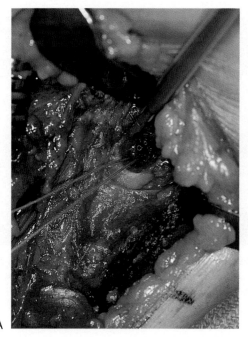

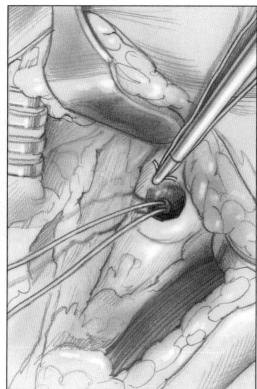

Figure 10-16. A,B: The tuberosity is excavated and two suture anchors are embedded in the tuberosity.

If a suture anchor is used, the tuberosity is excavated and two anchors are embedded in the base of the excavated bone (Fig. 10-16).

The sutures are passed through the end of the tendon and threaded proximally while the tendon is being teased distally into the prepared tuberosity bed (Fig. 10-17). The sutures are tied with the forearm in neutral rotation.

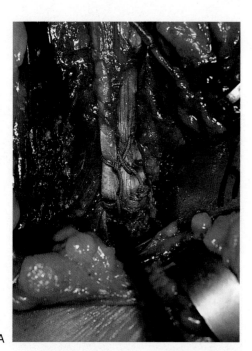

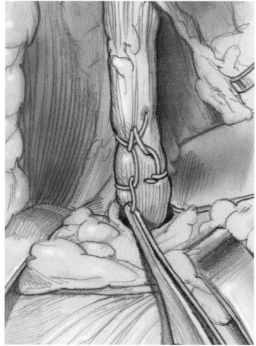

Figure 10-17. A crisscross or Krachow stitch is used to secure the tendon, which is then advanced into the tuberosity (**A,B**) as demonstrated radiographically (**C,D**). *(continued)*

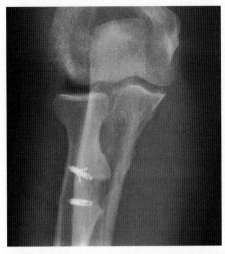
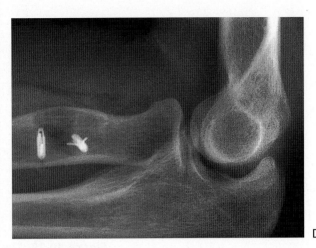

C   D

Figure 10-17. *Continued.*

DELAYED RECONSTRUCTION

When the tendon has retracted to the point that it cannot be reattached directly to the tuberosity, augmentation with an Achilles tendon allograft is our technique of choice.

Technique: Achilles Tendon Allograft

With the Achilles tendon allograft the exposure is more extensive, as the biceps muscle must be exposed (Fig. 10-18). After it is determined that the biceps tendon is inadequate for reattachment (Fig. 10-19), the tuberosity is exposed by blunt dissection and the curved hemostat identifies the site of the forearm incision (Fig. 10-20). The tuberosity is exposed and exca-

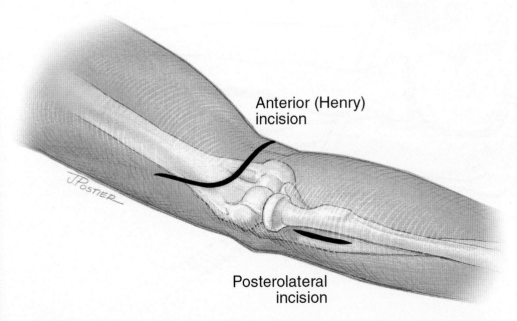

Anterior (Henry)
incision

Posterolateral
incision

Figure 10-18. The two-incision technique is used and employs a Henry-type incision in the antecubital space and a 4-cm incision over the posterolateral aspect of the proximal forearm. The anterior incision is extended as needed to expose the biceps muscle.

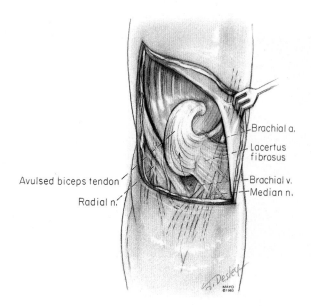

Figure 10-19. The tendon usually has recoiled and is of variable length, but the biceps stump is adequate to secure to the tendon allograft.

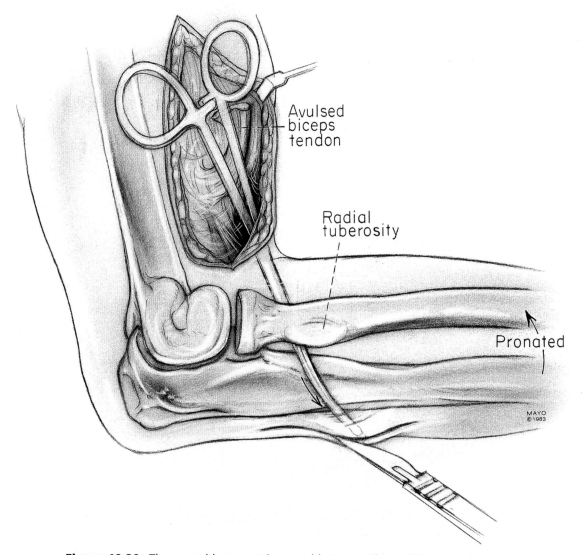

Figure 10-20. The curved hemostat is passed between the radial tuberosity and the ulna to emerge through the common extensor muscle mass and tent the skin on the proximal posterolateral aspect of the forearm.

vated as described earlier (Fig. 10-21). The calcaneal portion of the Achilles allograft composite is carefully trimmed sufficiently small to allow insertion into the tuberosity but taking care to maintain the tendon insertion to the calcaneus fleck of bone (Fig. 10-22). A No. 5 nonabsorbable suture is placed in the allograft tendon through holes in the small piece of calcaneus using a Krakow stitch. The tendon is then threaded from the anterior exposure into the forearm incision (Fig. 10-23). This is inserted into the tuberosity and secured through the holes in the tuberosity (Fig. 10-24). With the elbow at about 45 degrees of flexion the Achilles fascia is then secured around its margin to the biceps muscle, which has been retracted distally as much as possible to develop appropriate resting tension (Fig. 10-25).

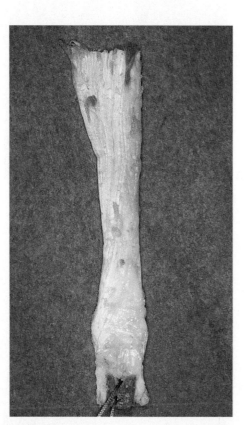

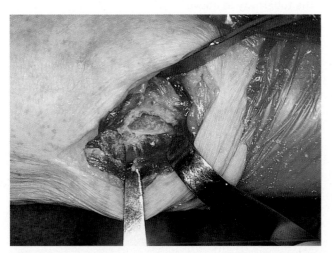

Figure 10-21. The exposure and preparation of the tuberosity are as described earlier.

Figure 10-22. The graft is prepared so the calcaneal attachment is intact and sufficiently small to fit into the prepared cavity in the tuberosity.

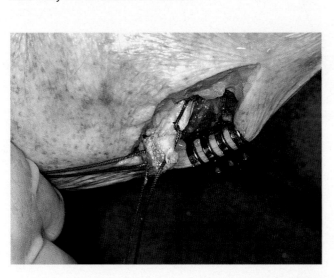

Figure 10-23. The stitch passes through a hole in the calcaneus and a Krachow stitch is used to secure the tendon.

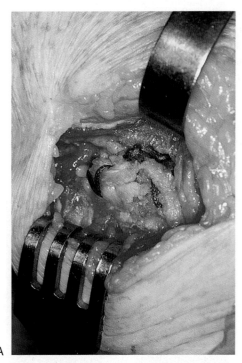

A

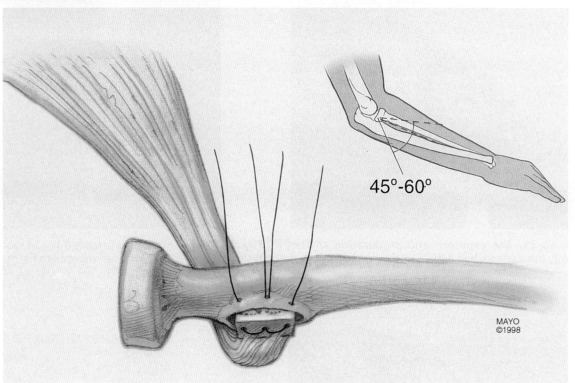

Figure 10-24. A,B: The fleck of bone is inserted into the tuberosity and secured with sutures placed through the margin of the tuberosity as above.

45°-60°

MAYO
©1998

B

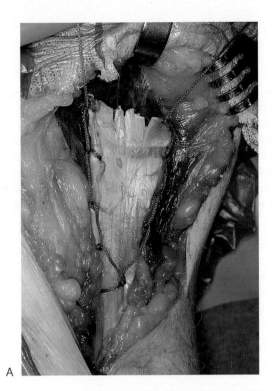

A

Figure 10-25. A,B: With the elbow at about 60 degrees of flexion, the biceps is "enveloped" with the Achilles fascia.

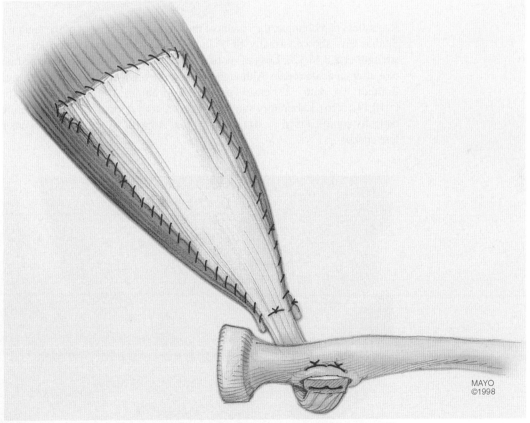

B

POSTOPERATIVE MANAGEMENT

Acute Repair

The patient is placed in a posterior splint with the elbow in 90 degrees of flexion and the forearm in neutral rotation. This is kept in place for 3 to 7 days.

At 1 week or less the posterior splint is removed and gentle passive flexion is allowed. Active extension to 30 degrees is allowed and encouraged from the first week after surgery. Full extension is allowed as tolerated and generally attained by the third week. Four weeks after surgery the patient is allowed to flex and extend against gravity as able. At 6 weeks a gentle flexion-strengthening program is allowed, starting with 1-kg weights. Activity as tolerated is permitted at 3 months. Full activity without restriction is allowed 6 months after surgery.

Allograft Reconstruction

The program is delayed somewhat when an allograft is used. The patient is placed in a CPM and protected for 3 weeks. Passive assisted motion is begun at 3 weeks and continued to 6 weeks. Full extension is avoided until the sixth week. Active motion for activities of daily living is allowed at 6 to 12 weeks. Activity as tolerated progresses from the third to the sixth month.

RESULTS

Regardless of technique, the results of immediate reattachment of the tendon are very good. Studies have shown virtually 100% improvement for restoration of flexion and supination strength (1,2,8,11,12). Loss of motion is not seen, and we have observed only one rerupture after an acute repair. Although popular, the clinical experience with suture anchors is limited. To date, 23 cases report no problem from several combined sources (5,10,14,15,16). Laboratory studies, however, not yet reported in the literature, reveal a statistically significant ($p < .01$) greater initial strength with the transosseous holes than suture anchor.

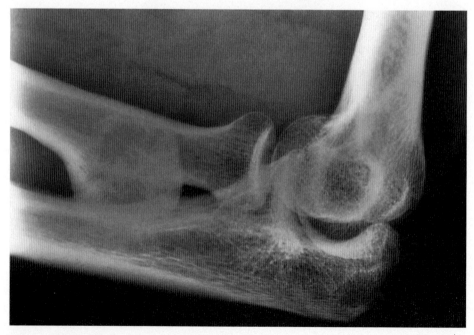

Figure 10-26. Ectopic bone bridging the proximal ulna and radius. The exposure of the radial tuberosity was across the periosteal surface of the ulna.

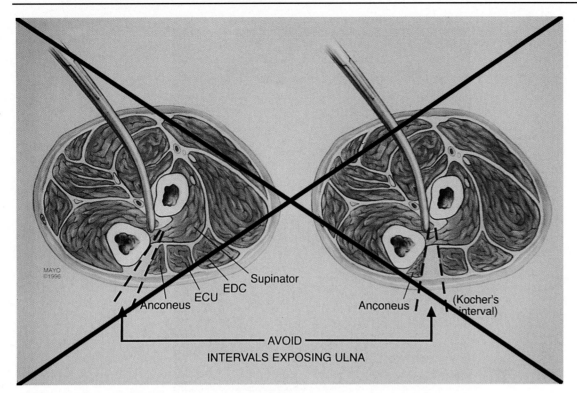

Figure 10-27. The forearm incision should **NOT** be through Kocher's interval or otherwise expose the periosteal surface of the proximal ulna.

COMPLICATIONS

Two major complications are associated with this procedure. Radial nerve injury has been reported and may be seen as often as 5% of the time after distal biceps tendon reattachment through anterior modified Henry approach (4,8). Ectopic bone is a recognized complication of the two-incision technique and bridges the proximal radius and ulna (Fig. 10-26). This, however, can be minimized or avoided by not exposing the periosteal surface of the ulna with the forearm incision (Fig. 10-27) and by splitting the muscle fibers as the tuberosity is exposed (Fig. 10-28)(6).

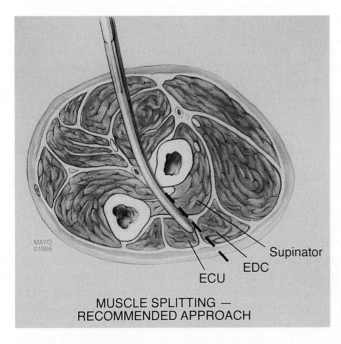

Figure 10-28. The forearm incision is a muscle-splitting approach.

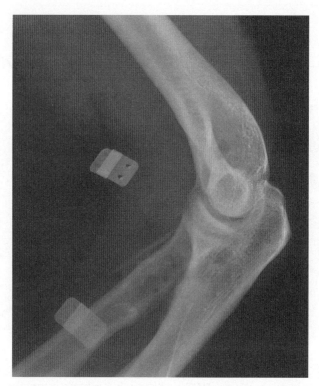

Figure 10-29. Removal of the ectopic bone restores functional forearm rotation in most patients. In this instance the tendon insertion was involved and required reattachment.

If a synostosis occurs it significantly limits function. After at least 6 months or when the radiograph demonstrates maturity, the osseous bar may be resected. The exposure is generally through the previously used forearm incision. Care should be taken during the exposure to avoid excessive retraction on the supinator muscle, which may injure the posterior interosseous nerve. Occasionally, the reattached biceps tendon itself is involved in the ectopic bone. In this instance the tendon may be released during the ectopic bone removal (Fig. 10-29) and is then reattached at the end of the excision.

MAYO EXPERIENCE

The Mayo experience with 88 procedures was recently reported by Kelly et al. Overall the satisfactory rate was over 90%. One rerupture occurred in a patient requiring wheelchair transfer. No synostosis occurred after 74 Mayo modified two-incision approaches. Of note is that the rate of complication doubles ($p < .05$) if a delay of more than 21 days occurs before surgery (9).

ILLUSTRATIVE CASE

This 55-year-old man sustained forced extension of the flexed elbow while trying to lift a freezer. He presented with obvious retraction of the distal aspect of the right dominant biceps muscle as he attempted to flex the arm (Fig. 10-30A). After discussion of the risks and benefits, a surgical procedure was undertaken and the biceps was found to have been avulsed from the radial tuberosity (Fig. 10-30B). The double Bunnell suture technique into the tuberosity through two incisions was carried out. Three weeks after the surgical procedure described earlier, he was placed in a flexion assist brace. At 6 months the patient had normal flexion (Fig. 10-30C) and extension (Fig. 10-30D). At 1 year his flexion and supination strength returned to normal.

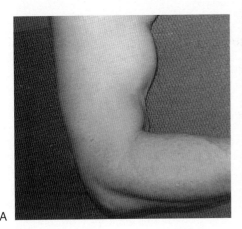

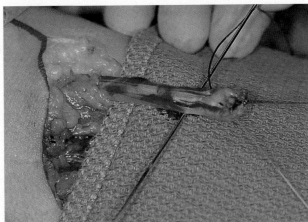

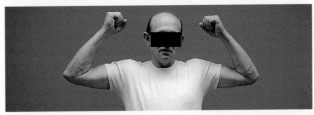

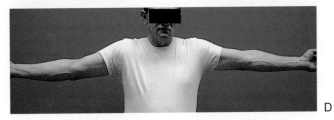

Figure 10-30. A: Proximal retraction of a ruptured distal biceps during resisted elbow flexion. **B:** The tendon is identified. The bulbous portion of the distal biceps has been trimmed, and nonabsorbable crisscross sutures have been placed. Six months after the procedure the patient has full range of flexion (**C**) and extension (**D**). His strength has returned to normal.

RECOMMENDED READINGS

1. Agins HJ, Chess JL, Hoekstra DV, et al. Rupture of the distal insertion of the biceps brachii tendon. *Clin Orthop* 1988;Sep(234):34.
2. Baker BE, Bierwagen D. Rupture of the distal tendon of the biceps brachii. *J Bone Joint Surg* 1985;67A:414.
3. Bourne MH, Morrey BF. Partial rupture of the distal biceps tendon. *Clin Orthop* 1991;Oct(271):143.
4. Boyd HB, Anderson MD. A method for reinsertion of the distal biceps brachii tendon. *J Bone Joint Surg* 1961;43A:1041.
5. Brunner F, Gelpke H, Hotz T, et al. Distal biceps tendon ruptures—experiences with soft tissue preserving reinsertion by bone anchors. *Swiss Surg* 1999;5:186–190.
6. Dobbie RP. Avulsion of the lower biceps brachii tendon: analysis of 51 previously reported cases. *Am J Surg* 1941;51:661.
7. Failla JM, Amadio PC, Morrey BF, et al. Proximal radioulnar synostosis after repair of distal biceps brachii rupture by the two-incision technique: report of four cases. *Clin Orthop* 1990;Apr(253):133.
8. Hovelius L, Josefsson G. Rupture of the distal biceps tendon. *Acta Orthop Scand* 1977;48:280.
9. Kelly E, O'Driscoll S, Morrey BF. Complications associated with distal biceps tendon reattachment. *J Bone Joint Surg* 2000;82A:1575–1581.
10. Lintner S, Fischer T. Repair of the distal biceps tendon using suture anchors and an anterior approach. *Clin Orthop* 1996;Jan(322):116–119.
11. Louis DS, Hankin FM, Eckenrode JF, et al. Distal biceps brachii tendon avulsion: a simplified method of operative repair. *Am J Sports Med* 1986;14:234.
12. Morrey BF, Askew LJ, An KN, et al. Rupture of the distal biceps tendon: biomechanical assessment of different treatment options. *J Bone Joint Surg* 1985;67A:418.
13. Norman WH. Repair of avulsion of insertion of biceps brachii tendon. *Clin Orthop* 1985;Mar(193):189.
14. Strauch RJ, Michelson H, Rosenwasser MP. Repair of rupture of the distal tendon of the biceps brachii. Review of the literature and report of three cases treated with a single anterior incision and suture anchors. *Am J Orthop* 1997;26:151–156.
15. Verhaven E, Huylebroek J, Van Nieuwenhuysen W, et al. Surgical treatment of acute biceps tendon ruptures with a suture anchor. *Acta Orthop Belgica* 1993;59:426–429.
16. Woods DA, Hoy G, Shimmin A. A safe technique for distal biceps repair using a suture anchor and a limited anterior approach. *Injury* 1999;30:233–237.

11

Triceps Tendon Repair and Reconstruction

Bernard F. Morrey

Addressing triceps insufficiency may be required in both acute and chronic settings. The treatment is different in each setting; thus the method of managing both of these conditions is presented.

INDICATIONS/CONTRAINDICATIONS

Triceps tendon repair is indicated in acute rupture when the patient has functional extension weakness, fatigue, or pain and the patient who requires extension strength. (This includes almost everybody.)

It is also indicated when a patient fails to regain extensor strength after several weeks of nonoperative management.

There are few contraindications if the patient is symptomatic and if the diagnosis has been confirmed.

If the patient is unwilling to perform rehabilitation, or ongoing or generalized enthesopathy and morbidity are present that will not be addressed by triceps reconstitution, other methods may be necessary.

In the case of reconstruction, surgery is indicated if weakness has become a major limitation of one's daily activities, if there has been no improvement over last 3 months, or if pain is rarely a major factor.

Reconstruction is contraindicated if the patient has unclear or unreasonable expectations of the reconstruction, or if he or she is unable or unwilling to participate in the postoperative program or to accept the period of postoperative recovery.

PREOPERATIVE PLANNING

The need for triceps tendon repair is often seen in body builders or middle-aged males or conversely, in debilitated states (1,6,7,9). Dominant extremity involved is only 33% in our experience (4). Approximately 80% have some residual active extension.

B.F. Morrey, M.D.: Mayo Medical School and Department of Orthopaedics, Mayo Clinic and Foundation, Rochester, Minnesota.

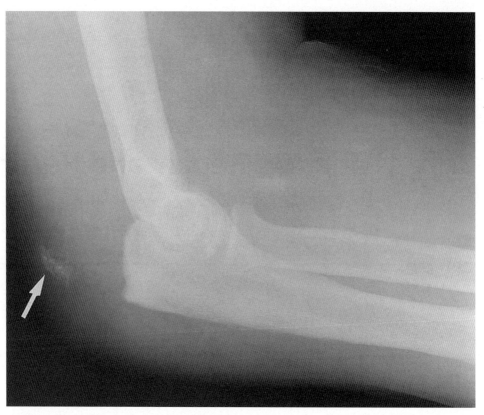

Figure 11-1. A radiograph with bone fleck signifying triceps avulsion is a helpful but uncommon finding.

Palpable central defect is present in about 67%. Some weakness is present in all, but complete loss of extension is observed in less than 20% if untreated. Acute avulsion with fleck of bone is seen in only about 15% (3,4). Pain subsides after 10 to 14 days, leaving residual weakness and fatigue pain as the major findings.

Observe for osseous fleck in the lateral radiograph (Fig. 11-1). An MR examination is not usually required to make the diagnosis. There may be some merit in localizing the disruption, which is usually at the site of attachment of the central slip (11). The defect is palpable in about two-thirds of cases.

Carefully assess the defect. Palpate the anconeus muscle as the patient extends against resistance. Usually, the anconeus expansion is intact, so some extension is possible. This is an important determination, as the muscle may be used for rotational reconstruction in chronic cases.

SURGERY

Acute Repair

The patient is placed supine on the operating table. The arm is prepped and draped but the tourniquet is not inflated. A straight posterior skin incision is made and centered just medial to the tip of the olecranon (Fig. 11-2). The dissection carries through the triceps fascia and the defect is identified. In most instances, the avulsion is from the central attachment to the olecranon. Cruciate drill holes are placed in the proximal ulna (Fig. 11-3). A No. 5 Mersilene suture is introduced from distal to proximal. The triceps disruption is mobilized and penetrated laterally by the suture. A Krachow type of stitch is then placed with three to four passes on each side of the triceps midtendinous locking region. The suture is then brought back through the opposite cruciate hole (Fig. 11-4). This results in a very firm and

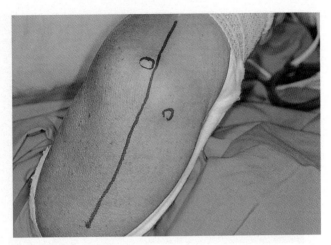

Figure 11-2. Midline incision showing tip of olecranon and medial epicondyle.

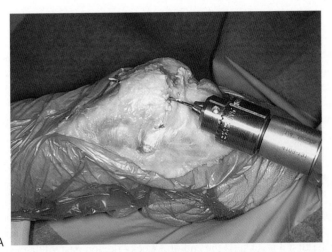

A

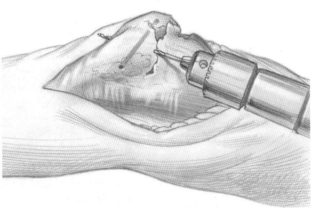

B

Figure 11-3. A,B: Cruciate drill holes are placed in the olecranon.

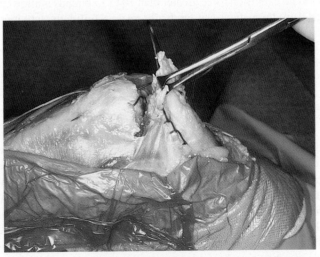

A

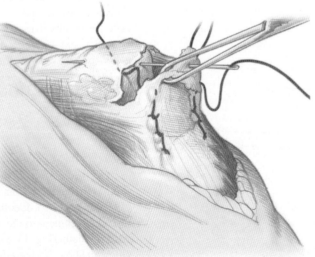

B

Figure 11-4. A,B: A Krachow stitch secures the tendon as the suture is being brought back across the olecranon. *Note:* The tissue is handled with an Allis clamp to avoid crush injury.

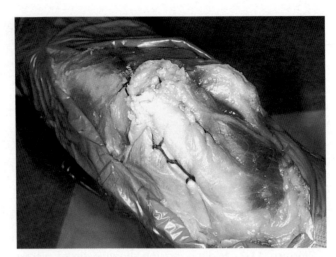

Figure 11-5. The completed repair is quite secure. Care is taken to tie the knot off the subcutaneous border to avoid irritation.

adequate repair, but a second transverse suture may be placed if there is any question about the security of the attachment. The precise site of disruption is roughened with a rongeur to enhance healing. Sutures are tied at the margin of the subcutaneous border of the ulna with the elbow in approximately 45 degrees of extension (Fig. 11-5).

The arm is elevated and an anterior splint is applied with the elbow in approximately 40 degrees of flexion.

POSTOPERATIVE MANAGEMENT

The elbow is placed in a posterior splint after the first or second day. This is maintained for approximately 4 or 5 days, after which gentle passive assisted motion is allowed. Flexion is limited to 90 degrees for the first 3 weeks. At the end of 3 weeks flexion past 90 degrees is encouraged and allowed by active assist. Passively assisted extension occurs with gravity and with the opposite extremity. At 4 to 6 weeks active flexion and extension are allowed but no forced extension is permitted for an additional 4 weeks. At 10 weeks routine daily activities are permitted but no extension force greater than 10 to 15 pounds is allowed. After 3 months if there is no pain, the patient can gradually resume full daily activities. Over the next 3 months, full extension strength is allowed.

RECONSTRUCTION

SURGERY

The prepping, draping, and initial skin incision for anconeus rotational reconstruction are as described earlier. If the residual tendon is contracted and cannot be advanced to bone (Fig. 11-6) but the anconeus is present, Kocher's interval is entered and the anconeus is mobilized (Fig. 11-7). Ideally, the translocated muscle is left intact distally and the proximal fascial attachment to the triceps is preserved. The muscle is elevated from the ulna and rotated medially (Fig. 11-8). The proximal ulna is prepared with cruciate drill holes. With the elbow in about 30 degrees of flexion, a No. 5 nonabsorbable suture is used to secure the rotated anconeus/triceps mechanism. Additional sutures are placed as necessary and the original defect is closed if possible (Fig. 11-9).

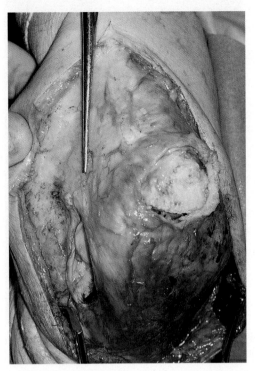

Figure 11-6. Large defect at the central attachment of the triceps in patient with total elbow arthroplasty.

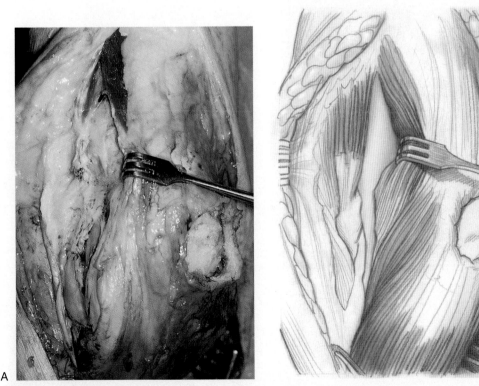

A   B

Figure 11-7. A,B: The anconeus is identified and separated from the extensor carpi ulnaris in Kocher's interval.

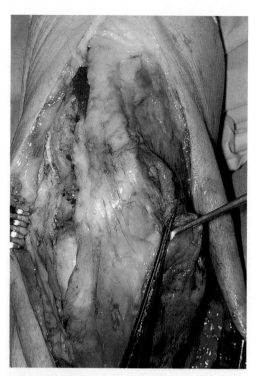

Figure 11-8. The anconeus is mobilized to cover the proximal ulna, leaving its distal attachment intact.

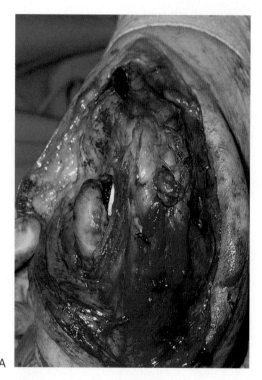

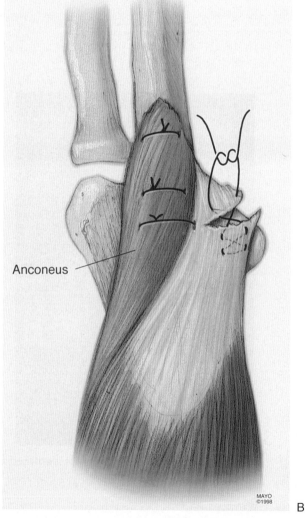

Anconeus

Figure 11-9. A,B: The anconeus is sutured with a crisscross stitch into bone. The defect is sewn to itself.

Achilles Tendon Allograft

If the defect is massive, the anconeus is inadequate, or the attachment to the triceps has been violated, an Achilles tendon allograft reconstruction is employed (Fig. 11-10). In this setting a chevron cut is made in the tip of the olecranon (Fig. 11-11). The calcaneal attachment of the Achilles tendon is then fashioned with the same angle (Fig. 11-12). Care is taken to dissect the tendon sufficiently to identify its precise insertion site on the calcaneus so the chevron cut in the calcaneus is precisely positioned. The calcaneus from the Achilles allograft is then fit within the V-shaped bed of the olecranon. Once the proper position has been obtained, it is secured with a single AO cancellous screw (Fig. 11-13). An additional suture is placed with a transverse drill placed through the proximal ulna, and a Krachow stitch is employed to further stabilize the tendon allograft to the host olecranon. After the distal at-

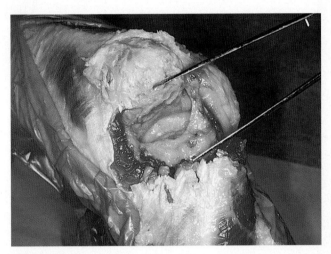

Figure 11-10. Large defect in the triceps does not allow direct repair to bone. Violation of the anconeus attachment precludes anconeus rotation as a solution.

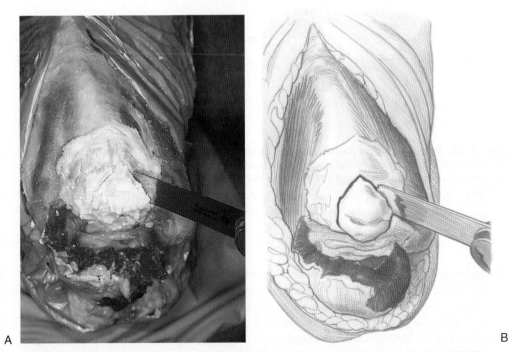

A   B

Figure 11-11. A,B: A chevron cut is made in the olecranon to receive the Achilles graft.

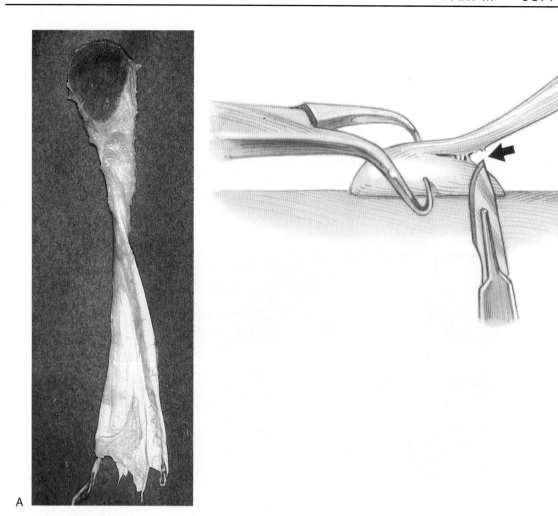

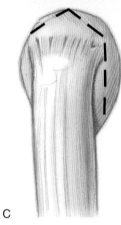

Figure 11-12. Achilles tendon allograft with calcaneus attached (**A**). Preparation for attachment to olecranon requires dissection so attachment is approximately the length of the resected olecranon (**B**). The chevron cut in the calcaneus matches that of the olecranon (**C**).

tachment has been secured, the triceps is mobilized as far distally as possible according to the dictates of the pathology. The central portion of the triceps, which contains the triceps tendon, is secured with a Krachow stitch, and the triceps is then attached to the tendon graft as far distally as possible with the elbow in about 30 degrees of extension (Fig. 11-14). Once this has been secured, the remainder of the Achilles graft is used to envelope the triceps musculature (Fig. 11-15). An absorbable No. O suture is used as a running stitch to secure the allograft over the triceps musculature.

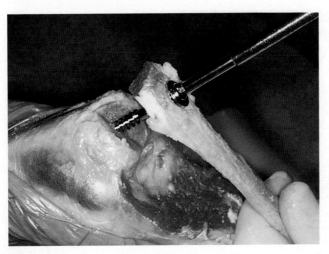

Figure 11-13. Calcaneus from the graft being secured with AO screw to the olecranon.

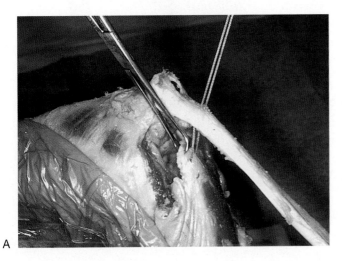

A

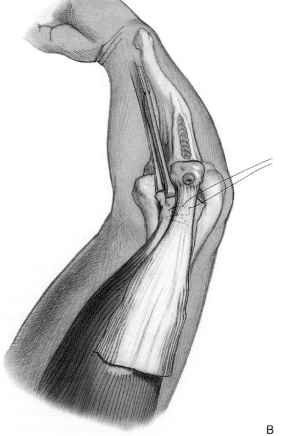

B

Figure 11-14. A,B: The triceps is mobilized and securely attached to the allograft with a No. 5 nonabsorbable suture and tied at about 30 degrees of flexion.

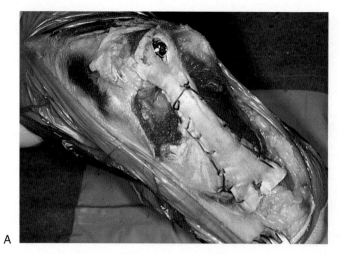

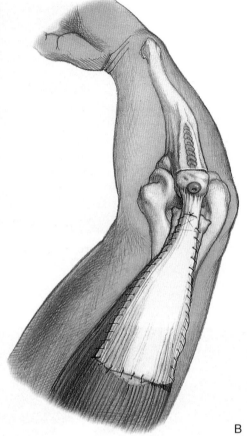

Figure 11-15. A,B: The triceps is enveloped with the remainder of the Achilles graft.

B

POSTOPERATIVE MANAGEMENT

Postoperative management is similar to that for the acute fracture.

RESULTS

There are few detailed results regarding surgical intervention for triceps deficiency. Most communiqués are case reports. If the avulsion includes a portion of bone, the AO tension band method of fixation generally allows virtually normal function (1,2,5,8,10).

We have recently reviewed the experience with 16 procedures. An acute repair was carried out in eight and a reconstructive procedure was done in the other eight (4). Of those repaired, strength returned to within an average of 90% of "normal" of the opposite extremity. In those with a reconstruction the mean strength recovery was about 85% of normal. Subjectively, all eight repairs and seven of eight reconstructions were satisfied with their outcome, and one had mild pain. Four of eight were noted as excellent results in the acute and two of eight were noted as excellent results in the reconstruction. The time to recovery was somewhat prolonged, however, averaging more than 6 months, with some reconstructions still demonstrating improvement a year after surgery.

COMPLICATIONS

In the Mayo experience with 16 procedures, one patient had a transient ulnar nerve palsy, one patient developed a rerupture, and one patient had persistent weakness and discomfort.

Note: These patients take a longer period for return of function than those with biceps tendon repair. In our experience, rarely is significant strength improvement noted before 6 months, and improvement continues for up to 1 year.

ILLUSTRATIVE CASE

A 38-year-old female developed a defect of the central attachment of the triceps to the olecranon after open reduction with internal fixation for a type II olecranon fracture treated by tension band wiring. The triceps tissue was scarred and contracted, not allowing direct suture repair (Fig. 11-16). Because the anconeus was intact, the extensor mechanism was re-

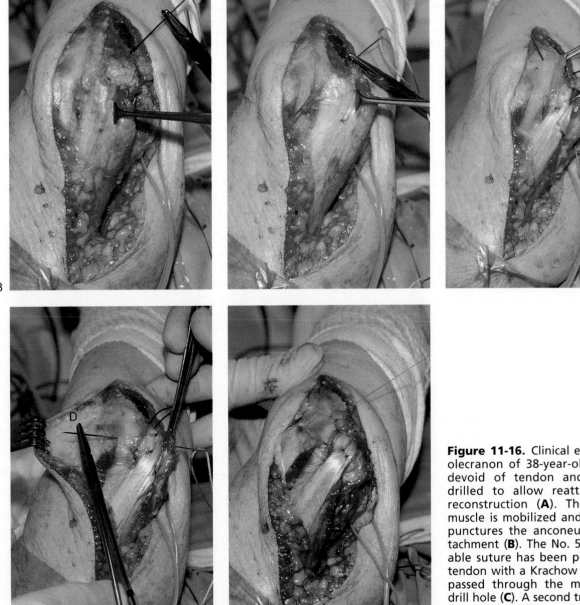

, B

C

D

, E

Figure 11-16. Clinical example. The olecranon of 38-year-old female is devoid of tendon and has been drilled to allow reattachment in reconstruction (**A**). The anconeus muscle is mobilized and the needle punctures the anconeus/triceps attachment (**B**). The No. 5 nonabsorbable suture has been placed in the tendon with a Krachow stitch and is passed through the midolecranon drill hole (**C**). A second transverse suture is placed (**D**). The repair was secure with restored continuity of the triceps mechanism (**E**).

constructed with an anconeus rotational flap. The reconstruction allowed excellent restoration of the triceps mechanism. The quality of the tissue and repair is well demonstrated in the illustration.

RECOMMENDED READINGS

1. Bach BR, Warren RF. Triceps rupture: a case report and literature review. *Am J Sports Med* 1987;15:285–289.
2. Clayton ML, Thirupathi RG. Rupture of the triceps tendon with olecranon bursitis: a case report with a new method of repair. *Clin Orthop* 1984;184:183–185.
3. Farrar EL, Lippert FG. Avulsion of the triceps tendon. *Clin Orthop* 1981;161:242–246.
4. Ho E, Morrey BF. Repair and reconstruction for triceps deficiency. Orlando, FL: AAOS, February 2000.
5. Inhofe PD, Moneim MS. Late presentation of triceps rupture: a case report and review of the literature. *Am J Orthop* 1996;25:790–792.
6. Louis DS, Peck, D. Triceps avulsion fracture in a weightlifter. *Orthopedics* 1992;15:207–208.
7. O'Driscoll SW. Intramuscular triceps rupture. *Can J Surg* 1992;35:203–207.
8. Pantazopoulos TH, Exarchou E, Stavrou Z, et al. Avulsion of the triceps tendon. *J Trauma* 1975;15:827–829.
9. Sherman OH, Snyder SJ, Fox JM. Triceps tendon avulsion in a professional body builder. *Am J Sports Med* 1984;12:328–329.
10. Tarnsey FF. Rupture and avulsion of the triceps. *Clin Orthop* 1972;83:177–183.
11. Zionts LE, Vachon LA. Demonstration of avulsion of the triceps tendon in an adolescent by magnetic resonance imaging. *Am J Orthop* 1997;26:489–490.

12

Lateral Epicondylitis (Tendinosis)

Robert P. Nirschl

Epicondylitis (tendinosis) occurs at least five times more commonly on the lateral than on the medial aspect of the joint. The selection factors to determine the candidates for surgery are similar for each process, yet there are some distinct features with regard to the surgical technique. Thus medial epicondylitis is discussed separately in Chapter 13.

INDICATIONS/CONTRAINDICATIONS

Pain is the major indication for surgery of lateral epicondylitis. There are three broad indications and a fourth feature to consider (7).

1. Pain is of significant intensity as to limit function and interferes with daily activity or occupation.
2. Localization is precisely at the lateral epicondyle and origin of the ECRB and EDC to the epicondyle.
3. A legitimate period of nonoperative management has been attempted. This typically includes at least 6 months of activity modification, forearm band, antiinflammatory agents, and a quality rehabilitation program;
4. Failure of cortisone injections is no longer considered an absolute necessity before offering surgical intervention. However, if injections have been used and the patient is no longer benefiting or has not benefited from them, then the patient is a candidate for a surgical procedure.

The contraindications to surgical intervention include an inadequate nonoperative program (10) and patients who have demonstrated lack of compliance with the recommendations, particularly that of activity modification. Individuals on worker's compensation disability should be assessed on several occasions to ensure that the preceding indications have been met.

R.P. Nirschl, M.D.: Director Nirschl Orthopedic Sports Medicine Clinic/Virginia Hospital Center Sports Medicine Fellowship Program, Arlington, Virginia. Associate Clinical Professor, Georgetown University Medical School Washington, D.C.

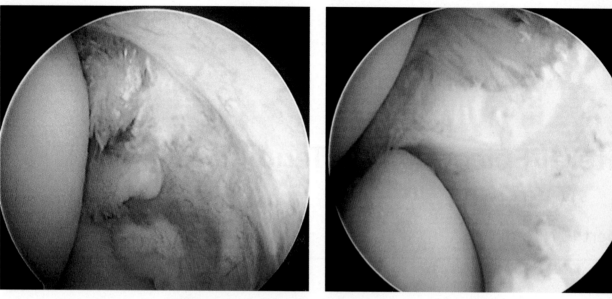

Figure 12-1. Arthroscopic identification of intraarticular pathology (**A**) was treated arthroscopically with relief of lateral epicondylitis symptoms (**B**).

PREOPERATIVE PLANNING

Physical findings include local tenderness to palpation over the tendon origin at the epicondyle. Provocative tests of pain with resisted wrist extension for lateral involvement are invariably positive, especially with the elbow in full extension (5). In some cases the symptoms may be aggravated by performing the test in elbow extension. If forearm pain is a component, examine for posterior interosseous nerve irritation. The most sensitive is pain on resistive supination (13).

The most commonly involved tissue, the pathologic process, and the principles of the surgical intervention should be reviewed before undertaking the surgical procedure (7,8,9,11).

The hallmarks of good surgical concept and technique include precise identification of the pathologic tissue, resection of all involved pathology, maintenance of normal tissue attachments, protection of normal tissue, enhancement of vascular supply, firm repair of the operative site, and quality postoperative rehabilitation.

The extensor carpi radialis brevis (100%) and the extensor communis (anterior edge) are the tissues most commonly involved laterally (100% and 35%, respectively) (1,2,3,4,9). Histologically, the pathologic tissue is devoid of inflammatory cells but has a characteristic pattern of fibroblasts and vascular elements (6,12). Recent electron microscopic evidence reveals lack of extracellular cross-linkage (6). Furthermore, approximately 20% of surgical cases have been noted to have some form of bony exostosis at the lateral epicondyle. Less common pathologic changes include calcification in the soft-tissue elements (extensor communis and radial collateral ligament). Intraarticular changes, including synovitis and orbicular ligament abnormality, are being recognized with increasing frequency with the advent of elbow arthroscopy as a therapeutic tool (Fig. 12-1).

SURGERY

Lateral Epicondylitis

The described technique and illustrations apply for the large majority of cases. It should be noted, however, that individual variations can and do occur. In these instances, the pathologic variations should be addressed as identified.

Arthroscopy

The data on arthroscopic debridement are incomplete at this time to draw a conclusion or to recommend this treatment. The topic is addressed in Chapter 2.

Technique

After anesthesia (general or arm block), the arm is draped free with a nonsterile tourniquet and placed on an arm board.

The incision extends from 1 to 2 cm proximal and just anteromedial to the lateral epicondyle just to the level of the joint (i.e., 1 cm distal to the epicondyle) (Fig. 12-3). The sub-

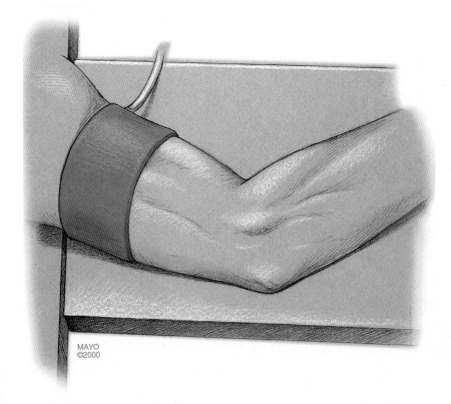

MAYO
©2000

Figure 12-2. All illustrations are of a right elbow. The arm was draped with a nonsterile tourniquet and placed on an arm board.

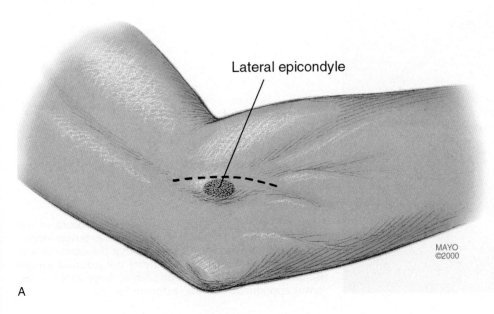

Lateral epicondyle

MAYO
©2000

A

Figure 12-3. The skin incision extends from 1 to 2 cm proximal and just anterior to the lateral epicondyle distally 1 cm just to the level of the elbow joint (**A**). *(continued)*

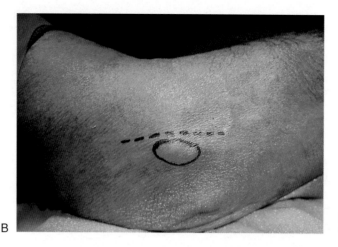

B

Figure 12-3. *Continued.* Circled area identifies lateral epicondyle (**B**).

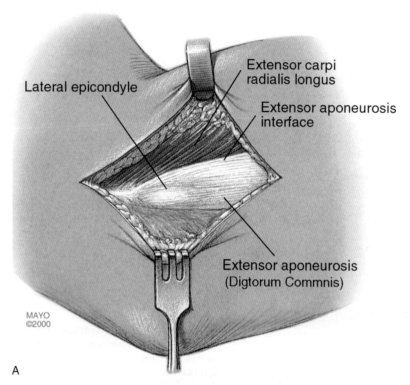

Lateral epicondyle

Extensor carpi radialis longus

Extensor aponeurosis interface

Extensor aponeurosis (Digtorum Commnis)

MAYO
©2000

A

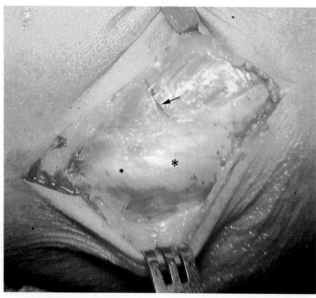

B

Figure 12-4. Identification of tendons. Exposure of the lateral epicondyle and interface between extensor longus and extensor aponeurosis (**A**). Note that the extensor brevis is not visible as it is hidden under the extensor longus (**B**). *Small asterisk,* lateral epicondyle; *large asterisk,* extensor aponeurosis; *arrow,* extensor longus.

cutaneous tissue and superficial fascia are incised and retracted, locating the interface between the extensor longus muscle and the firm anterior edge of the extensor aponeurosis. A palpable crevice is present at this interface as the fascia over the extensor longus is thin and the anterior edge of the aponeurosis is firm and thick (Fig. 12-4). A splitting incision 2 to 3 mm in depth is made between the extensor longus and the extensor aponeurosis in the identified interface extending from 1 to 2 cm proximal to the lateral epicondyle distally to the level of the joint line. The extensor longus is released by scalpel dissection and retracted anteromedially to 2 to 3 cm. This retraction brings the extensor brevis into direct view (Fig. 12-5).

Technical note: A common error in the incision at the extensor longus interface is to penetrate too deeply by vertical dissection. As noted, the extensor longus is only 2 to 3 mm thick at this level. Once the 2- to 3-mm depth is reached, the dissection is primarily horizontal progressing medially. This technical subtlety is important to avoid iatrogenic distortion as well as to bypass the body of the extensor brevis tendon. Such iatrogenic distortion can easily complicate the identification of the pathologic regions.

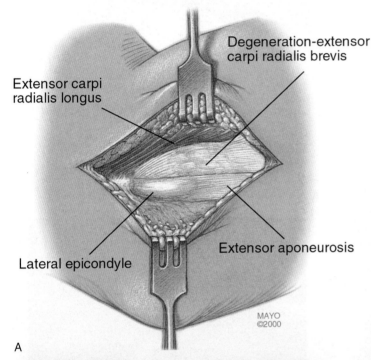

A

Figure 12-5. An incision in the extensor longus/extensor aponeurosis interface with anteromedial retraction of extensor longus exposes the pathologic origin of the extensor brevis (**A**). A key technical point is not to incise too deeply but more medially as the extensor longus is only 2 to 3 mm in depth at this level. Variations in pathoanatomic damage include degeneration of the extensor brevis origin (**B**) and a full avulsion rupture of the extensor brevis origin, as shown in a world-class tennis player (**C**). *Small asterisk*, lateral epicondyle; *large asterisk*, extensor aponeurosis; *double asterisks*, extensor longus; *arrow*, brevis tendinosis.

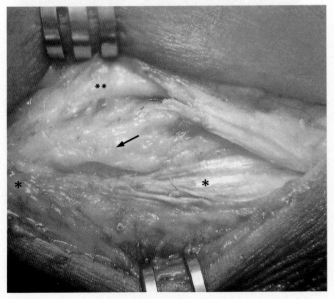

B

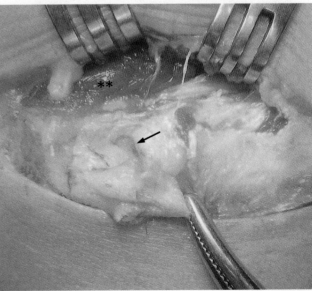

C

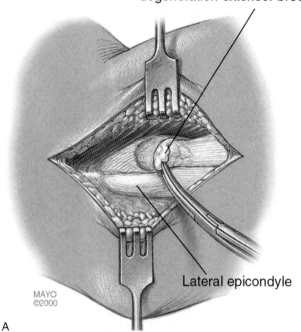

Removal, angio-fibroblastic
degeneration extensor brevis

Lateral epicondyle

MAYO
©2000

A

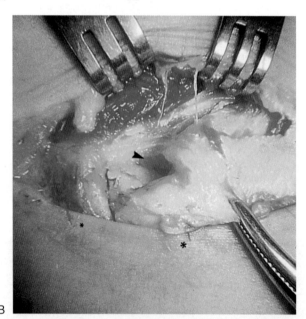

B

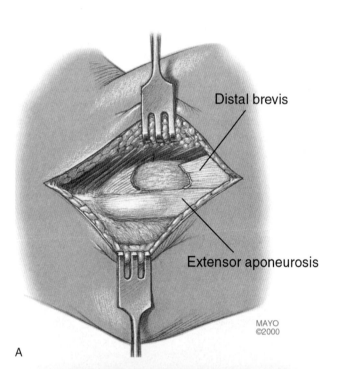

Distal brevis

Extensor aponeurosis

MAYO
©2000

A

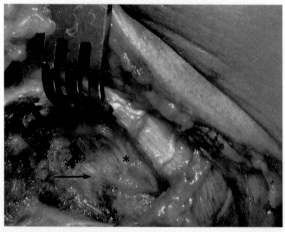

B

Figure 12-6. Resection of pathologic tissue. Resection of pathologic sections (histologically termed *angiofibroblastic tendinosis*) of extensor brevis origin. In this rendering, 100% of the origin is involved and a partial rupture is depicted (**A**). In no circumstance is the extensor aponeurosis totally released from the epicondyle. Surgical photograph of resection of pathologic extensor brevis origin (**B**) shows major tendinosis with an underside rupture. Note a small strip of normal tendon at the edge of the extensor longus muscle. The remaining pathologic alteration has a dull-grayish edematous gross appearance typical of angiofibroblastic tendinosis. (*Small asterisk,* lateral epicondyle; below skin; *large asterisk,* extensor aponeurosis; *arrow,* tear.)

Figure 12-7. Completed resection of pathologic tissue. Resected pathologic section of the entire extensor brevis tendon (**A**). Surgical photograph depicting completed resection of the degenerated extensor brevis origin (**B**). *Arrow,* defect left after brevis resection; *asterisk,* healthy fascia over retracted longus.

With proper case selection and appropriate exposure, the entire origin of the extensor brevis will be easily identified. The gross appearance of the pathologic change is dull-grayish tissue, often edematous and friable, and, on occasion, ruptured (Fig. 12-5). Normal tissue in contrast is shiny, is firm, and has a slightly yellowish-white hue. The pathologic tissue often encompasses the entire origin of the extensor brevis, and in our series the anterior 10% edge of the extensor aponeurosis is abnormal in approximately 35% of cases.

Excision of all pathologic tissue in the extensor brevis origin is performed en bloc. This tissue block is somewhat triangular in shape with the base distal (Fig. 12-6). The typical size of tissue is 2 × 1 cm (Fig. 12-6). It should be noted that the brevis origin is released from the lateral epicondyle and the anterior edge of the extensor aponeurosis. If the anterior aponeurosis has pathologic alteration, the pathologic tissue is also removed (but not normal tendon).

Pathologic tissue is easily identified by its visual appearance and confirmed by the "Nirschl scratch test." This makes use of the friability of pathologic tissue, which easily peels off by utilizing a scratching motion with the scalpel. When healthy tissue is reached, it no longer peels off with the scratching motion. This technique is especially helpful when removing the pathologic changes in the anterior edge of the aponeurosis.

In the 20% of cases that present with an exostosis or prominence of the lateral epicondyle, the proximal edge of the aponeurosis is temporarily peeled off the epicondyle for adequate exposure and the exostosis is removed by rongeur and smoothed by a rasp.

Once the pathologic tissue is adequately resected, a defect is present in the prior area of the extensor brevis tendon origin. The more distal aspect of the extensor brevis is still attached to the orbicular ligament, distal anterior aponeurosis, and underside of the extensor longus (Fig. 12-7). The brevis therefore does not retract distally to any appreciable degree, thereby maintaining an essentially normal working length of the entire extensor brevis muscle-tendon unit (i.e., from elbow to wrist). If a segment of the anterior edge of the extensor aponeurosis or a bone exostosis is present on the lateral epicondyle, these abnormalities are resected at this time. Firm repair of the aponeurosis is always undertaken in these circumstances. The goal of the operation is resection of all pathologic tissue, not tendon release.

A small synovial opening may be made at this time to inspect the anterolateral joint compartment. Unless the patient presents with clear intraarticular signs and symptoms preoperatively, it is uncommon to find meaningful intraarticular changes.

To enhance vascular supply, two to three 5/64-inch holes are drilled through cortical bone in the resected area. This technique is theorized to encourage rapid replacement of this triangular tissue void with healthy fibrotendinous tissue (Fig. 12-8).

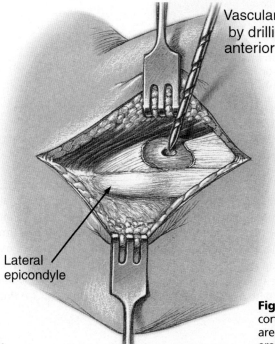

Vascular enhancement
by drilling
anterior lateral condyle

Lateral
epicondyle

A

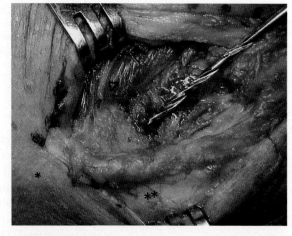

B

Figure 12-8. A,B: Enhancement of revascularization by cortical drilling. The cortical bone is drilled with a 5/64-inch bit to enhance revascularization of the area. (*Asterisk,* lateral epicondyle.) Note: do not drill the tip area of the lateral epicondyle as bony disturbance here causes increased post-op pain.

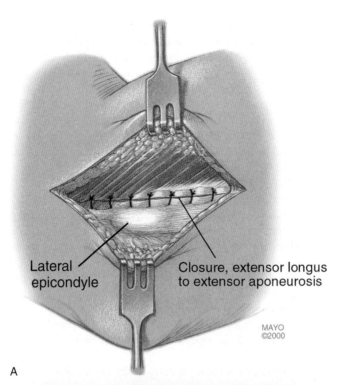

Lateral
epicondyle

Closure, extensor longus
to extensor aponeurosis

MAYO
©2000

A

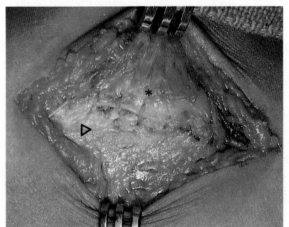

B

Figure 12-9. A,B: Repair of tendon interface. In all cases the interface between the extensor longus and the extensor aponeurosis is firmly closed. It is theorized that blood clot transformed to biologically healthy fibrous tissue (painless) replaces the proximal defect of the resected brevis area further reinforcing the security of the ultimate brevis origin. *Arrow,* lateral epicondyle; *asterisk,* extensor longus.

The interface between the posterior edge of the extensor longus and the remaining anterior edge of the extensor aponeurosis is now firmly closed (Fig. 12-9). I use a simple running stitch of No. 1 PDS. It is unnecessary to suture the distal extensor brevis since a firm attachment is retained to the orbicular ligament, distal aponeurosis, and underside of extensor longus distally. The extensor aponeurosis is firmly repaired anteriorly, and its proximal attachment is largely undisturbed; thus rapid mobilization postoperatively is possible and encouraged. The skin is closed with 3-0 subcutaneous cat gut, subcuticular 3-0 Prolene and supporting Steri-strips.

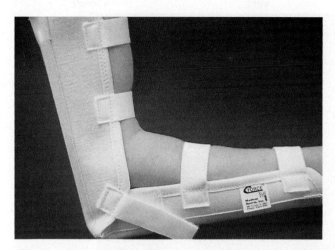

Figure 12-10. Light elbow immobilizer with Velcro straps provides comfortable support in the immediate postoperative period. Motion exercises are usually started 48 hours postoperative but intermittent immobilizer protection is usually maintained for 5 to 6 days. (Courtesy of Medical Sports, Inc., Arlington, VA.)

POSTOPERATIVE MANAGEMENT

The arm is placed in an elbow immobilizer with four Velcro straps (Fig. 12-10). The joint is at 90 degrees flexion, the forearm is in neutral, and the wrist and hand are free. I use full immobilization for 2 days. Motion exercises are usually started within 48 hours following surgery (tendon and/or tendon with nerve surgery when combined medial and lateral surgery is done).

Intermittent immobilizer protection is usually maintained for 5 to 6 days, at which time normal activities of daily living are resumed. Counterforce support (forearm band) providing protective function is utilized thereafter until full forearm strength returns (usually 3 to 6 months). The brace is used at times of forearm and shoulder rehabilitation exercise and more vigorous forearm activities such as heavier household activities. A gradual return to sports such as tennis and golf often is initiated at 8 to 10 weeks with brace protection.

RESULTS

After lateral surgery, approximately 85% to 90% of patients may be anticipated to expect full return of all prior activities (1,2,9). In the remainder, improvement is usually seen, but not adequate to allow the person to return to all sport activity levels. In less than 5% no improvement is observed, and in rare instances the patient's condition has deteriorated. Thus less than 5% of patients are considered failures.

COMPLICATIONS

The most frequent complication after surgery for tennis elbow is residual pain of varying degrees. This is not common in our experience and occurs in fewer than 10% of patients. When pain after surgery is present, a logical analysis is conducted and the following determinations must be considered (7,11):

1. Has there been sufficient time and/or proper rehabilitation to allow adequate healing?
2. Did the proper diagnosis exist before the surgical intervention?

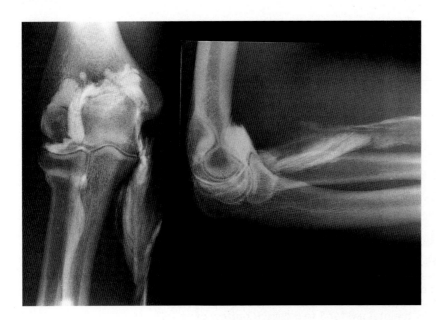

Figure 12-11. Arthrogram reveals extravasation of contrast material in forearm musculature after ill advised tennis elbow surgery technique.

3. Did something occur at the time of surgery to cause iatrogenic symptoms.
4. Was the true patho-anatomy adequately addressed?

An inadequate surgical excision leaving behind some of the pathologic tendinosis tissue is implicated most commonly as the cause of failure. In this case, a second surgical procedure should be considered (7,11). Worker's compensation may affect an individual's motivation and should be considered during the rehabilitation phase.

An aggressive release of the common tendon from the lateral or medial epicondyle can result in a release of the collateral ligament and resulting joint instability (7,11). Occasionally, instability is manifested as residual pain and not as laxity. This is diagnosed by stress view radiographs and occasionally by an arthrogram (Fig. 12-11). The treatment is collateral ligament repair or reconstruction.

ILLUSTRATIVE CASE

A world-class tennis player had lateral epicondylitis for 6 months. She had not responded to activity modification and counterforce bracing. At surgery a complete rupture of the de-

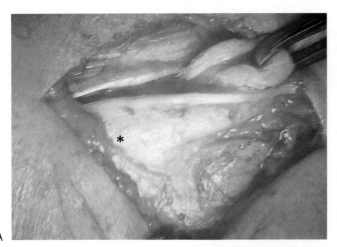

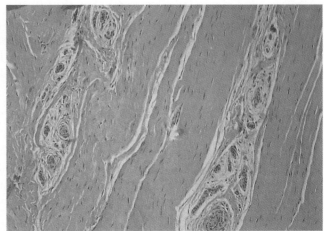

Figure 12-12. Complete rupture of brevis tendon in a professional tennis player (**A**). Histologic examination confirmed this to be a degenerative, rather than inflammatory, process (**B**). *Asterisk,* lateral epicondyle.

generated brevis origin was identified and resected (Fig. 12-12). Effectiveness was slightly altered but good enough to reach the quarter-finals of the U.S. Open 9 months after surgery and to achieve a ranking thereafter in the world's top 10.

RECOMMENDED READINGS

1. Boyd HB, McLeod AC. Tennis elbow. *J Bone Joint Surg* 1973;55A:1183.
2. Coonrad RW, Hooper WR. Tennis elbow: its course, natural history, conservative and surgical management. *J Bone Joint Surg* 1973;55A:1177.
3. Cryiax JH. The pathology and treatment of tennis elbow. *J Bone Joint Surg* 1936;18:921.
4. Goldie I. Epicondylitis lateralis humeri (epicondylalgia or tennis elbow): a pathogenetical study. *Acta Chir Scand Suppl* 1964;339.
5. Kraushaar BS, Nirschl RP. Pearls: handshake lends epicondylitis cures. *Phys Sportsmed* 1996;24:15.
6. Kraushaar B., Nirschl R.: Tendinosis of the Elbow (Tennis Elbow) Clinical Features and Findings of Histological Immunohostochemical and Electron Microscopy Studies, *J Bone Joint Surg* Vol. 81-A (2)1999:259–278.
7. Morrey BF. Reoperation for failed surgical treatment of refractory lateral epicondylitis. *J Shoulder Elbow Surg* 1992;1:47–55.
8. Nirschl RP. Sports and overuse injuries to the elbow. Muscle and tendon trauma; medial and lateral tennis elbow. In: Morrey BF, ed. *The elbow and its disorders,* 3rd ed. Philadelphia: WB Saunders; 2000.
9. Nirschl RP, Pettrone F. Tennis elbow: the surgical treatment of lateral epicondylitis. *J Bone Joint Surg* 1979;61A:832.
10. Nirschl RP, Sobel J. Conservative treatment of tennis elbow. *Phys Sports Med* 1981;9:42.
11. Organ S., Nirschl R., Kraushaar B., Guidi E.: Salvage Surgery for Lateral Tennis Elbow. *Am J Sports Med* 1997;25:746–750.
12. Regan W, Wold LE, Coonrad R, Morrey BF. Microscopic histopathology of lateral epicondylitis. *Am J Sports Med* 1992;20:746–749.
13. Werner CO. Lateral elbow pain and posterior interosseous nerve entrapment. *Acta Orthop Scand Suppl* 1979;174:1.

13

Medial Epicondylitis

Gerard T. Gabel and Robert P. Nirschl

Medial epicondylitis is a consequence of acute or chronic loads applied to the flexor pronator mass of the forearm resulting in activity-related medial and elbow proximal forearm pain (6). It is approximately one-fourth as common as lateral epicondylitis and has a similar demographic profile. The concomitant presence of ulnar neuropathy at the elbow is seen in 30% to 50% of patients and may be the primary management concern (3,5,9). Physical examination reveals direct epicondylar tenderness and indirect tenderness with resisted pronation. Ulnar nerve examination may demonstrate a positive Tinel's sign, elbow flexion test, or nerve compression test. Valgus stress examination is essential to assess medial instability either as an associated concern or as the primary process. Subluxation of the medial head of the triceps and medial antebrachial cutaneous neuropathy should be ruled out as well (1,7).

Plain radiographs are required to evaluate additional diagnoses, most commonly degenerative arthritis (which may require diagnostic xylocaine injection of the elbow to differentiate an intraarticular or extraarticular source of symptoms). Valgus stress radiographs should be obtained if indicated. Magnetic resonance imaging is usually not required, as this is primarily a clinical diagnosis.

Medial epicondylitis is classified with a combined epicondylitis and ulnar neuropathy classification system (3). To simplify the original classification, type I is an isolated medial epicondylitis and type II is medial epicondylitis with an associated ulnar neuropathy. This may be further classified as of minimal or moderate severity.

The initial management of type I medial epicondylitis is similar to that of lateral epicondylitis, including corticosteroid injection, counterforce bracing, wrist splinting, and a conditioning program. Injections should be placed at the anterior aspect of the epicondyle with the elbow in extension to avoid the ulnar nerve (8) as well as the anterior oblique fragment. Instances of type I medial epicondylitis that fail to respond to nonoperative management and all type II medial epicondylitis are indications for surgical intervention.

G.T. Gabel, M.D.: Department of Orhopedic Surgery, Baylor College of Medicine, Houston, Texas.

R.P. Nirschl, M.D.: Department of Orthopedic Surgery, Georgetown University Medical School, Washington, D.C.; and Arlington Hospital/Nirschl Orthopedic Sports Medicine Clinic, Arlington, Virginia.

INDICATIONS/CONTRAINDICATIONS

As with lateral epicondylitis, the indications for surgery are pain that limits daily activity and/or interrupts sleep. The duration of nonoperative management is a minimum of 6 to 9 months and ideally at least 12 months. All conservative measures should have been tried. At least one cortisone injection is helpful to isolate the lesion, and failure of this therapy strengthens the indications for surgery.

The most significant contraindication is a history and physical that does not accurately coincide with expectations of medial epicondylitis. Poor motivation, worker's compensation, and unrealistic expectations are also issues of concern and to be considered before surgical intervention is carried out. Individuals who are improving or who have had symptoms less than 6 months are generally not considered candidates for surgery.

PREOPERATIVE PLANNING

The surgical procedure of choice relates to the classification of medial epicondylitis. Operative management of type I medial epicondylitis involves medial epicondylar debridement alone. The type II medial epicondylitis may require ulnar nerve decompression, including cubital tunnel release if symptoms are mild (A) or medial epicondylar debridement and ulnar nerve transposition if nerve symptoms predominate (B). Medial epicondylitis should be avoided, as anterior epicondylar removal (for the medial epicondylitis) and posterior epicondylar removal (for the ulnar nerve) may result in compromise of the anterior oblique ligament origin. When medial epicondylar debridement is carried out, the flexor pronator mass is already violated, so submuscular translocation is logical.

Valgus instability, if present, may be operatively treated at the same setting with anterior oblique ligament reconstruction (4) in association with submuscular ulnar nerve transposition and medial epicondylar debridement. The obvious concern of elevation of the active medial elbow stabilizer (the flexor pronator mass) at the same time as the passive ligamentous restraint (the anterior oblique ligament) can be obviated by formal repair of the flexor pronator origin in addition to the anterior oblique ligament (AOL) reconstruction.

The medial conjoint tendon (MCT) is the primary anatomic focus in medial epicondylitis. The MCT is the perpendicularly oriented septum originating on the anterior aspect of the medial epicondyle and separates the common flexor and pronator teres origins (Fig. 13-1). It lies immediately anterior to the anterior oblique ligament with, in most cases, no identifiable interval between these two structures. The MCT serves as the intramuscular tendon origin for the flexor pronator mass musculature, including the flexor carpi radialis, the pronator teres, the palmaris longus, and the flexor digitorum sublimis. At the level of the medial epicondyle the tendon is fully conjoint and remains so for the first 2 cm, at which point the MCT splits into two septae separated by the muscle belly of the flexor carpi radialis. The anterior oblique ligament remains along the posterior border of the MCT throughout the course of the anterior oblique ligament. The medial conjoint tendon extends distally 10 to 12 cm into the forearm. Gross pathologic involvement of the tendon is seen within the proximal 2 to 3 cm of the tendon, the level where it is conjoint. It is at this level that the surgical debridement in medial epicondylitis is conducted.

SURGERY

Type I Medial Epicondylitis

After induction of a general anesthetic, the arm is prepped and draped in usual fashion. A longitudinal incision is created starting 1 cm anterior to the proximal margin of the medial epicondyle and extending distally for 3 to 4 cm (Fig. 13-2). Blunt subcutaneous dissection is performed to allow for identification and protection of the posterior branch of the medial

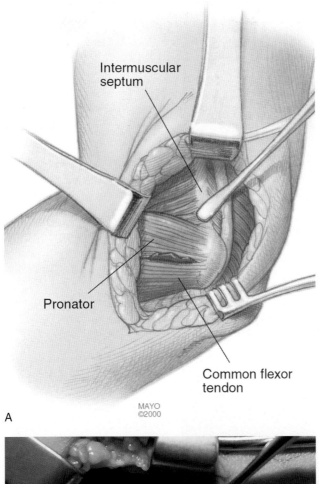

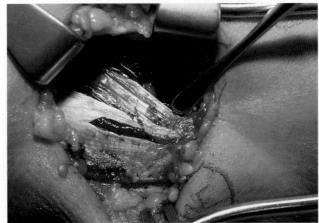

Figure 13-1. A,B: The medial conjoint tendon within the flexor pronator mass. This is the tendinous origin of the flexor carpi radialis, pronator teres, palmaris longus, and flexor digitorum sublimis. It lies immediately anterior to the anterior oblique ligament.

antebrachial cutaneous nerve (Fig. 13-3). The flexor pronator fascia is discretely exposed from the proximal margin of the pronator teres origin at the superior aspect of the medial epicondyle extending distally to a level approximately 3 cm distal to the inferior aspect of the medial epicondyle. The superficial fascia of the flexor pronator mass is incised starting at its proximal (pronator teres) edge leaving a 3- to 4-mm rim attached to the epicondyle. This initially involves elevation of the pronator teres muscle off the anterior aspect of the medial epicondyle, but as dissection extends distally to the anterior inferior margin of the epicondyle, the proximal border of the medial conjoint tendon is encountered. The superficial fascia of

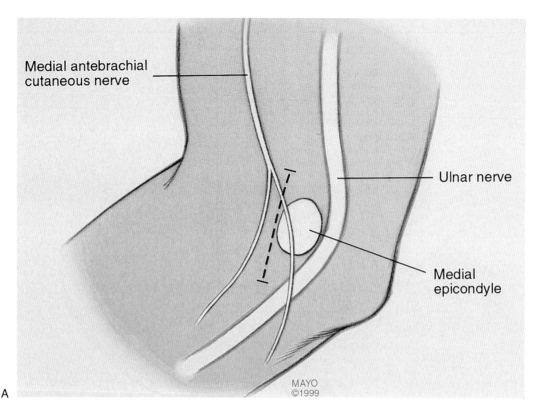

Medial antebrachial
cutaneous nerve

Ulnar nerve

Medial
epicondyle

MAYO
©1999

A

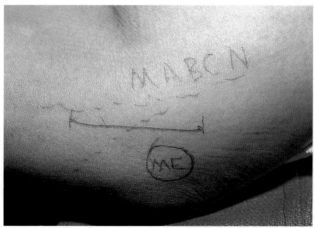

B

Figure 13-2. A,B: Incision for medial epicondylar debridement with or without cubital tunnel release. This incision can be extended proximally and distally for conversion to a transposition procedure if necessary.

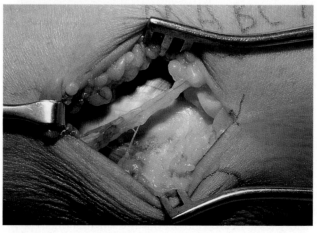

Figure 13-3. Exposure of flexor pronator mass. Note the posterior branch of the medial antebrachial cutaneous nerve, which can be easily identified and protected.

the flexor pronator mass is incised longitudinally along the anterior edge of the medial conjoint tendon. Pronator teres elevation continues in a proximal-to-distal manner off the anterior margin of the medial conjoint tendon with tenotomy scissors to discretely expose the proximal 2 to 3 cm of the medial conjoint tendon. The medial conjoint tendon is usually 2 to 3 mm thick from anterior to posterior, and the posterior margin can be readily identified using a freer elevator or tenotomy scissors to expose this posterior margin (Fig. 13-4).

Large lesions are immediately evident at this site (Fig. 13-5). If a degenerative nidus is present it is usually seen at the proximal aspect of the medial conjoint tendon along its anterior margin extending at times to the posterior aspect of the tendon. The anterior oblique ligament can be seen and palpated with a freer elevator immediately posterior to the medial conjoint tendon (Fig. 13-6). The interval between these two structures can be developed by passing the freer elevator down along the posterior margin of the medial conjoint tendon, creating an interval at the corner formed by the anterior oblique ligament and the medial conjoint tendon. Once the anterior oblique ligament is identified, debridement of the medial conjoint tendon can be safely and fully performed. Tenotomy scissors or a scapula are used to elevate the origin of the medial conjoint tendon of the anterior aspect of the epicondyle, leaving the anterior oblique ligament. The tendon is elevated off the epicondyle flush with the anterior oblique ligament and elevation continues distally, again flush with the ligament for 2 to 3 cm. At this point, the proximal 2 to 3 cm of the medial conjoint tendon have been isolated and are excised with tenotomy scissors (Fig. 13-7). The anterior

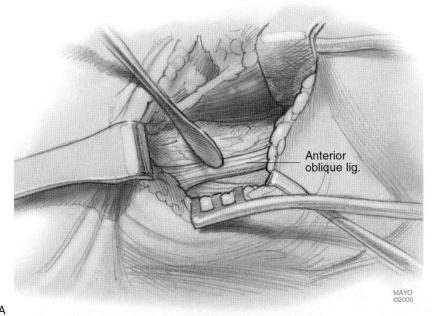

Anterior
oblique lig.

MAYO
©2000

A

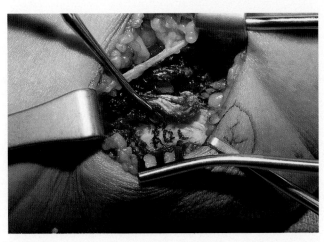

B

Figure 13-4. A,B: Elevation of pronator teres muscle from the anterior aspect of the medial epicondyle and from the anterior aspect of the medial conjoint tendon. The probe marks the proximal anterior margin of the medial conjoint tendon.

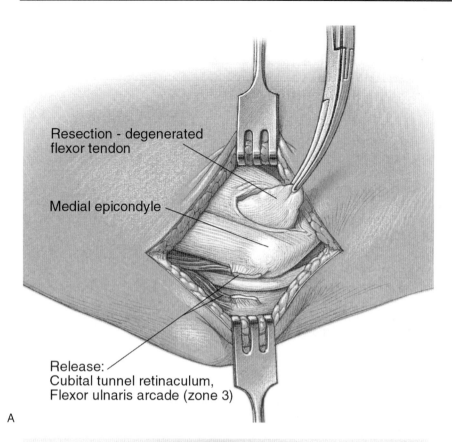

Resection - degenerated flexor tendon

Medial epicondyle

Release:
Cubital tunnel retinaculum,
Flexor ulnaris arcade (zone 3)

A

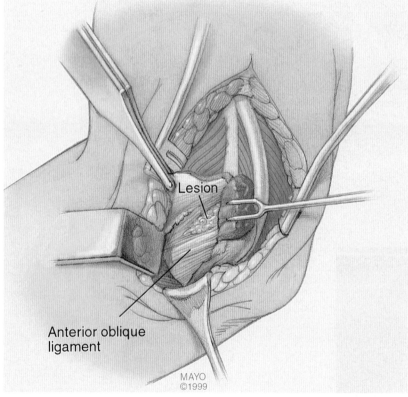

Lesion

Anterior oblique ligament

MAYO
©1999

B

Figure 13-5. A,B: Extensive degenerative lesion and disruption of the common flexor pronator origin at the medial conjoined tendon.

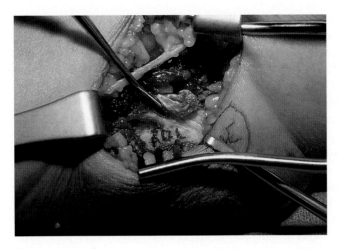

Figure 13-6. Posterior dissection along the medial conjoint tendon exposes the anterior oblique ligament contiguously along the posterior border of the medial conjoint tendon. There is typically no anatomic interval, but a surgical interval can be identified (at the level of the probe) to allow excision.

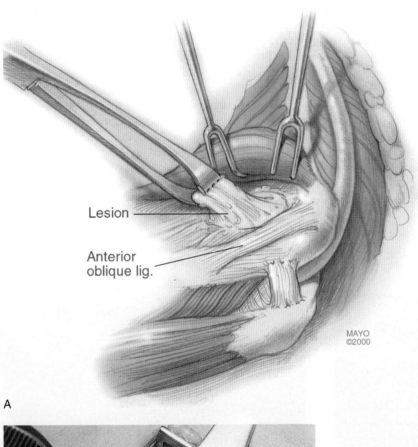

Lesion

Anterior
oblique lig.

MAYO
©2000

A

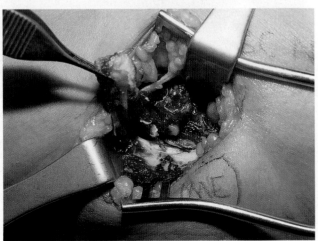

B

Figure 13-7. A,B: Isolation and excision of the medial conjoint tendon. The tendon is elevated directly off the medial epicondyle with a scalpel turning distally immediately superficial to the anterior oblique ligament. The proximal 2 to 3 cm of the medial conjoint tendon should be excised. The superficial fascia of the flexor pronator mass is then closed in an anatomic fashion.

oblique ligament can be inspected but is usually grossly normal except in chronic valgus loading situations. (This is usually anticipated preoperatively on physical examination.)

At this time the anterior aspect of the epicondyle can be "freshened up" with a rongeur, and the superficial fascia of the flexor pronator fascia is closed with a 2-0 vicryl suture side to side and to the remnant attached to the epicondyle. Skin closure is completed and a bulky dressing is applied, followed by application of a single sugar tong splint with the wrist and forearm at neutral.

Type II Medial Epicondylitis

In cases with mild associated ulnar neuropathy (IIA) the most common side of impingement is the so-called zone 3 of Nirschl. Cubital tunnel release can be performed in this setting or submuscular transposition can be elected. Cubital tunnel release is acceptable only when the environs of the ulnar nerve at the cubital tunnel are pristine (i.e., no prior trauma, good nerve gliding without scarring, and no subluxation with flexion either before or following cubital tunnel release). The procedure of debriding the medial conjoint tendon is identical to that given earlier but is performed after the nerve status has been assessed, and if submuscular transposition is felt to be required, the debridement occurs with tendon origin release. The initial skin incision is the same as that for isolated medial epicondylar debridement. Attention is directed posteriorly to the cubital tunnel before violating the flexor pronator fascia. The posterior margin of the medial epicondyle is identified and the flexor carpi ulnaris fascia is exposed (Fig. 13-8). The fascia overlying the nerve is opened with tenotomy scissors at the posterior/inferior corner of the medial epicondyle. The fascia is then incised for 4 to 5 cm, exposing the two heads of the flexor carpi ulnaris muscle. These two heads are bluntly spread apart, exposing the deep fascia of the flexor carpi ulnaris, which lies directly on the ulnar nerve (Fig. 13-9). This fascia layer must be released as well to complete the cubital tunnel release.

The ulnar nerve is then examined without disturbing its bed. If there is any structural abnormality of the cubital tunnel (e.g., adhesions, exostoses), then conversion to a submuscular transposition is initiated.

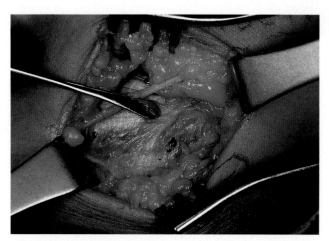

Figure 13-8. Posterior dissection to expose cubital tunnel region. Identify the posterior inferior corner of the medial epicondyle.

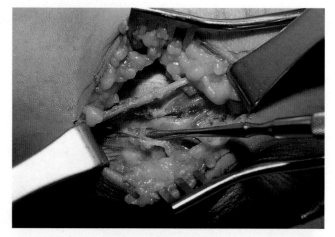

Figure 13-9. Cubital tunnel release is performed starting at the posterior inferior corner of the medial epicondyle, incising the flexor carpi ulnaris arcade, bluntly creating the interval between the two heads of the flexor carpi ulnaris muscle and releasing the deep fascia of the flexor carpi ulnaris immediately superficial to the ulnar nerve. If examination of the nerve reveals any significant abnormality, conversion to a submuscular transposition is elected.

For medial epicondyle debridement and submuscular translocation a 12- to 15-cm incision over the course of the ulnar nerve is created. The medial antebrachial cutaneous nerve is identified and protected distally in the wound. Attention is directed proximally, incising the brachial fascia overlying the nerve posterior to the medial intermuscular septum, proximal to the medial epicondyle. The fascia is incised proximally, releasing the arcade of Struthers in the process. With the elbow in relative extension to relax the nerve, the fascia is incised distally, ultimately extending into the fascia of the flexor carpi ulnaris. The deep flexor pronator aponeurosis within the flexor pronator mass is bluntly decompressed by placing metzenbaum scissors, tips up, on the ulnar nerve and gently advancing immediately superficial to the nerve and deep to the flexor pronator aponeurosis. This completes the decompression.

Mobilization of the nerve is performed, preserving the longitudinal vascularity as described in Chapter 16. The first motor branch, to the ulnar head of the flexor carpi ulnaris, is mobilized by performing an intramuscular neurolysis to gain 1 to 2 cm of length to allow the ulnar nerve to translate anteriorly without kinking.

Once the nerve has been mobilized, the flexor pronator mass is elevated, leaving a 2- to 3-mm tuft of fascia attached to the epicondyle (Fig. 13-10). The lacertus fibrosis is incised to free up the proximal margin of the pronator teres. The flexor pronator is elevated distally, exposing the medial conjoint tendon within the muscle mass. The medial conjoint tendon is isolated for its proximal 3 to 4 cm (Fig. 13-11) and incised along the anterior margin of the anterior oblique ligament (similar to debridement alone). It is then excised, to debride the tendon origin, but also to prevent fascial compression of the nerve with repair of the flexor pronator mass. Elevation of the flexor pronator mass continues posterior to the MCT, again with care not to violate the anterior oblique ligament. The posterior fascia of the humeral head of the flexor carpi ulnaris is incised to allow reentry of the ulnar nerve into the flexor pronator mass without impingement on this fascial structure.

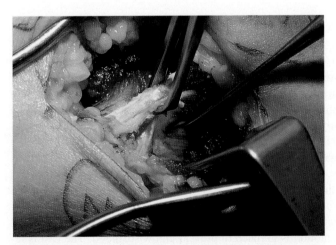

Figure 13-10. Submuscular transposition involves the standard decompression and nerve mobilization as in pure ulnar neuropathy. Flexor pronator mass elevation consists of pronator teres evaluation and isolation of the medial conjoint tendon.

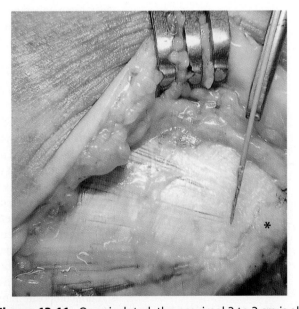

Figure 13-11. Once isolated, the proximal 2 to 3 cm is elevated, being careful to avoid the anterior oblique ligament. This portion of the tendon is resected to address the medial epicondylitis as well as to allow placement of the ulnar nerve deep to the flexor pronator mass without secondary compression.

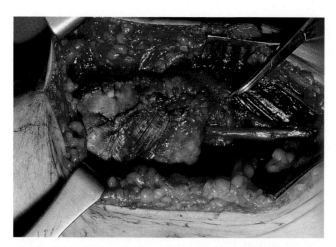

Figure 13-12. The flexor pronator mass is repaired with approximately 1 cm of lengthening to provide more room for the ulnar nerve as well as to functionally lengthen the muscle group (pointer is at original proximal margin of FP mass). The superficial fascia is repaired at the flexor carpi ulnaris arcade as well as at the level of the conjoint tendon.

The ulnar nerve is then brought beneath the flexor pronator mass and the alignment is assessed proximally and distally for new levels of compression or acute angulation. Further release is performed as needed to prevent new levels of compression in the nerves' newly transposed position. The flexor pronator fascia is repaired in a lengthened fashion repairing the fascia 1 cm distal to its anatomic position. This allows for more room beneath the flexor pronator mass for the ulnar nerve and minimizes the risk of recurrent impingement. The fascial closure includes the flexor carpi ulnaris (FCU) arcade, as the nerve is now deep to this layer and the repair allows for more secure repair of the fascia and provides more coverage of the nerve (Fig. 13-12). Skin closure is completed and the arm is placed into a single sugar tong splint, well padded at the posterior elbow to prevent splint irritation of the wound.

POSTOPERATIVE MANAGEMENT

As with lateral procedures for type I or IIA, the arm is placed in an elbow immobilizer at 90 degrees of flexion, the forearm is in neutral, and the wrist and hand are free. After 2 days, gentle active assisted motion exercises are usually started (tendon and/or tendon with nerve surgery). Intermittent immobilizer protection is usually continued for 6 to 7 days, at which time normal activities of daily living are resumed. Counterforce support providing protective function is utilized until full forearm strength returns (usually 3 to 6 months). The brace is used at times of rehabilitation exercise and more vigorous forearm activities, such as heavier household activities. A gradual return to sports often is initiated at 8 to 10 weeks with brace protection. For the type IIB procedure, sutures are removed at 10 days and a Muenster cast is applied for an additional 2 weeks in all cases except if a concomitant lateral epicondylar debridement has been performed (in which case a wrist splint is applied and noncomposite range of motion is initiated to prevent elbow stiffness). The cast is removed after an additional 2 weeks and noncomposite range of motion is started, progressing to composite range of motion at week 5 or 6. Strengthening is started at 6 weeks, if tolerated, and a flexor pronator program is continued until symmetric pain-free strength is gained. A counterforce brace is continued until after full strength is restored and full-duty status is reserved until the same point in time. This takes a minimum of 3 to 6 months on the average.

RESULTS

An emerging body of evidence has clarified the expectations of surgery for medial epicondylitis. Three recent reports all reveal a greater than 90% satisfaction with this surgery (3,6,9). However, both Gabel and Morrey, and Kurvers and Verlan emphasize the poor prognosis associated with ulnar nerve involvement. Final outcome is realized in 6 months in most but may take more than a year to fully recover in some.

COMPLICATIONS AND SURGICAL FAILURE

The most frequent complication after surgery for tennis elbow is residual pain. This is not common in the Mayo or Jobe experience and occurs in fewer than 10% of patients. However, Kurvers et al. report a significantly worse prognosis with medial epicondylitis than with lateral epicondylitis.

Complications relate to nerve as well as flexor pronator concerns. Medial antebrachial cutaneous neuropathy (MABCN) may result from avulsion, traction, or transection of the nerve. If this is recognized intraoperatively, the nerve should be mobilized proximally and transposed into the brachialis muscle belly. If the neuropathy is identified postoperatively, a desensitization program as well as neurogenic pain medication, such as nortriptyline™ or neurontin™, is started. A corticosteroid injection at the point of maximum Tinel's may be useful if the neuropathic pain persists. Sympathetic mediated pain may result from MABCN injury, but is not synonymous. If other hallmarks of a sympathetic mediated pain process are identified, pain management consultation may be indicated.

Transient exacerbation of the ulnar neuropathy symptoms is not uncommon, especially if a transposition has been performed. Objective incomplete loss of function of the ulnar nerve is uncommon but usually also resolves spontaneously. Complete loss of nerve function is quite rare and may indicate compression from a hematoma, fibrous band, or acute angulation. Complete loss of function requires early reexploration but may be associated with no objective level of compression, indicating a possible intraneural vascular event. Recovery is usually seen even in these circumstances but is typically incomplete.

Medial collateral ligament injury can occur and may result in medial instability of the elbow. If this occurs, anterior oblique ligament reconstruction may prove to be necessary to alleviate symptoms.

Persistent medial epicondylitis symptoms may indicate a prolonged recovery rather than a failure of the procedure. Symptoms that recur or continue after 6 months should be managed in a manner similar to that of the preoperative program. If injections are used after a transposition procedure, they should be kept well medial on the epicondyle to avoid intraneural injection of the ulnar nerve. Significant epicondylar symptoms that persist beyond 18 to 24 months may require revision, but this is the case in fewer than 2% to 3% of medial epicondylitis cases. Persistent ulnar nerve symptoms are more common but still rarely require revision, especially following a submuscular transposition. Cubital tunnel release may be associated with persistent or increased ulnar nerve symptoms and may be revised to a submuscular transposition (2) if indicated.

ILLUSTRATIVE CASE

A recreational tennis player presented with chronic symptoms for 1 year without response to conservative management. Ulnar nerve irritation to palpation was present in zone 3. At surgery the pathology was identified at the interval between the flexor carpi radialis and

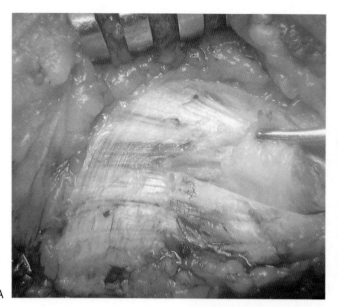 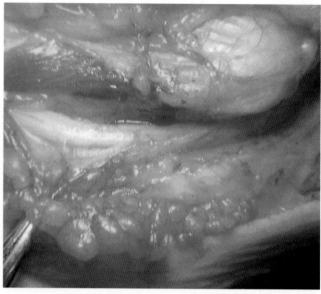

A   B

Figure 13-13. Exploration of flexor pronator origin revealed amorphous tissue at the medial conjoined tendon at the interval between the flexor carpi radialis and the pronator origin (**A**). Because ulnar nerve symptoms were present, the nerve has been decompressed distally (**B**).

pronator teres muscle origin (Fig. 13-13). The ulnar nerve was decompressed and the patient had a full recovery.

RECOMMENDED READINGS

1. Baumgard SH, Schwartz DR. Percutaneous release of the epicondylar muscles for humeral epicondylitis. *Am J Sports Med* 1982;10;233–236.
2. Gabel GT, Amadio PC. Reoperative for failed decompression of the ulnar nerve in the region of the elbow. *J Bone Joint Surg* 1990;72A:213–219.
3. Gabel GT, Morrey BF. Operative treatment of medial epicondylitis: influence of concomitant ulnar neuropathy at the elbow. *J Bone Joint Surg* 1995;77A:1065–1069.
4. Jobe FW, Stark H, Lombardo SJ. Reconstruction of the ulnar collateral ligament in athletes. *J Bone Joint Surg* 1986;68A:1158–1163.
5. Kurvers H, Verhaar J. The results of operative treatment of medial epicondylitis. *J Bone Joint Surg* 1995;77A:1374–1379.
6. Ollivierre CO, Nirschl RP, Pettrone FA. Resection and repair for medial tennis elbow: a prospective analysis. *Am J Sports Med* 1995;23:214–221.
7. Spinner RJ, Goldner RD. Surgery of the medial head of the triceps and recurrent dislocation of the ulnar nerve: anatomical and dynamic factors. *J Bone Joint Surg* 1998;80A:239.
8. Stahl S, Kaufman T. Ulnar nerve injury at the elbow after steroid injection for medial epicondylitis. *J Hand Surg* 1997;21B:69–70.
9. Vangsness T, Jobe F. The surgical treatment of medial epicondylitis. *J Bone Joint Surg* 1991;73B:409–411.

14

Treatment of Ulnar Collateral Ligament Injuries in Athletes

Neal S. ElAttrache and Frank W. Jobe

The anterior bundle of the ulnar collateral ligament is the primary structure resisting valgus stress at the elbow (Fig. 14-1) (7,11). Interestingly, trauma to this ligament rarely leads to symptomatic instability of the elbow in the majority of those injured (5,11). However, athletes participating in overhead or throwing sports place repetitive high valgus stress upon the medial aspect of the elbow joint (9). This may result in symptomatic valgus instability due to ulnar collateral ligament injury, occasionally requiring operative treatment to restore overhead athletic function.

INDICATIONS/CONTRAINDICATIONS

A history of pain after repetitive overhand throwing activities is the most common presentation. Pain is localized to the medial side of the elbow, especially during the late cocking or acceleration phases of the throwing motion (Fig. 14-2). Significant injury requiring intervention may follow one of three scenarios: the experience of an acute "pop" or sharp pain on the medial aspect of the elbow leading to the inability to throw further, the gradual onset of medial elbow pain over time with throwing, or pain following an episode of heavy throwing with the inability on successive attempts to throw above 50% to 75% of full function. The patient may report associated recurrent pain or paresthesia radiating onto the ulnar aspect of the forearm, hand, and fourth and fifth fingers, especially with throwing.

Valgus stability of the elbow is best examined with the patient seated and the hand and wrist held securely between the examiner's forearm and trunk (Fig. 14-3). The patient's elbow is flexed beyond 25 degrees to unlock the olecranon from its fossa and minimize the bony contribution to joint stability. The ulnar collateral ligament is palpated while simulta-

---

N.S. ElAttrache, M.D.: Department of Orthopaedic Surgery, University of Southern California School of Medicine, Kerlan-Jobe Orthopaedic Clinic, Los Angeles, California.

F.W. Jobe, M.D.: Department of Orthopaedic Surgery, University of Southern California School of Medicine, Los Angeles, California.

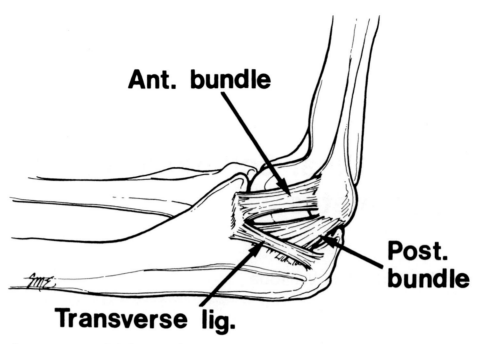

Figure 14-1. Medial ulnar collateral ligament complex, right arm. Anterior bundle has an eccentric location across medial joint. It attaches to the coronoid tubercle and the base of the medial epicondyle.

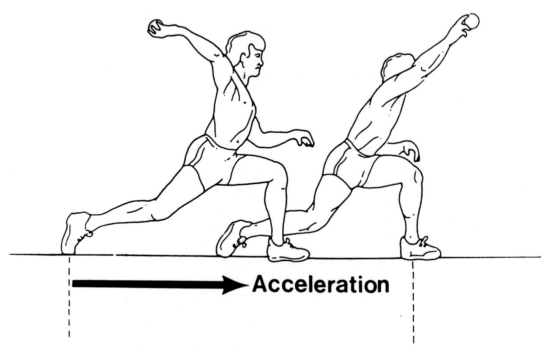

Figure 14-2. Arm and elbow position during acceleration phase of throwing resulting in high valgus force.

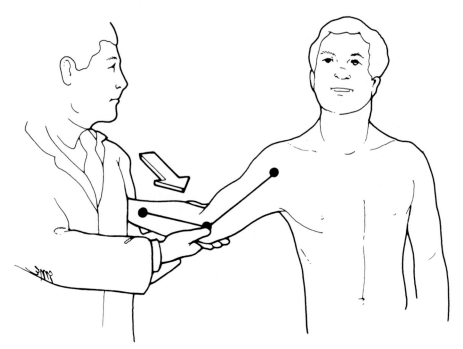

Figure 14-3. Valgus stress test produces pain and tenderness over ulnar collateral ligament.

neously applying a valgus stress. Local pain, tenderness, and end-point laxity are characterized with this maneuver. The "milking test" is a sensitive test for damage to the ulnar collateral ligament and is performed with the elbow at 70 to 90 degrees of flexion (Fig. 14-4).When the valgus instability leads to degenerative or traumatic arthritis with the formation of osteophytes and loose bodies posteriorly and medially, surgical intervention is appropriate (6).

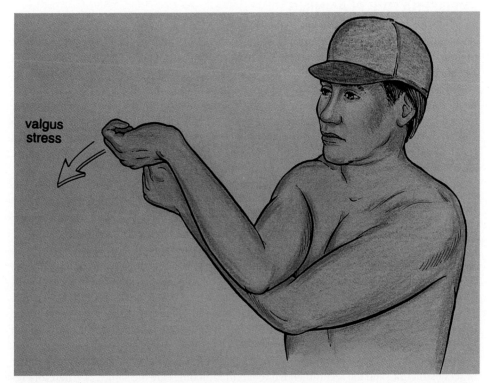

Figure 14-4. O'Brien's "milking test." The elbow is flexed at 70 to 90 degrees and traction is placed on the thumb in a radial direction imparting a valgus force on the elbow.

Rest and nonoperative management, including nonsteroidal antiinflammatory medications, alternating ice and heat, and other physical therapy modalities applied in the early symptomatic period, may arrest the progression of instability and allow return to full function without surgery (1). We have not found steroid injection to be helpful. Rest periods with rehabilitation of up to 3 months should be attempted and repeated at least once, especially in those patients who have not experienced an acute rupture.

If joint stability and pain relief are the main goal, nonoperative treatment usually suffices. However, if the patient desires to return to highly competitive overhead or throwing sports and has failed to improve despite nonoperative treatment, surgical intervention is indicated.

Surgical management consists of two types: repair of the ligament and reconstruction using tendon graft. In our experience, the indications for repair of the ulnar collateral ligament are limited. This technique is reserved for those patients with an acute proximal avulsion of the ulnar collateral ligament from its humeral attachment. The avulsed ligament should be of good quality and without calcifications presented within it. In this case, repair may be attempted. However, this presentation occurs rarely (2).

Symptoms of ulnar nerve impairment also justify stabilization. These symptoms are present in more than 40% of patients with ulnar collateral ligament insufficiency (2). Symptoms of ulnar neuropathy may also be caused by traction, friction, and compression of the nerve (3,4). The medial joint instability under valgus loading and the cubitus valgus deformity lead to nerve traction injury, whereas friction injuries result from recurrent subluxation of the nerve or abrasion by posteromedial osteophytes. Elbow flexion deformities are often found but usually do not adversely affect performance, since the throwing motion involves elbow positions between 120 degrees and 20 degrees of flexion (8). Calcifications within the injured ligament are also common but of themselves are not justification for surgery.

In noncompetitive, occupational circumstances, reconstruction should not be performed until a trial of work modification has been performed.

PREOPERATIVE PLANNING

A detailed history and physical examination are the key to making the correct diagnosis of ulnar collateral ligament insufficiency. It is important to record previous elbow injuries and treatment.

Physical examination may reveal tenderness to palpation over the ulnar collateral ligament complex, depending upon the degree of inflammation at the time of examination. Such inflammation may also irritate or compress the ulnar nerve locally as it traverses the cubital tunnel (3). A positive Tinel's sign along the cubital tunnel is an indication of this focal ulnar nerve irritability. A careful neurologic examination of the upper extremity should be performed.

Radiographic tests are helpful if positive, but a negative study should not rule out the diagnosis of ulnar collateral ligament insufficiency. The importance of radiographs is to ensure there is no associated pathology that may need to be addressed at the time of surgery. Standard radiographs may identify ossification within the ulnar collateral ligament, loose bodies in the posterior compartment, marginal osteophytes about the radiocapitellar or the ulnohumeral articulations, olecranon and condylar hypertrophy, or osteochondrotic lesions of the capitellum. Stress radiographs can show excessive medial joint line opening, indicating ligament laxity (Fig. 14-5).

We have found MRI to be helpful in demonstrating both acute and chronic injury to the ulnar collateral ligament. Intraarticular injection of contrast can increase sensitivity of the test (Fig. 14-6).

The frequency of postoperative ulnar nerve symptoms has been similar following repair or reconstruction, and the recommended rehabilitation times are the same (2). Therefore reconstruction of the insufficient ulnar collateral ligament with free autologous tendon graft is our surgical treatment of choice.

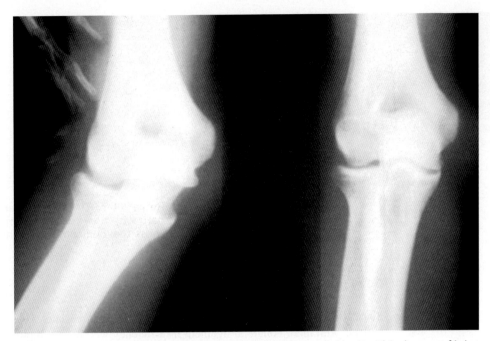

Figure 14-5. Valgus stress radiograph showing gross medial laxity. This degree of joint space opening is frequently absent.

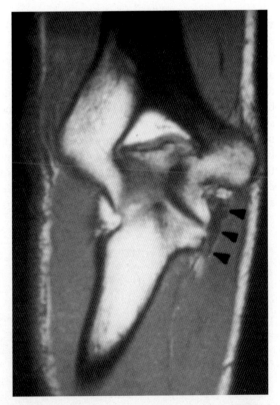

Figure 14-6. Magnetic resonance imaging (MRI) showing edema and fiber injury in the ulnar collateral ligament (*arrowheads*).

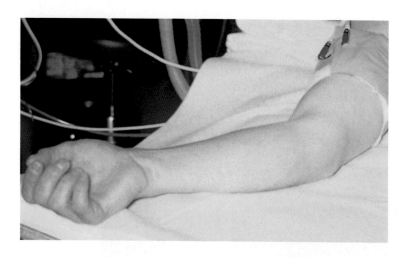

Figure 14-7. The arm is placed on an arm board with the shoulder externally rotated to expose the medial aspect of the elbow.

SURGERY

Since 1987 we have performed a reconstruction utilizing free autologous tendon graft in all patients with ulnar collateral ligament insufficiency who have symptomatic valgus instability unresponsive to nonoperative treatment.

With a pneumatic tourniquet on the upper arm, the patient is given a general anesthetic and is placed supine with the arm abducted to the side on a Parker arm board (Fig. 14-7).

Technique

A 10-cm incision centered over the medial epicondyle is used to expose the myofascia and aponeurosis of the flexor pronator muscle mass, the medial epicondyle, and the medial intermuscular septum of the brachium (Fig. 14-8). Care is taken to protect the medial antebrachial cutaneous nerve as it passes through the medial aspect of the forearm across the surgical field (Fig. 14-9). If there has been a previous anterior transposition of the ulnar nerve, the nerve should be identified and protected before exposure of the ulnar collateral ligament. For this exposure, a longitudinal split is made in the myofascia, the underlying flexor pronator aponeurosis and muscle mass at its more anterior origin from the medial epicondyle. Retraction of the flexor mass to both sides provides access and exposure to the anterior portion of the ulnar collateral ligament (Fig. 14-10).

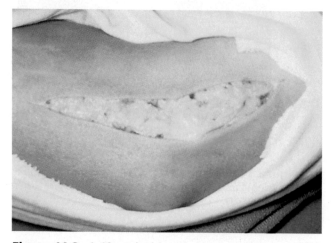

Figure 14-8. A 12-cm incision is centered over the distal aspect of the medial epicondyle and just anterior to it.

A longitudinal incision is made into the ligament itself to inspect the medial aspect of the elbow joint. The elbow is flexed to 20 to 30 degrees and a valgus stress is applied. With insufficiency of the medial collateral ligament, the medial joint should easily open several millimeters (Fig. 14-11).

A primary repair may be performed in a few patients with adequate ligamentous tissue remaining after debridement of calcific deposits from the ligament, or in those with an acute injury causing an avulsion of the ligament from the medial epicondyle. However, we feel this is the exception and not the rule, especially in overhead and throwing athletes. Usually it is necessary to reconstruct the ligament.

If the ligament does permit primary repair, it should be debrided and reattached to the periosteum of the medial epicondyle or any substantial proximal remnant of ligamentous tissue. Slack in the ligament can be imbricated and tightened by using a figure-of-eight suture on both sides of the longitudinal split and then suturing the two halves of the ligament together. An avulsion of the ligament from its attachment to the medial epicondyle can be

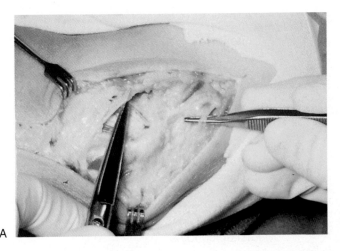

A

Figure 14-9. A,B: The medial antebrachial cutaneous nerve is identified and protected as it crosses the surgical field. The common flexor pronator tendon is observed directly deep to the nerve.

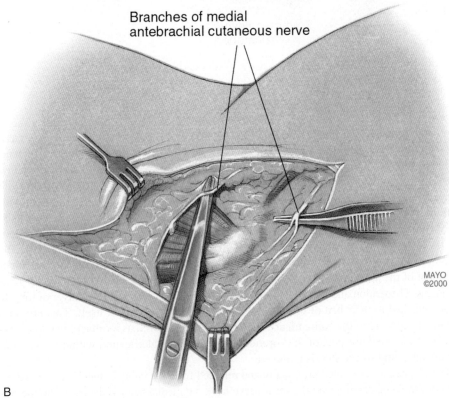

Branches of medial
antebrachial cutaneous nerve

MAYO
©2000

B

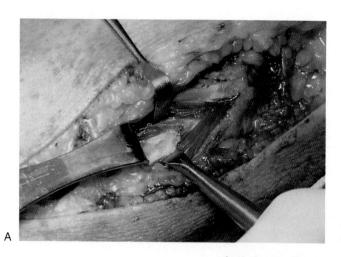

A

Figure 14-10. A,B: Ulnar collateral ligament exposed through a longitudinal split in the flexor muscle mass at the base of the medial epicondyle.

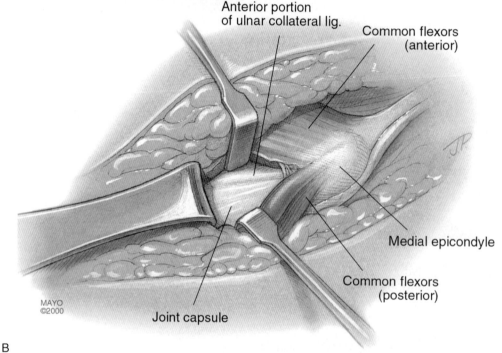

Anterior portion
of ulnar collateral lig.

Common flexors
(anterior)

Medial epicondyle

Common flexors
(posterior)

Joint capsule

MAYO
©2000

B

repaired by placing a Bunnell-type stitch through the body of the ligament and then passing the two free ends of the suture through drill holes in the medial epicondyle. The reattachment site should be prepared well with a rongeur to provide a good base for healing. The sutures are then tied securely on the posterior aspect of the medial epicondyle, with care taken to protect the ulnar nerve.

In most patients reconstruction of the ligament is necessary. In patients with associated preoperative ulnar motor neuropathy or evidence suggesting posterior compartment osteophytes or loose bodies, preparation is made to transpose the ulnar nerve anteriorly. The tendinous origin of the flexor pronator muscle bundle is transected 1 cm distal to the attachment of the aponeurosis on the medial epicondyle, leaving a stump of tendon for reattachment. The tendon and muscle are then reflected distally, leaving a thin layer of muscle fibers attached to their bed of origin on the ulnar collateral ligament itself. This provides excellent exposure of the entire ulnar collateral ligament as well as its attachment to the tubercle on the medial aspect of the coronoid process. Any calcification within the remaining ligament and soft tissues is removed.

The ulnar nerve is located proximally and released from the cubital tunnel. The fascial arcade of Struthers, passing over the ulnar nerve from the medial head of the triceps to the medial intermuscular septum, is identified and released. The nerve is dissected free and carefully

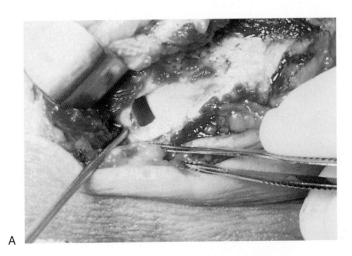

A

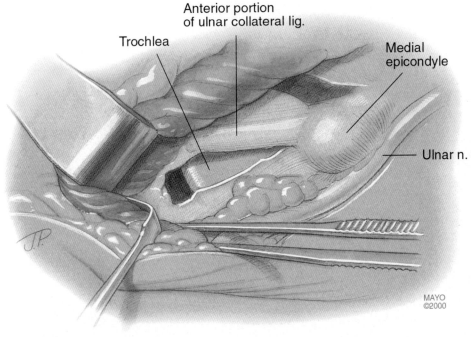

B

Figure 14-11. A,B: Longitudinal incision in the ulnar collateral ligament, revealing medial joint opening with valgus stress.

Trochlea

Anterior portion
of ulnar collateral lig.

Medial
epicondyle

Ulnar n.

mobilized proximally from the level of the arcade of Struthers and distally to the interval between the two heads of the flexor carpi ulnaris. A loop of 6.4-mm Penrose drain is placed about the nerve to protect it and to manipulate it during mobilization (Fig. 14-12). Care is taken to preserve any blood vessels intimately coursing with the nerve, and as many vascular tributaries as possible to minimize segmental devascularization of the nerve (8). The articular branches of the nerve are sacrificed, but its motor branches to the flexor carpi ulnaris muscle are preserved. A portion of the medial intermuscular septum in the brachium is excised sufficiently, allowing the transposed nerve to course anterior to the epicondyle without contacting any remaining sharp edges of septum. With the nerve anteriorly transposed, the posterior compartment of the elbow is easily accessible through a thin veil of capsular tissue, and any posterior loose bodies or osteophytes on the posteromedial margin of the olecranon can be removed.

Divergent 3.2-mm drill holes are then made in the medial epicondyle, creating bone tunnels though which the graft will be passed. A single entry hole is made anteriorly near the base of the epicondyle. The drill holes diverge and exit separately in the cubital tunnel posteriorly (Fig. 14-13).

Convergent 3.2-mm drill holes are made in the ulna located at the level of the tubercle on the medial aspect of the coronoid process. These holes are separated by approximately 1 cm (Fig. 14-13).

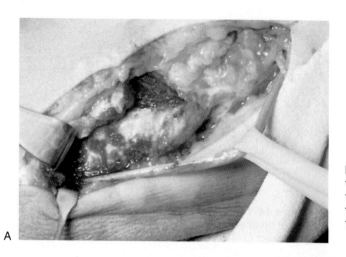

Figure 14-12. A,B: Flexor pronator conjoint tendon transected 1 cm distal to epicondylar attachment and reflected distally. Muscle fibers can be seen originating from the ligament itself. The ulnar nerve is shown retracted from the cubital tunnel with a Penrose tubing.

A

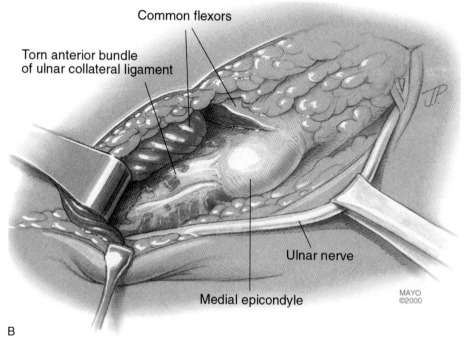

Common flexors

Torn anterior bundle
of ulnar collateral ligament

Ulnar nerve

Medial epicondyle

MAYO
©2000

B

At this point, attention is turned to harvesting suitable tendon for autologous graft tissue. We prefer to use the ipsilateral palmaris longus tendon for the free graft if available; however, the contralateral tendon, the plantaris tendon, a 3- to 5-mm medial strip of Achilles tendon, or tendon from lesser toe extensors may be used. The palmaris longus tendon has been shown to fail at higher loads with nearly four times the ultimate strength as compared with the anterior band of the ulnar collateral ligament (10). In our experience, the removal of palmaris tendon for reconstruction of the ulnar collateral ligament causes minimal morbidity with superior overall results as compared with repair of the ulnar collateral ligament. The presence of a palmaris longus tendon must be documented preoperatively. If absent, alternative autologous graft tissue may be used as mentioned earlier.

The palmaris longus tendon is harvested by first creating a 2-cm transverse skin incision at the level of the distal flexor crease of the wrist. The median nerve and its palmar cutaneous branch are protected by isolating the tendon and identifying the tendinous insertion into the palmar fascia. A second transverse skin incision is made 10 cm proximal to the wrist at the level of the palmaris longus musculotendinous junction. The tendon is then transected distally and brought out through the proximal incision. It is divided at the musculotendinous junction, providing a free autogenous graft approximately 15 cm in length (Fig. 14-14). These incisions are irrigated and closed routinely.

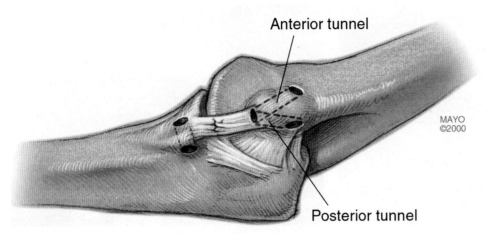

Anterior tunnel

Posterior tunnel

MAYO
©2000

Figure 14-13. Drill hole orientation in the coronoid tubercle distally and epicondyle proximally.

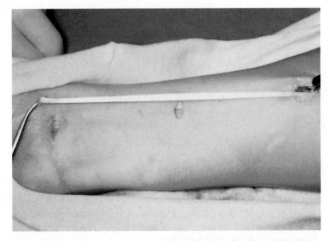

Figure 14-14. A 15- to 20-cm segment of palmaris longus tendon is harvested through three small incisions.

A No. 1 nonabsorbable braided suture is placed in one end of the graft, and a flexible suture passer is used to thread the tendon through the bone tunnels in a figure-of-eight fashion. With the elbow held in 45 degrees of flexion and neutral varus/valgus position, the graft is pulled taut and sutured to itself (Fig. 14-15). The graft is also sutured to the tough tissue of the intermuscular septum near the epicondyle and to any remnants of the ulnar collateral ligament. The elbow is then brought through a full passive range of motion to verify isometricity and checked for abrasion of the graft on the joint line. A gentle valgus stress is applied with the elbow in 30 and 70 degrees of flexion to test stability. A stable reconstruction will prevent medial joint line opening.

The flexor pronator muscle group is reattached to the medial epicondyle superficial to the anteriorly transposed ulnar nerve (Fig. 14-16). A surgical drain is also placed beneath the flexor pronator mass.

In patients without ulnar neuropathy, posterior osteophytes, or loose bodies, the ulnar nerve is not transposed. This avoids the risk of perioperative nerve impairment caused by segmental devascularization, intraoperative traction, or compression in the transposed position. Also, the flexor pronator aponeurosis origin on the medial epicondyle can be preserved.

Alternative methods of ulnar collateral reconstruction under current study attempt to facilitate easier graft placement tensioning and fixation (Figs. 14-17 and 14-18).

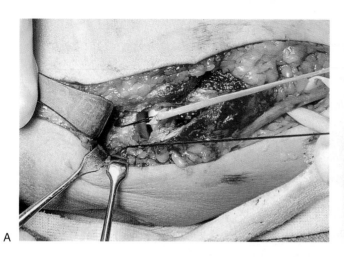
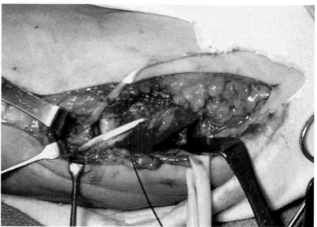

A   B

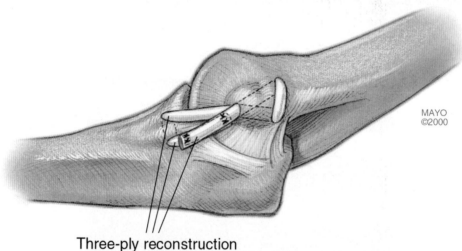

MAYO
©2000

C

Three-ply reconstruction

Figure 14-15. A,B: The graft is secured at one end with nonabsorbable suture and pulled through the bone tunnels with a suture passer **(C)**. The graft is placed in a figure-of-eight fashion and sutured to itself. It can also be reinforced by suturing it to soft tissue around the epicondyle.

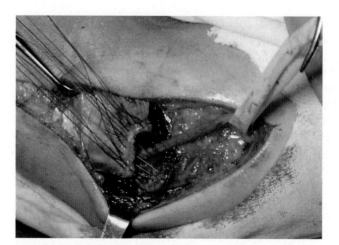

Figure 14-16. The conjoint tendon is repaired to the 1-cm cuff of tendon on the epicondyle with the ulnar nerve transposed anteriorly in the submuscular position when indicated (see text).

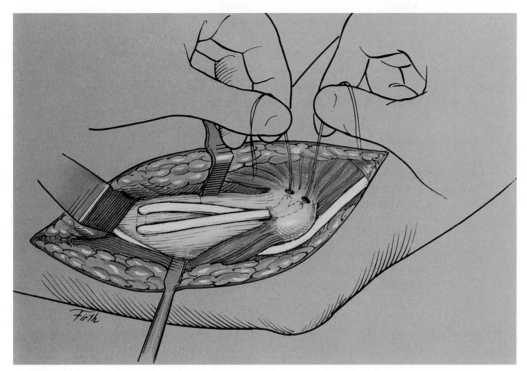

Figure 14-17. The "docking procedure." A two- or three-ply graft is placed through drill holes anterior and posterior to the ulnar tubercle. Then the proximal ends are "docked" into the epicondylar drill hole with attached sutures tensioned and tied over a proximal epicondylar bone bridge.

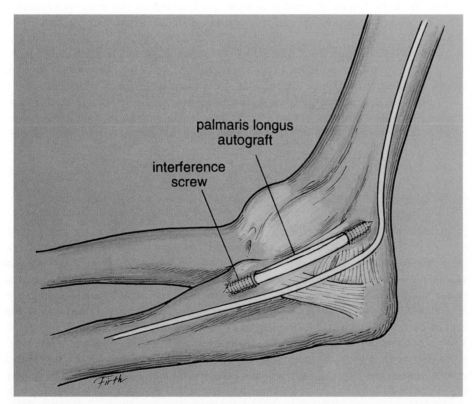

Figure 14-18. Anatomic interference reconstruction. A three- or four-ply graft is inserted and fixed distally into a 4.0 drill hole with an interference screw. Then it is tensioned and fixed proximally into the epicondyle with a second screw.

POSTOPERATIVE MANAGEMENT

The postoperative regimens for repair and reconstruction of the ulnar collateral ligament are identical. The patient begins gentle hand grip exercises squeezing a sponge or soft ball on the first postoperative day or as soon as it is comfortable to do so. The patient is discharged from the hospital on the second postoperative day.

Rehabilitation

Immobilization is discontinued at 10 days, at which time active elbow and shoulder and wrist range-of-motion exercises are started. After 4 to 6 weeks, muscle-strengthening exercises of the wrist and forearm are initiated, including flexion, extension, pronation, and supination of the hand and wrist. At 6 weeks, elbow-strengthening exercises are begun while avoiding valgus stress until 4 months after the operation. Shoulder exercises, including those for strengthening and maintaining the rotator cuff, are continued throughout the rehabilitative period.

At 3 to 4 months, the patient may toss a ball without a wind-up motion for a distance of 30 to 40 feet two to three times per week for about 10 to 15 minutes per session. At 5 months after surgery, the patient may increase the tossing distance to 60 feet and at 6 months the patient may perform an easy wind-up. Thereafter the patient may perform exercises and tossing on alternate days. Ice is used following all workouts to decrease swelling and inflammation.

At 7 months, a graduated program of range-of-motion and strengthening exercises, as well as total body conditioning is performed. Throwers and pitchers are carefully supervised, limiting throwing to one-half full speed while gradually increasing the duration of their sessions to 25 to 30 minutes. Pitchers are permitted to return to the mound and progress to 70% of maximum velocity during the eighth or ninth month.

Over the next 2 months, careful attention is focused on the body mechanics of throwing, including the lower extremities and torso. Duration of throwing sessions and velocity is slowly increased to eventually simulate a game situation. Throwing in competition is permitted at 1 year if the shoulder, elbow, and forearm are pain-free while throwing and have returned to normal strength and range of motion. Rhythm, proprioception, and accuracy are the last skills to be regained in overhead athletes following reconstruction of the ulnar collateral ligament of the elbow. In a professional pitcher, it may require more than 18 months to regain preoperative ability and competitive level, with relatively shorter periods required for other player positions or overhead sports (4).

RESULTS

Reconstruction of the ulnar collateral ligament in overhead or throwing athletes unable to compete due to valgus instability of the elbow has been successful in returning most patients to their previous level of participation (2,4). Of 70 operations on 68 patients with valgus instability of the elbow treated at the Kerlan-Jobe Orthopaedic Clinic, 14 had direct repair and 56 had a reconstruction of the torn or incompetent ligament, using a free tendon graft (2). These patients were followed for 6.3 years postoperatively. Fifty percent of the repair group and 68% of the reconstruction group returned to their previous level of participation. The mean time to return to competition was 9 months in the repair group and 12 months in the reconstruction group. Twelve of 16 major league baseball players who underwent reconstruction without previous elbow surgery returned to playing in the major leagues. Two of seven major league players who had a direct repair as their primary procedure returned to that level. Previous operations on the elbow were shown to decrease the patients' chances of return to their preinjury level of participation in their sport.

If specific sport participation and player position are considered, it appears that baseball pitchers are the most difficult patients to return to their previous competitive level, with 62% showing excellent results in the reconstruction group.

The length of time from onset of symptoms to operation, the mode of onset of symptoms (acute versus insidious), and the type of ligament injury (avulsion versus attenuation) did not affect the postoperative outcome. Also, postoperative flexion deformities of the elbow up to 25 degrees may not decrease a thrower's performance, especially if present preoperatively.

COMPLICATIONS

Postoperative problems involving the cutaneous nerves or the ulnar nerve constitute the most common complication following ulnar collateral ligament repair or reconstruction in conjunction with nerve transposition and may occur in up to 25% of patients (2). Careful subcutaneous dissection may prevent inadvertent transection of cutaneous nerves causing local paresthesia or painful neuroma formation. Also, meticulous hemostasis and placement of surgical drains help to prevent compression of the ulnar nerve secondary to hematoma formation. Segmental devascularization of the transposed ulnar nerve may play a major role in the occurrence of postoperative ulnar nerve palsy (8,12). Therefore in patients requiring ulnar nerve transposition, gentle handling of the ulnar nerve and preservation of as much of its vascular leash as possible may limit the incidence of this problem. To address the incidence of postoperative ulnar nerve problems, dissection and anterior transposition of the nerve are now performed only when symptoms of ulnar neuropathy are present or when pathology in the posterior compartment requires exposure through the cubital tunnel. Rupture or stretch of the reconstruction is possible but is uncommon if three strands of the graft cross the joint. If the joint becomes dysfunctional, reoperation is indicated and a new autogenous graft is used to construct the deficiency ligament.

ILLUSTRATIVE CASE

A competitive athlete presented with medial insufficiency but no ulnar nerve symptoms. The approach and exposure of the flexor pronator conjoint tendon is the same as described earlier. The conjoint tendon and muscle fibers of the flexor pronator group are split longitudinally and retracted to expose the ulnar collateral ligament. The ulnar nerve is not exposed and is left in position in the cubital tunnel. The flexor pronator tendon origin is also left intact, not transecting it at the epicondyle. The drill holes in the coronoid tubercle of the ulna are fashioned as described earlier. However, care should be taken to protect the ulnar nerve and its muscular branches at the level of the coronoid tubercle as it courses within the muscle fibers on the inferior and medial aspect of the exposure. The nerve may be visible at this level (Fig. 14-19). The initial drill hole at the humeral epicondylar attachment of the ligament is made and angled more superiorly and anteriorly than the procedure described earlier. Two drill holes are then made on the superior and anterior surface of the epicondyle approximately 1 cm apart with both placed anterior to the intermuscular septum. They are angled so that they communicate with each other and with the initial entry hole within the substance of the epicondyle (Fig. 14-20). In this way, the cubital tunnel is not penetrated and the ulnar nerve is not disturbed. The tendon graft is harvested and placed through the bone tunnels as described earlier (Figs. 14-21 and 14-22).

The graft is tensioned and sutured to itself with the ends buried within the bone tunnels. The longitudinal split in the flexor pronator wad may then be repaired if desired by simply closing the superficial myofascia with absorbable suture.

The tourniquet is then released, hemostasis is obtained with electrocautery, and the wound is closed in routine fashion (Fig. 14-23). A long-arm posterior plaster splint is used to immobilize the elbow in 90 degrees of flexion and neutral rotation, leaving the wrist and hand free.

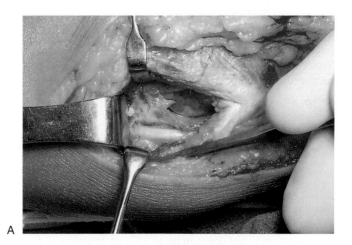

A

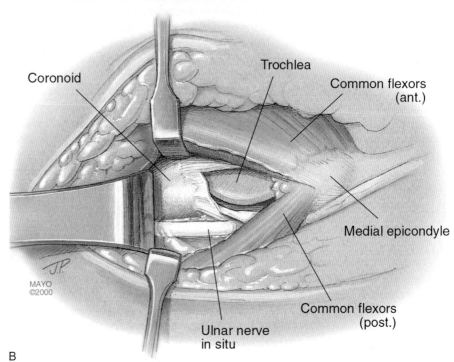

B

Figure 14-19. A,B: When ulnar nerve transposition is not required, the procedure is performed through a longitudinal incision in the conjoint tendon and muscle instead of transecting the epicondylar attachment. Above, the calcified ligament that had been debrided and the coronoid tubercle is exposed for drilling. Note the ulnar nerve on the lower aspect of the exposed tubercle.

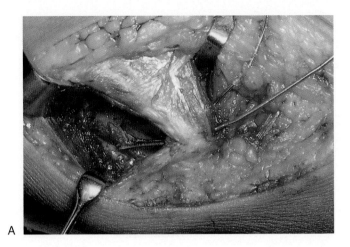

A

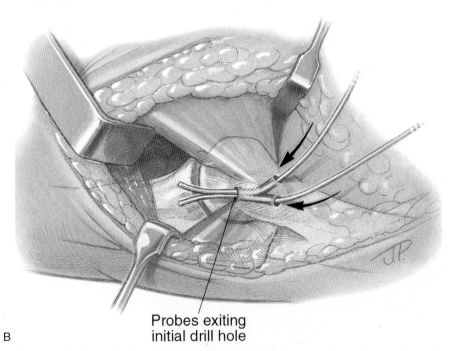

Probes exiting
initial drill hole

B

Figure 14-20. A,B: Epicondylar drill holes oriented anterior and superior to the intermuscular septum. Shown above with probes through the holes.

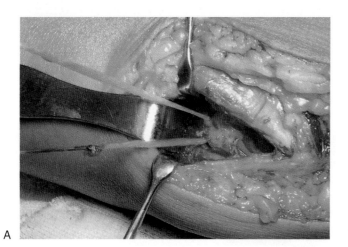

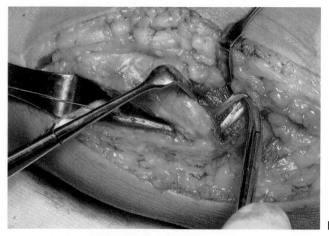

A

B

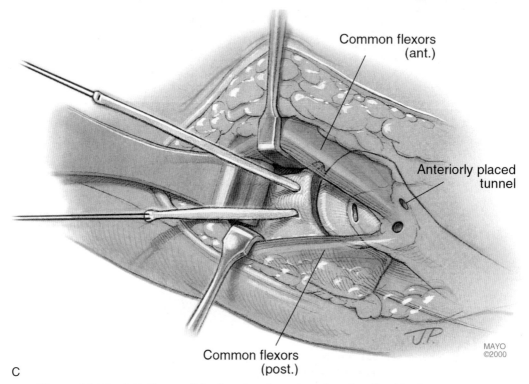

Common flexors
(ant.)

Anteriorly placed
tunnel

Common flexors
(post.)

C

Figure 14-21. A-C: The graft is placed and tensioned as described in the text.

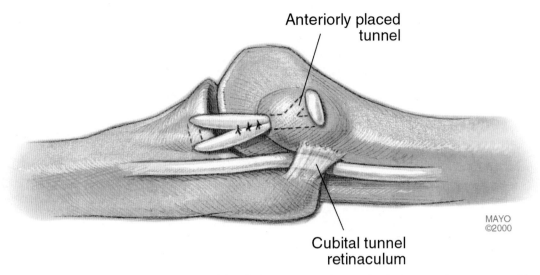

Figure 14-22. The epicondylar holes are anterior to the intermuscular septum with the ulnar nerve left in position in the cubital tunnel.

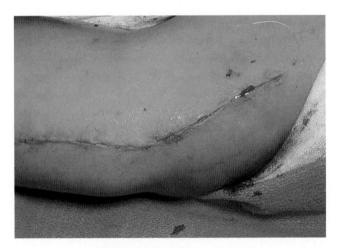

Figure 14-23. Skin closure.

RECOMMENDED READINGS

1. Barnes PA, Tullos HS. An analysis of 100 symptomatic baseball players. *Am J Sports Med* 1978;6:63.
2. Conway JE, Jobe FW, Glousman RE, Pink, M. Medial instability of the elbow in throwing athletes: surgical treatment by ulnar collateral ligament repair or reconstruction. *J Bone Joint Surg* 1992;74:67–83.
3. Jobe FW, Kvitne RS. Elbow instability in the athlete. *Instr Course Lect* 1991;40:17.
4. Jobe FW, Start H, Lombardo SF. Reconstruction of the ulnar collateral ligament in athletes. *J Bone Joint Surg* 1986;68A:1158.
5. Josefsson PO, Johnell O, Gentz CF. Long term sequelae of simple dislocations of the elbow. *J Bone Joint Surg* 1984;66A:927.
6. King JW, Brelsford HJ, Tullois HS. Analysis of the pitching arm of the professional baseball pitcher. *Clin Orthop* 1969;67:116.
7. Morrey BF, An KN. Articular and ligamentous contributions to the stability of the elbow joint. *Am J Sports Med* 1983;11:315.
8. Ogata K, Naito M. Blood flow of peripheral nerve effects of dissection, stretching, and compression. *J Hand Surg* 1986;11B:10.
9. Pappas AM, Zawacki RM, Sullivan TJ. Biomechanics of baseball pitching: a preliminary report. *Am J Sports Med* 1985;13:216.
10. Regan WD, Korinek SF, Morrey BF, et al. Biomechanical study of ligaments around the elbow joint. *Clin Orthop* 1991;271:170–179.
11. Schwab GH, Bennet JB, Woods GW, et al. Biomechanics of elbow instability: the role of the medial collateral ligament. *Clin Orthop* 1980;146:42.
12. Starkweather RJ, Nevaiser RJ, Adams JP, et al. The effect of devascularization on the regeneration of lacerated peripheral nerves: an experimental study. *J Hand Surg* 1978;3:163.

15

Surgical Reconstruction of the Lateral Collateral Ligament

Shawn W. O'Driscoll and Bernard F. Morrey

The mechanics of elbow dislocation is now recognized to involve a common pathway that begins as a posterolateral rotatory subluxation. In virtually all cases of complete dislocation, the essential lesion is disruption of the ulnar part of the lateral collateral ligament (6,8–10). The medial collateral ligament may be intact. The annular ligament remains unaffected. This pattern of instability involves rotatory ulnohumeral subluxation accompanied by posterolateral subluxation or dislocation of the radiohumeral joint, with the ulna and radius rotating off the humerus together as a unit (Fig. 15-1). We have now come to recognize that possibly the most common clinical expression of lateral ulnar collateral ligament (LUCL) deficiency relates to exposure and treatment of radial head pathology associated with elbow distraction.

INDICATIONS/CONTRAINDICATIONS

Surgery is indicated in patients with symptomatic instability. We are not aware of any nonsurgical means of treating this condition once established except for the permanent use of an elbow brace. This is cumbersome and not always effective, especially in obese patients. Osborne and Cotterill (11) suggested that the lax tissues around the elbows of young children with instability might tighten with growth and prevent recurrences of their instability. We have no data to substantiate this thought, although it is an attractive proposition.

We are not aware of any absolute contraindications to reconstruction. There are several relative ones. Children with open epiphyseal plates should not have their ligaments reconstructed with tendon grafts that cross the physis. Instead, the existing lateral collateral ligament (LCL) tissues are imbricated and reattached to bone isometrically. Our youngest pa-

S.W. O'Driscoll, M.D., PH.D.: Orthopedic Surgery, Mayo Medical School, Mayo Foundation, Rochester, Minnesota.

B.F. Morrey, M.D.: Mayo Medical School and Department of Orthopaedics, Mayo Clinic and Mayo Foundation, Rochester, Minnesota.

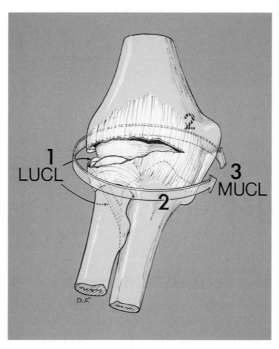

Figure 15-1. We have now come to recognize that the spectrum of elbow ligament/capsule disruption is imitated by description of the LCL.

tient, who was 4 years old at the time of surgery, was the victim of child abuse and repeatedly injured herself by falling. Her repair has failed and her parent has been advised that she should not be reoperated until her mental development and family circumstances improve. The absence of a radial head adversely affects the prognosis but is not a contraindication to surgery.

PREOPERATIVE PLANNING

The preoperative planning for surgical reconstruction of the lateral ligament of the elbow involves assessment of the findings on history and physical examination but is based first on the prerequisite understanding of the functional anatomy as well as the pathoanatomy and etiology of elbow instability.

Because this condition is not fully appreciated by all, an explanation of the anatomy and pathology is appropriate here. On the lateral side of the elbow, an ulnar insertion has been variably illustrated in the anatomy literature (1,3–5,7,14). We identified this ligament as part of the lateral capsuloligamentous complex in 17 of 17 fresh-frozen cadaver elbows (Fig. 15-2) (9). Lack of awareness in the past is probably due to the fact that it blends with the fibers of the lateral collateral complex from which it is indistinguishable (7). It originates from the lateral epicondyle. As it courses superficially over the annular ligament it blends with it and then curves posteriorly and ulnarward to insert on the tubercle of the supinator crest of the ulna (4,14). Its fibers are distinct at its insertion but are hidden beneath the fascia covering the supinator and the extensor carpi ulnaris muscles. It can be palpated at its insertion by applying a varus or supination moment to the elbow.

Posterolateral rotatory instability of the elbow is usually posttraumatic, with about one-half of patients having a history of a documented dislocation requiring reduction (6). The remainder of the posttraumatic cases have experienced injuries such as "sprains" or fractures of the radial head or coronoid. Finally, this condition can also be iatrogenic, caused by violation of the ulnar part of the LCL during lateral release for lateral epicondylitis or radial head excision (6,8). It should be noted that the ulnar part of the LCL passes around

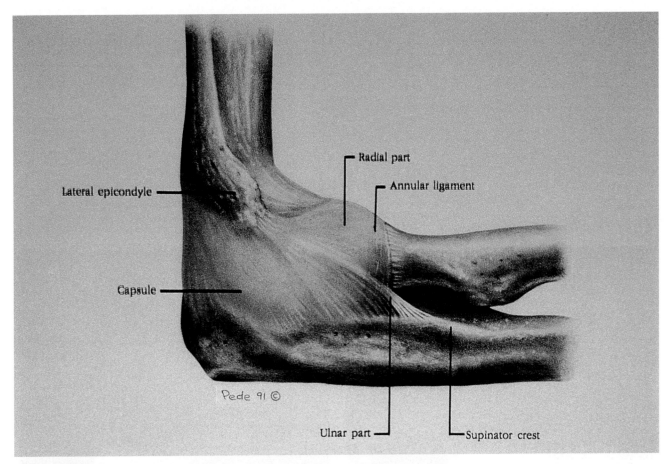

Lateral epicondyle

Capsule

Radial part

Annular ligament

Pede 91 ©

Ulnar part

Supinator crest

Figure 15-2. The lateral collateral ligament (LCL) is a complex of fibers consisting of the radial part, the ulnar part, and the annular ligament, all of which blend together. The ulnar part is indistinct at its origin on the lateral epicondyle. In fact, the common extensor origin also blends with this but has been excised for the purpose of this illustration. The ulnar part of the LCL arches over the annular ligament, with which it is closely integrated. It is most distinct along its anterior border as it inserts on the tubercle of the supinator crest. There is an additional fan-shaped insertion posterior to this, along the base of the annular ligament and just proximal to it. This gradually thins out until only the capsule remains. (Reprinted from O'Driscoll SW, Horii E, Morrey BF, et al. Anatomy of the ulnar part of the lateral collateral ligament of the elbow. *Clin Anat* 1992;5:296–303, with permission.)

the radial head, which augments tension in the ligament (7). Removal of the radial head can cause slight laxity.

Diagnosis

Patients typically present with a history of recurrent catching or locking of the elbow. Careful interrogation reveals that this occurs in the extension half of the arc of motion with the forearm in supination. The physical examination may be unremarkable. Valgus stress may show some laxity. However, the classic physical finding is that of a positive pivot shift maneuver (8) (Fig. 15-3). The elbow is supinated by applying torque at the wrist, and a valgus moment is applied to the elbow during flexion. This results in a typical apprehension response with reproduction of the patient's symptoms and a sense that the elbow is about to dislocate. Reproducing the actual subluxation and the clunk that occurs with reduction can usually be accomplished only with the patient under general anesthetic or occasionally af-

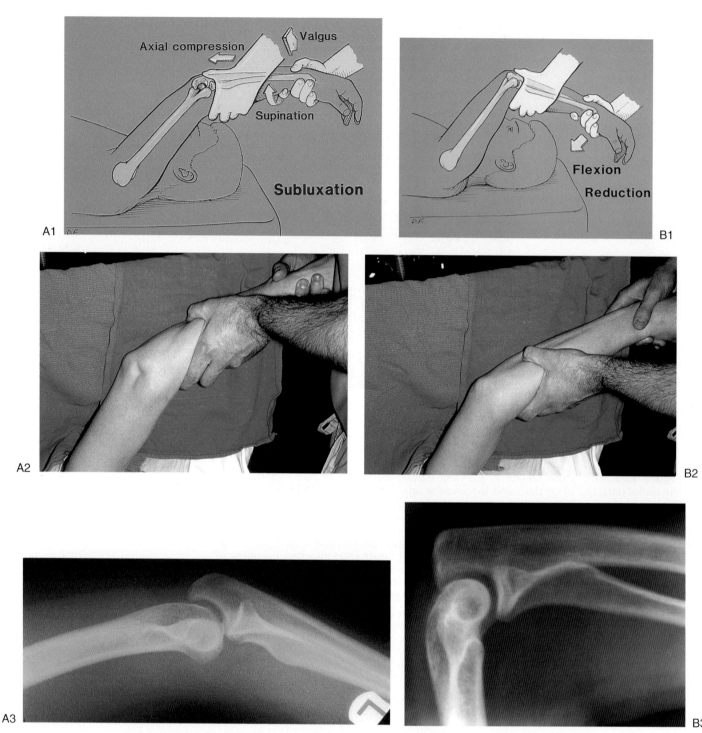

Figure 15-3. The lateral pivot-shift test of the elbow. **A:** The lateral pivot-shift test is most easily performed with the arm overhead. (We now use this method routinely.) Full external rotation of the shoulder provides a counterforce for the forearm supination and leaves one hand free to control valgus. The posterolateral dislocation of the radio-humeral joint produces a bony prominence and an obvious dimple, where the skin is "sucked in" just proximal to the dislocated radial head. On the lateral radiograph the radiohumeral joint is dislocated posterolaterally and there is a rotatory subluxation of the ulnohumeral joint; the semilunar notch of the ulna is rotated away from the trochlea. **B:** Reduction occurs with elbow flexion or sometimes simply with forearm pronation. The dimple disappears laterally and the lateral radiograph is normal.

ter injecting local anesthetic into the elbow joint. The lateral pivot shift test performed in that manner results in subluxation of the radius and ulna off the humerus, which causes a prominence posterolaterally over the radial head and a dimple between the radial head and the capitellum. As the elbow is flexed past approximately 40 to 60 degrees, reduction of the ulna and radius together on the humerus occurs suddenly with a palpable visible clunk. It is the reduction that is apparent. It should be emphasized that the lateral pivot-shift test for posterolateral rotatory instability is not easy to learn or teach and is readily demonstrable only in the extreme case.

Arthroscopy also may be useful in some cases. In some a subtle instability is insufficient to demonstrate with the pivot-shift test. In those patients with symptoms strongly suggestive of recurrent subluxations, arthroscopy reveals an excessive degree of widening of the ulno-humeral articulation with forced supination or widening of the lateral ulnohumeral joints.

SURGERY

The patient is positioned supine with the affected limb prepped and draped from the tourniquet on the upper arm distally to include the hand. If no palmaris longus is present, the leg is prepped and draped to permit access to the knee region for obtaining the semitendinosus tendon. The elbow is operated on with the arm on the patient's chest.

Surgical correction is performed by reattaching the avulsed lateral ulnar collateral ligament or reconstructing it with a tendon graft. Avulsion has been observed in children and in a few cases of acute fracture-subluxations of the elbow. Repair of the lateral complex must be meticulously performed when closing the capsule after treating the radial head in the fracture dislocation. In general, one can safely assume that in chronic cases the damaged ligament will be attenuated and require substitution with a graft. Our first choice is the ipsilateral palmaris longus, which is obtained through a 1-cm transverse incision in the wrist crease, using a long tendon stripper. At least 20 cm of length is required for the tendon reconstruction. If the patient does not have a palmaris longus, the semitendinosus or plantaris can be used. The larger tendons can be split to reconstruct both the medial and lateral ligaments when necessary.

In many instances the radiohumeral joint is being addressed surgically for a variety of pathologic states of variable extent when the lateral collateral ligament is released. This occurs usually by reflection from the humerus. The inadequate or inconsistent repair of this structure is one of the most common reasons for lateral collateral ligament insufficiency, which frequently leads to subtle clinical presentation of posterolateral rotatory instability.

In instances in which there is adequate soft tissue a drill hole is placed in the midportion of the lateral epicondyle, which is the center of the projected curvature of the capitellum and is coincident with the origin of the lateral collateral ligament. A No. 2 or No. 5 Mersilene suture is employed in a running locked fashion distally to the tubercle of the supinator crest. The purchase in the ulna is through a drill hole at that site or through the remnant of the ligament as it attaches to the tubercle. The suture is then brought proximally through a second drill hole again in the anatomic origin of the lateral collateral ligament (Fig. 15-4). The forearm is pronated and is immobilized between 60 and 90 degrees of flexion.

Technique

A 10-cm Kocher-type skin incision is used, passing between the epicondyle and olecranon (Fig. 15-5). The deep fascia is incised along the supracondylar ridge and distally between the anconeus and extensor carpi ulnaris muscles (Fig. 15-6). The triceps is reflected off the posterolateral aspect of the distal humerus in continuity with the anconeus, which is reflected off the lateral side of the ulna and capsule (Fig. 15-7). The common extensor origin is partially reflected to expose the capsule. Capsuloligamentous attenuation is assessed and laxity is confirmed. This is usually proximal to the annular ligament, and the capsular laxity is best appreciated by varus stress or performing the pivot-shift maneuver.

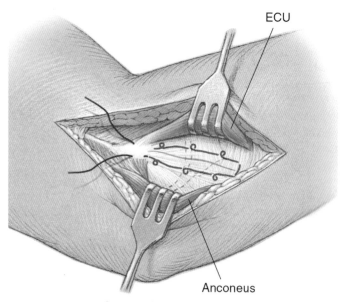
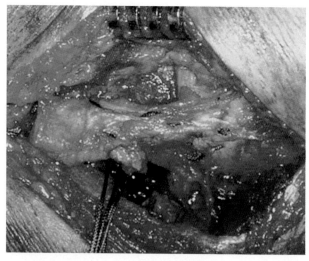

ECU

Anconeus

Figure 15-4. Insufficient LUCL is repaired by a suture placed through a bone tunnel at the lateral epicondyle. A running locked (Krachow) stitch is used to repair/reconstruct this deficiency. The proximal suture is also placed through a bone hole.

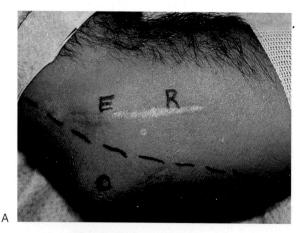
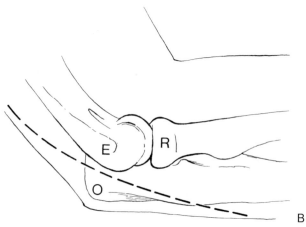

A

B

Figure 15-5. A,B: A 10-cm Kocher-type skin incision is used, passing between the epicondylar and olecranon.

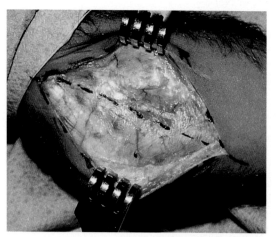
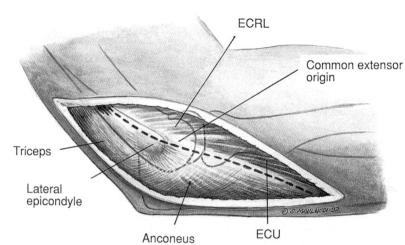

ECRL

Common extensor origin

Triceps

Lateral epicondyle

Anconeus

ECU

A

B

Figure 15-6. A,B: The deep fascia is incised along the supracondylar ridge and distally between the anconeus and extensor carpi ulnaris muscles. The interval is best identified by palpation.

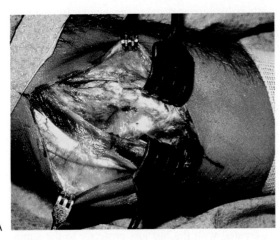

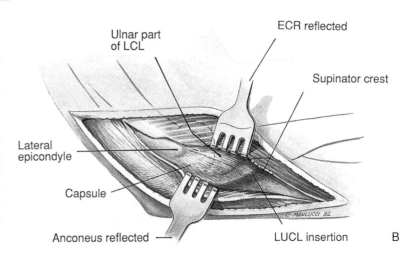

Ulnar part
of LCL

ECR reflected

Supinator crest

Lateral
epicondyle

Capsule

Anconeus reflected

LUCL insertion

A   B

Figure 15-7. A,B: The triceps and anconeus are reflected in continuity off the posterior humerus and capsule, exposing the lateral side of the ulna. The common extensor origin is partially reflected to expose the capsule. Capsuloligamentous attenuation is assessed and laxity confirmed.

The capsule is opened along the capitellum in an arc to permit inspection of the joint and later imbrication of the capsule (Fig. 15-8). An alternative is to open the capsule either posterior or anterior to be in line with the flow of the ligament. The insertion site for the tendon graft is then prepared by creating 3- to 4-mm drill holes in the ulna, one near the tu-

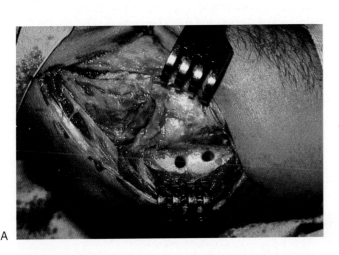

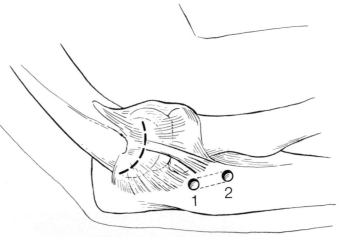

A   B

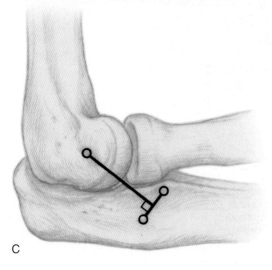

C

Figure 15-8. A,B: The capsule is opened along the capitellum in an arc to permit inspection of the joint and later imbrication of the capsule. An alternative approach is to open the capsule obliquely from the epicondyle to just posterior to the annular ligament. The insertion site for the tendon graft is then prepared by creating two drill holes in the ulna, one near the tubercle on the supinator crest (which is felt by stressing the elbow in varus or supination) and the other 1.25 cm proximally at the base of the annular ligament. The underlying bone is channeled with a curved awl from the Bankart set of instruments. **C:** The ulnar holes are sometimes made so the line connecting these holes is perpendicular to the line of the collateral ligament.

bercle on the supinator crest, which is easily palpated just distal to the annular ligament attachment on the ulna. The other is 1 cm posterior/proximal to the first and on a line perpendicular to the line of the graft (Fig. 15-8C). The underlying bone is channeled with a curved awl or curette.

The isometric point of attachment of the LCL is in the center of the capitellum (viewed from the lateral side). A No. 1 suture is passed through these two holes and grasped with a hemostat at the estimated isometric center of rotation of the elbow (Fig. 15-9). The isometric ligament origin is then determined by flexing and extending the elbow to see if the suture moves. No movement occurs if the suture and hemostat are on the isometric point. The entry site for the graft, hole No. 3, is then burred into the humerus at that point. Two technical points are worth noting. First, since the instability is most noted in extension, the ligament must be tight in extension. Hence if there is any question, the hole is made more anterior than expected. Finally, once the starting point is identified, it should be expanded to be about 5 to 6 mm. This enlargement takes place superior/anterior, *not* posterior/distal (Fig. 15-10). An exit site, hole No. 4, is created with the bur just posterior to the supracondylar ridge about 1.5 cm proximally and a tunnel created between the two with the curved awls or curettes (Fig. 15-10). A reentry site, hole No. 5, is created with the bur distally so that a bridge of bone, 1.25 cm, spans the two holes, and a tunnel is created from this site to the original entry site at the epicondyle, where the tendon will exit again.

The tendon graft is then brought through the first two holes in the ulna, holes No. 1 and No. 2, and sutured to itself (Fig. 15-9). It is then passed into the entry site, hole No. 3, in the lateral epicondyle, which represents the isometric origin of the ligament being reconstructed, out through the exit site, hole No. 4, proximally, down the posterior surface of the distal humerus, back into the bone through the reentry site, hole No. 5, to emerge at the isometric origin at hole No. 3 (Fig. 15-11). It is tensioned (Fig. 15-12) and sutured down to itself with the elbow in 30 to 40 degrees of flexion and forced pronation (Fig. 15-13). The

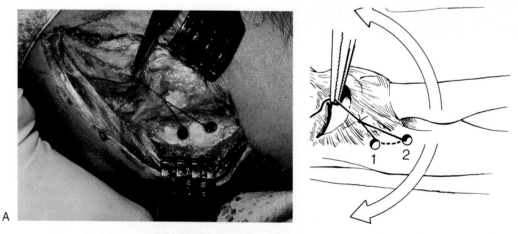

Figure 15-9. A,B: A No. 1 suture is passed through these two holes and grasped with a hemostat at the estimated isometric center of rotation of the elbow. The isometric ligament insertion is then determined by flexing and extending the elbow to see if the suture moves. No movement occurs if the suture and hemostat are on the isometric point. This point is usually more anterior than might be thought.

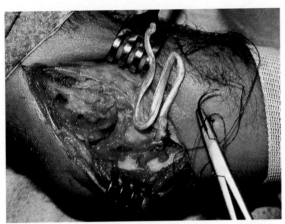
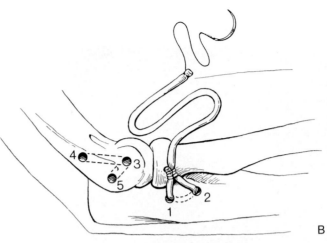

A   B

Figure 15-10. A,B: An entry site for the graft, hole No. 3, is then burred into the humerus at that point. Since the hole is bigger than the tip of the hemostat, one should make the hole posterior and proximal to the hemostat point (Fig. 15-8B inset). If it is placed distal or posterior, the tendon graft will be lax in extension and tight in flexion or vice versa. An exit site, hole No. 4, is created with the bur just posterior to the supracondylar ridge about 1.5 cm proximally and a tunnel created between the two with the curved and straight awls. A reentry site, hole No. 5, is created with the bur distally so that a bridge of bone, 1.25 cm, spans the two holes, and a tunnel is created from this site to the original entry site at the epicondyle where the tendon will exit again (hole No. 3). The tendon graft is then brought through the first two holes in the ulna, holes 1 and 2, and sutured to itself.

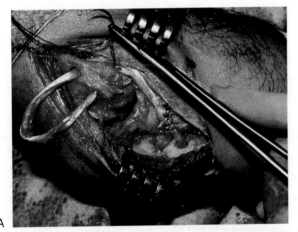
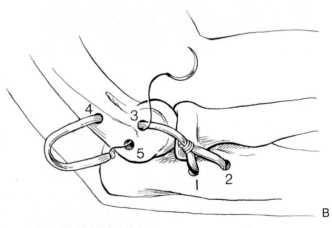

A   B

Figure 15-11. A,B: The graft is then passed into the entry site, hole 3, in the lateral epicondyle, which represents the isometric origin of the ligament being reconstructed, out through the exit site, proximally, hole 4, down the posterior surface of the distal humerus, back into the bone through reentry site, hole 5, to emerge at the isometric origin at hole 3.

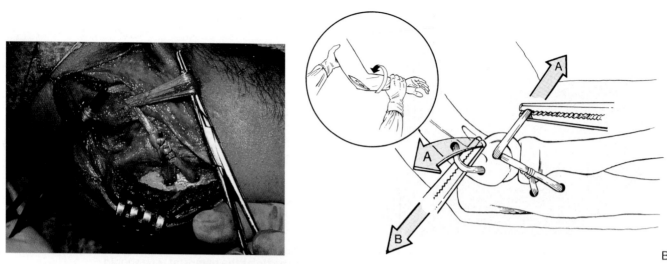

Figure 15-12. A,B: The graft is tensioned by pulling the proximal loop with a hemostat while pulling on the free end.

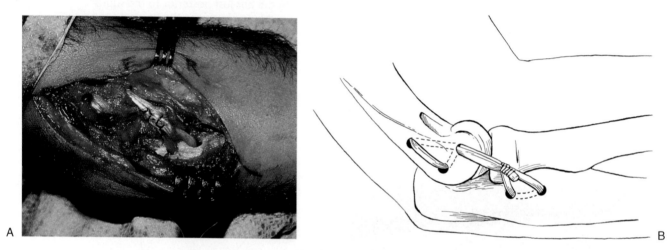

Figure 15-13. A,B: The free end is sutured to the remainder of the graft with the elbow in 40 degrees of flexion and forced pronation.

reconstruction can be augmented by passing a heavy No. 2 absorbable (Dexon) suture through the same course as the tendon graft (Fig. 15-14). If the capsule has been opened longitudinally, the suture should be woven through the capsule in an arch and not permitted to fall deep to the capsule because it will rub on the side of the capitellum and radial head. The capsule is closed and plicated, and the original arch of the ulnar part of the LCL is restored by pulling the graft anteriorly and suturing it to the capsule (Fig. 15-15). This also prevents the graft from slipping posterior to the radial head and permits optimum testing. The capsule must be closed under the graft to prevent it from rubbing on the radial head or capitellum. If further tension is desirable, this can be accomplished by closing the distal triangular gap between the two limbs of the graft (Fig. 15-16).

Subsequent Modifications

A modification of the procedure that we have performed in some patients is to make a minimal arthrotomy in line with the ulnar part of the LCL but just near the epicondyle. This provides access to the origin of the LCL where the graft must be attached to the humerus but minimizes the dissection and arthrotomy. The rest of the procedure is the same except the capsule is plicated only from anterior to posterior, rather than from distal to proximal. The advantage of this modification is that it obviates the tedious task of closing the capsule

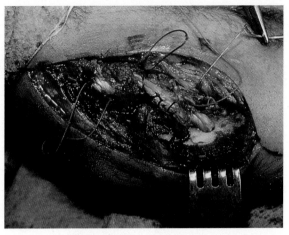
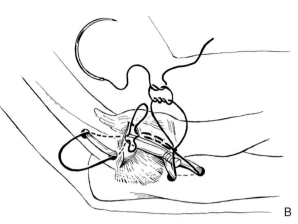

A   B

Figure 15-14. A,B: The reconstruction can be augmented by passing a heavy No. 2 absorbable (Dexon) suture through the same course as the tendon graft. If this is done, the suture should be woven through the capsule in an arch and not permitted to fall deep to the capsule. This is particularly important when a longitudinal arthrotomy is used because the tendon will rub on the side of the capitellum and radial head.

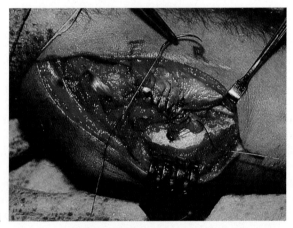
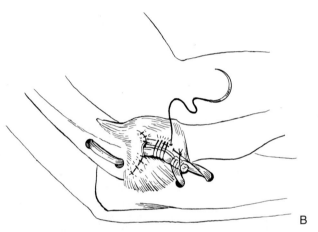

A   B

Figure 15-15. A,B: The capsule is closed and plicated, and the original arch of the ulnar part of the LCL is restored by pulling the graft anteriorly and suturing it to the capsule. This also prevents the graft from slipping posterior to the radial head. The capsule must be closed under the graft to prevent it from rubbing on the radial head or capitellum.

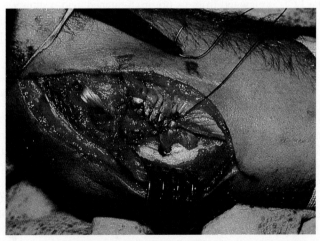
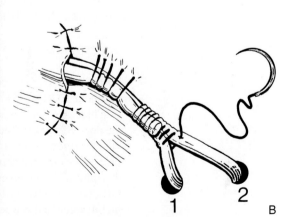

A   B

Figure 15-16. A,B: If further tension is desirable, this can be accomplished by closing the distal triangular opening between the two limbs of the graft. The closure is routine and the forearm is held pronated until the limb is immobilized.

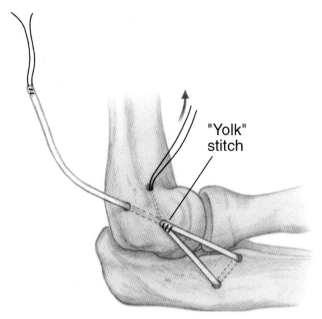

Figure 15-17. The short arm of the graft is secured to the long arm with a "yolk" stitch so both enter the isometric hole.

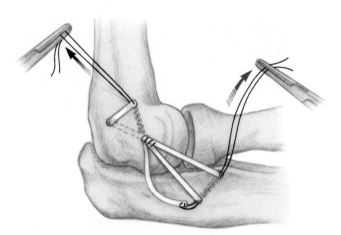

Figure 15-18. The long arm is looped through the humeral tunnels. Tension is maintained on the "yolk" stitch, which is drawn through the humeral hole for this purpose. If length allows and clinical goals require a third "arm," the graft is brought back through the ulnar tunnel.

beneath the graft, and it is quicker. The former is necessary to prevent the graft from rubbing on the joint margins or slipping posterior to the radial head.

More recently, the author (BFM) makes the distal holes in the ulna on a line perpendicular to the LUCL reconstruction (Fig. 15-8C). Proximally, we have also been making hole No. 5 the distal posterior hole on the humerus anterior to the supracondylar ridge. This permits wrapping the tendon over the strong bone in the supracondylar ridge. Finally, we have also been employing a yolk stitch. By suturing the end of the ligament to the rest of the graft so both "arms" of the reconstruction enter the isometric hole, tension is placed on the suture that is not yet cut, as well as on the long arm of the graft (Fig. 15-17). The long end is then wrapped around the supracondylar ridge and then distally to enter the ulna tunnel (Fig. 15-18).

The closure in both the standard and modified procedure is routine and the forearm is kept in full pronation to protect the repair until the limb is immobilized.

In children with open epiphyseal plates, the graft would cross the physis, so we do not do this operation. Instead the LCL is elevated from its origin, tightened, and resutured to the isometric point on the lateral epicondyle with heavy sutures that pass through bone but not through the physis. The method is similar to that described by Osborne and Cotterill (11).

POSTOPERATIVE MANAGEMENT

Postoperatively, the elbow is usually immobilized in a locked hinge brace in full pronation for about 10 days. Then protected motion is allowed in the brace with a 30-degree extension block for 3 to 6 weeks. The period of immobilization and bracing varies depending on the degree of generalized laxity of the patient, the security of the repair, the history of previous episodes of immobilization (and whether or not they caused stiffness), and the attitude of the surgeon about the appropriateness of immobilizing an elbow. We have varied this quite a bit ourselves, ranging from immediate motion in a brace for 6 weeks to immobilization for 6 weeks followed by bracing for up to 3 months. In general, 10 days of immobilization and 6 weeks of protected motion are used. Children and those patients who have previously undergone prolonged immobilization for up to 6 weeks without developing contractures are thought to be at less risk of developing contractures and are immobilized for 3 to 6 weeks. As our experience and follow-up accumulate, these guidelines will certainly change.

RESULTS

In general, the results of surgery have been rewarding. Osborne and Cotterill (11) reported that eight patients treated for recurrent elbow dislocations during a 4-year period by imbrication and reattachment of the LCL did not experience any recurrences. Our initial experience with reconstruction in patients ranging from 4 to 49 years of age has just been recently updated by Sanchez-Sotelo et al. In the group of 42 patients, stability was restored in about 90%, and excellent results (no pain, no loss of motion, no instability) occur in about 60% (6). As noted in the original report, the update confirms that. If arthritis was present or the radial head had been excised, the outcome was less predictable (6,12). The other 40% complain of either some pain or loss of motion, although this could be related to the fact that they typically have had one or more previous operations. In the primary case of untreated instability, the results are highly successful.

COMPLICATIONS

Complications to date have included one case of rupture of the palmaris longus tendon during harvesting, one case in which the length of tendon harvested was suboptimal (the repair was not as secure, although the patient's instability has not yet recurred), one saphenous nerve neuroma from the semitendinosus donor site, and one deep vein thrombosis (DVT) in a patient with a prior history of DVTs. There has been one instance of fracture of the humeral tunnel site.

ILLUSTRATIVE CASE

A 20-year-old woman experienced an elbow dislocation 4 years earlier. She had been immobilized for almost 3 weeks. Her presenting complaint was that the elbow slipped out of joint with certain stress, especially when the elbow was extended and supinated. The lateral rotatory stress test showed posterior lateral rotatory instability, as did the varus stress test (Fig. 15-19). A palmaris longus tendon was harvested (Fig. 15-20) and the lateral complex was reconstructed as described earlier (Fig. 15-21). One year later her motion was normal and the joint was stable (Fig. 15-22).

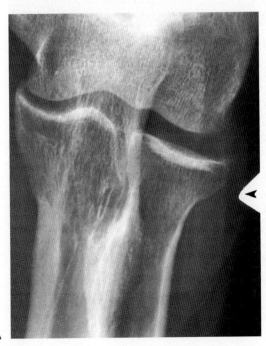
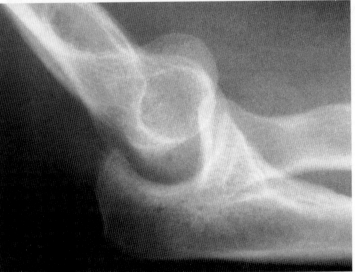

A

B

Figure 15-19. A,B: Stress radiographs reveal a deficiency of the lateral collateral ligament with varus and posterolateral rotary stress.

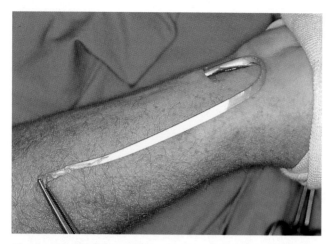

Figure 15-20. The ipsilateral palmaris longus tendon has been harvested.

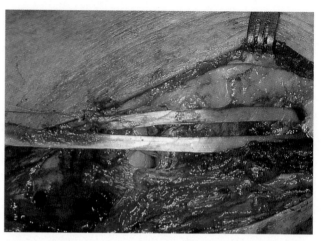

Figure 15-21. The graft is placed in the isometric position as described in Fig. 15-9.

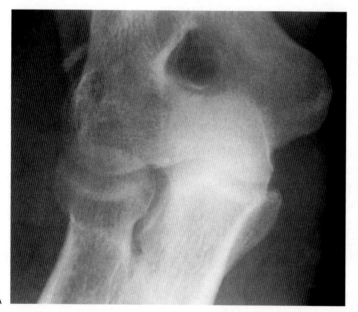

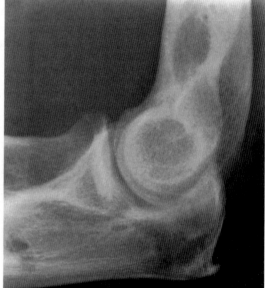

A   B

Figure 15-22. A,B: One year later the joint is painless and stable.

Acknowledgment We are grateful to Gino Mallucci, B.Sc.B.M.C., and Paul Pede, B.Sc.B.M.C. for the medical illustrations.

RECOMMENDED READINGS

1. Grant JCB. *An atlas of anatomy.* Baltimore: Williams & Wilkins; 1972:49–57.
2. Kinast C, Jakob RP. Differentialdiagnostik bei Ellbogenge-lenksblockierungen—die Subluxationsstressaufnahmetechnik. *Hefte Zur Unfallheilkunde* 1986;181:339–341.
3. Langman J, Woerdeman MW. *Atlas of medical anatomy.* Philadelphia: WB Saunders; 1978:266.
4. Martin BF. The annular ligament of the superior radio-ulnar joint. *J Anat* 1959;92:473–481.
5. Morrey BF. Anatomy of the elbow joint. In: Morrey B, ed. *The elbow and its disorders.* Philadelphia: WB Saunders; 1985:21–22.
6. Nestor BJ, O'Driscoll SW, Morrey BF. Ligamentous reconstruction for posterolateral instability of the elbow. *J Bone Joint Surg* 1992;74A:1235–1241.
7. Netter FH. Musculoskeletal system. Part I: Anatomy, physiology, and metabolic disorders. *The Ciba Collection of Medical Illustrations.* Summit, MJ: Ciba-Geigy; 1987;197:43.

8. O'Driscoll SW, Bell DF, Morrey BF. Posterolateral rotatory instability of the elbow. *J Bone Joint Surg* 1991;73A:440–446.

9. O'Driscoll SW, Horii E, Morrey BF, et al. Anatomy of the ulnar part of the lateral collateral ligament of the elbow. *Clin Anat* 1992;5:296–303.

10. O'Driscoll SW, Morrey BF, Korinek S, et al. Elbow subluxation and dislocation: a spectrum of instability. *Clin Orthop* 1992;280:17–28.

11. Osborne G, Cotterill P. Recurrent dislocation of the elbow. *J Bone Joint Surg* 1965;48B:340–346.

12. Sanchez-Sotelo J, Morrey BF, O'Driscoll S. Reconstruction of the lateral ulnar collateral ligament. (Submitted)

13. Schwab GH, Bennett JB, Woods GW, et al. Biomechanics of elbow instability: the role of the medial collateral ligament. *Clin Orthop* 1980;146:42–52.

14. Spalteholz W. *Hand atlas of human anatomy,* Barker LF, trans. Philadelphia: JB Lippincott; 1923:183.

15. Tullos HS, Schwab G, Bennett JB, et al. Factors influencing elbow instability. *Instr Course Lect* 1981;30:185–199.

16

Nerve Decompression

Morton Spinner and Robert J. Spinner

ULNAR NERVE

INDICATIONS/CONTRAINDICATIONS

In recent years the trend has been away from early surgery for ulnar nerve compression lesions at the elbow. Although conservative management may be appropriate for spontaneous ulnar neuritis, it is not indicated in certain instances associated with fractures or dislocations. If the ulnar nerve is entrapped or impaled by fracture fragments, or trapped in the joint following reduction of a dislocation, early surgery is appropriate. If an open injury exists or if open reduction of the fracture is necessary, then primary concomitant surgical evaluation and management of the ulnar nerve should be performed.

Conservative management is appropriate when progressive objective signs of neuropathy are not present. The conservative management consists of instructing the patient to avoid leaning on the elbow on the inner aspect and prolonged elbow flexion. A long arm splint with the elbow at 70 degrees of flexion, the forearm in midposition, and the wrist in neutral position is worn full-time for approximately 4 to 6 weeks. With improvement, the splint is then used only at night for an additional 2 to 3 months. If the patient improves with this management, as happens in about 50% of cases, surgery can be avoided.

The patient is followed clinically for his or her subjective complaints. Often the numbness that is in the little finger improves after 10 days; on occasion, symptoms are relieved within a day or two. Weakness of the hand is a common finding in ulnar paresis. Even without clawing of the fingers, there may be weakness of the intrinsic muscles. In our experience, the pinch dynamometer mirrors the electromyographic studies. If the strength improves, so does the electrical conduction across the elbow.

With clinical improvement, the conservative treatment is continued, usually for 3 months. After removal of the night splint, the patient is instructed not to sleep with the el-

M. Spinner, M.D.: Department of Orthopaedic Surgery, Albert Einstein College of Medicine, New York, New York.

R.J. Spinner, M.D.: Departments of Neurologic Surgery and Orthopedics, Mayo Medical School, Mayo Foundation, Rochester, Minnesota.

bow fully flexed, but rather to put it out straight or on a pillow at night. If necessary a 70-degree flexion splint can be worn. Certainly if the condition recurs and there is no evidence of atrophy of the intrinsic muscles, the splint can be worn for an additional 6- to 8-week period.

Surgery is indicated when the sensory loss does not subside, and if there is progressive atrophy of the intrinsic muscles and weakness as observed with the pinch dynamometer. Serial electrodiagnostic studies in this instance, if performed, reveal slowing of conduction of the ulnar nerve across the elbow, and fibrillations and sharp waves in the ulnar nerve innervated intrinsic muscles.

If confusing variables exist, such as worker's compensation or pending litigation, surgical intervention should be considered very carefully and reluctantly.

PREOPERATIVE PLANNING

The correct localization of the lesion is vital. The patient can have a pure ulnar nerve lesion at the elbow or a double-crush lesion, most frequently at the elbow and the neck. Fibrillations on electromyographic studies in the cervical paravertebral muscle region would suggest a more proximal lesion. A conduction block across the elbow would confirm and localize the lesion to the elbow. Nevertheless, one can have a lesion at both regions in a double-crush lesion.

The usual sensory symptomatology of ulnar nerve compression at the elbow is numbness in the dorsal and palmar aspects of the little finger and half of the ring finger. For clinical localization of the neural lesion to the elbow level, sensory loss on the dorsoulnar aspect of the hand is a characteristic finding. With more proximal neural involvement (i.e., in the chest, thoracic outlet, or neck), a different pattern of sensory disturbance involving the forearm or arm would be present. However, when the little finger is numb only on the palmar side, the ulnar nerve compression is usually at the level of the canal of Guyon.

Motor involvement from an elbow level localization may result in paresis or paralysis of the flexor carpi ulnaris, flexor digitorum profundus of the ring and little fingers, and the ulnar-innervated hand intrinsics. A positive percussion sign helps localize the problem to the elbow, but false-positives are not uncommon findings in patients with "irritable" nerves. Dislocation of the ulnar nerve, with or without snapping on elbow flexion, is often associated with a positive percussion sign at the elbow level. It is also important to be sure that the patient who has a symptomatic dislocating and snapping ulnar nerve does not have a coexistent snapping medial triceps. The dislocating ulnar nerve and snapping triceps can be diagnosed clinically preoperatively (and typically intraoperatively); it can be embarrassing to translocate the ulnar nerve anteriorly and have persistence of the snapping postoperatively with elbow flexion due to a triceps snap.

SURGERY

Indications for specific types of ulnar nerve procedures remain controversial. In our practice, we have attempted to correlate electromyographic studies to the type of operative procedure. The simple release of the arcade and the cubital tunnel retinaculum can be utilized in those cases in which the compression is at that site and the patient has persistent symptoms of mild ulnar neuropathy with minimal or no electrical findings after appropriate conservative care fails. It should not be utilized with a dislocating ulnar nerve.

When ulnar nerve symptoms are caused by a dislocating ulnar nerve, it is best to perform anterior translocation, since the soft-tissue restraints typically released in an *in situ* decompression are not present. A completely dislocating ulnar nerve, in contrast to a subluxating nerve, rarely causes problems. However, thin patients with minimal subcutaneous fat may especially become symptomatic. A dislocating nerve may be vulnerable to friction over the medial epicondyle; a subluxating nerve may be susceptible to compression against the epicondyle or by direct trauma.

Anterior translocation of the ulnar nerve is a commonly practiced surgical procedure. We prefer the anterior translocation, either subcutaneous or submuscular, over *in situ* decompression, when there is electrical indication confirming the patient's more severe ulnar nerve involvement, especially when axonal degeneration is present. Of subcutaneous and submuscular transposition, we prefer the submuscular transposition.

Additional techniques are advocated by some other authors. We have not been placing the nerve intramuscularly, as we have often treated patients with recurrent neurologic symptoms. We do not recommend the modification of the Learmonth procedure in which the flexor pronator muscles are detached directly from the epicondyle and reattached to it, or when the epicondyle is osteotomized. In addition, we do not perform medial epicondylectomy.

Isolated Decompression Without Translocation

A general anesthesia is given and the extremity is placed on an arm board after preparation and draping (Fig. 16-1). The arm is externally rotated and a few folded sheets are placed under the elbow to elevate it. The medial aspect of the elbow is in view, with the medial epicondyle prominent. When the ulnar nerve is not to be translocated, a longitudinal incision 6 to 8 cm long is made centered at the region of the cubital tunnel retinaculum. The terminal branches of the medial cutaneous nerve of the arm and the crossing branches of the medial cutaneous nerve of the forearm in the region of the olecranon should be preserved. They are found deep to the fat just superficial to the fascia overlying the flexor carpi ulnaris (Fig. 16-2). A rubber band is placed about each of them so they can be retracted. The ulnar nerve, which passes longitudinally just deep to the aponeurotic origin of the flexor carpi ulnaris, can be palpated.

The aponeurosis is incised (Fig. 16-3). The cubital tunnel retinaculum (Fig. 16-4), which is about 4 mm wide, is released. Hemostasis is obtained with a Malis hyfrecator; an epineurotomy of the ulnar nerve is usually not necessary. If, after release of the soft-tissue restraints, the ulnar nerve dislocates with elbow flexion, an anterior transposition should be performed. The wound is closed.

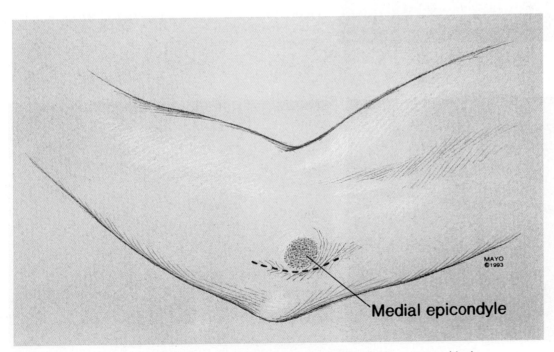

Figure 16-1. The arm is draped free and placed on an arm board. The proposed incision for an *in situ* decompression is demonstrated.

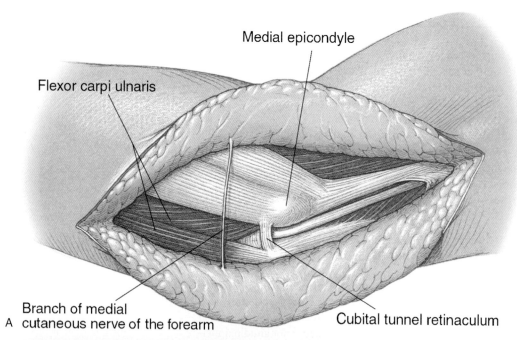

Medial epicondyle

Flexor carpi ulnaris

Branch of medial
A cutaneous nerve of the forearm

Cubital tunnel retinaculum

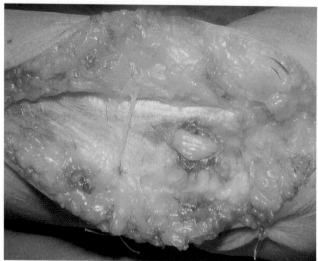

B

Figure 16-2. A,B: Typical appearance of the nerve at the cubital tunnel. Note the crossing branch of medial cutaneous nerve of forearm.

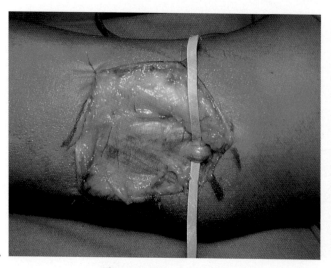

A

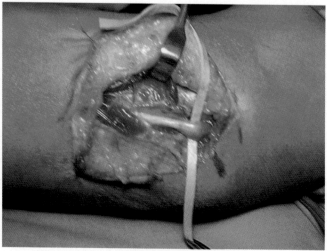

B

Figure 16-3. Compression of the nerve at this level (**A**) is seen clearly following release of the cubital tunnel retinaculum (**B**).

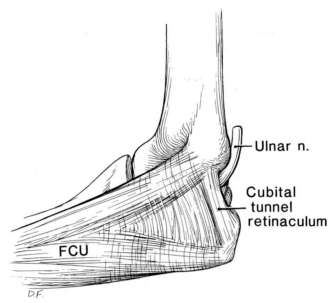

Figure 16-4. A schematic representation of the cubital tunnel.

Subcutaneous Translocation

The patient is usually under general anesthesia in a supine position, and a tourniquet is in place (Fig. 16-1). In a primary case, an approximately 15-cm-long incision is made, curved posterior to the medial epicondyle, centered on the epicondyle. The medial cutaneous nerves of the arm and forearm are identified and preserved. The ulnar nerve is identified in virgin tissue proximal to the elbow and mobilized with its extrinsic vasculature. The arcade of Struthers is released when it is found 8 cm proximal to the epicondyle (Fig. 16-5A,B). An anatomic point for the presence of the arcade is in the appearance of muscle fibers of the medial head of the triceps crossing superficial to the ulnar nerve (Fig. 16-5C). The arcade is released (Fig. 16-5D,E), and the medial intermuscular septum is freed and excised (Fig. 16-6).

The ulnar nerve is traced distally. The cubital tunnel retinaculum is released, as is the flexor carpi ulnaris aponeurosis. Just distal to the elbow joint, the articular branch is encountered and should be released. The motor branches to the flexor carpi ulnaris and the flexor digitorum profundus branch should be preserved. These branches are mobilized microsurgically from the ulnar nerve as much as necessary to permit the anterior neural transposition. These steps permit the ulnar nerve to be easily brought forward over the epicondyle.

The nerve is transposed straight without sharp bends in either plane to prevent kinking of the ulnar nerve distal to the epicondyle by the common aponeurosis between the flexor digitorum superficialis of the ring finger and the humeral head of the flexor carpi ulnaris (Fig. 16-7). When the nerve is translocated anteriorly in the subcutaneous plane (Fig. 16-8), it therefore runs a straight course.

During closure, the fascia of the skin flap is sutured to the antebrachial fascia just lateral to the epicondyle. This maintains the ulnar nerve anteriorly. A fascial sling can be utilized alternatively to stabilize the nerve in an anterior position.

Learmonth Submuscular Transposition

The first half of the procedure is similar to that described in the subcutaneous technique. It differs in that the incision is longer, being 8–10 cm proximal and distal to the epicondyle. Furthermore, a sterile tourniquet is utilized.

The second half of the procedure is not difficult, but it is technically demanding with two principles in mind. First, the ulnar nerve must pass in a straight line. The longitudinal extrinsic vascular supply should be maintained during mobilization of the ulnar nerve. This should be preserved as far distally as possible by ligating the muscular communicating branches, thus keeping the extraneural vascular supply with the ulnar nerve. One can usually maintain the full length of the venae commitantes to the elbow level. The vascular variations about the elbow usually prevent full maintenance of the extrinsic vascular supply. On rare occasion, the senior author has seen an ulnar nerve that had only an intrinsic vascular supply and he mobilized it as necessary to perform the procedure without difficulty. Second, the ulnar nerve must run parallel to the median nerve in a good soft tissue bed. If the deep bed is inadequate, as in severe arthrosis or with bad articular fractures, especially

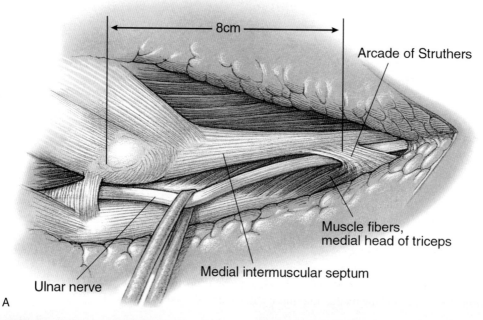

A

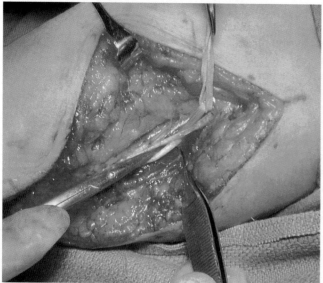

B

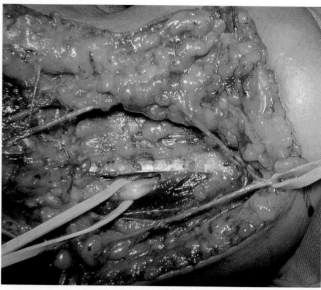

C

Figure 16-5. The arcade of Struthers is demonstrated with the ulnar nerve passing through it. It arises about 8 cm proximal to the epicondyle (**A,B**). Muscular fibers of the medial head of the triceps are seen when an arcade is present (as in approximately 70% of limbs) (**C**). *(continued)*

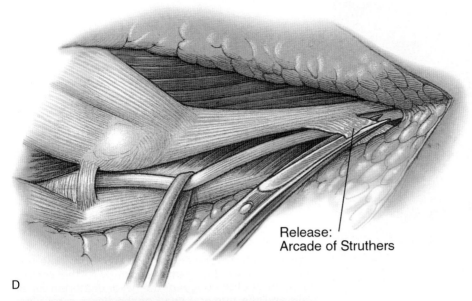

Release:
Arcade of Struthers

D

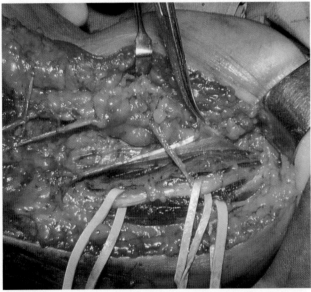

E

Figure 16-5. *Continued.* Release of the arcade of Struthers is necessary when translocating the ulnar nerve anteriorly (**D,E**).

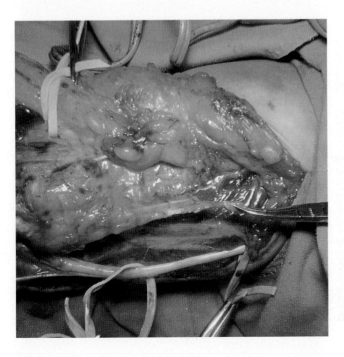

Figure 16-6. The medial intermusuclar septum (in the hemostat) is being removed.

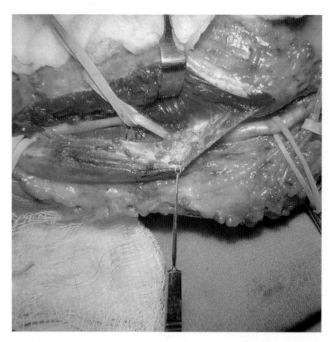

Figure 16-7. To prevent an entrapment of the ulnar nerve distal to the medial epicondyle, the common aponeurosis of the origin of the flexor digitorum superficialis and the humeral head of the flexor carpi ulnaris must be released.

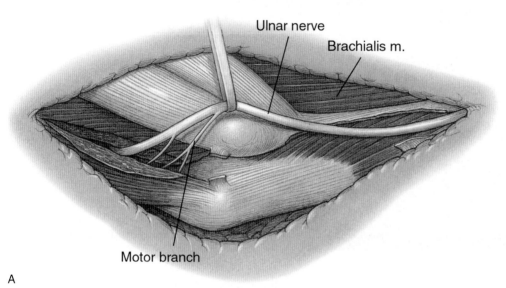

Ulnar nerve

Brachialis m.

Motor branch

A

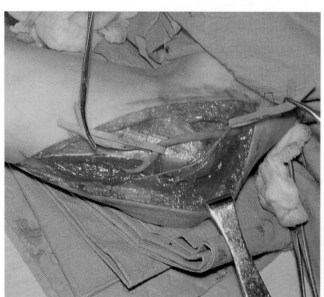

B

Figure 16-8. Subcutaneous anterior translocation of the ulnar nerve is seen with the nerve in a straight line. The articular branch has been released. The muscular branches are preserved (**A,B**).

of the medial half of the elbow joint, a subcutaneous transposition of the ulnar nerve is a better choice.

In the next phase of the dissection, the lacertus fibrosus is visualized by elevating the lateral skin flap. The cutaneous nerves are preserved. The median nerve is identified deep to the lacertus. A rubber band is placed about it and the overlying fascia is released. The limits of the flexor pronator muscles are clearly in view. The median nerve is lateral to it and the ulnar nerve is medial. A large tonsillar hemostat is inserted just distal to the epicondyle from the lateral side deep to the flexor pronator muscles, avoiding the recurrent vessels. The flexor pronator group of muscles is severed 1.5 to 2 cm distal to the medial epicondyle (Fig. 16-9). The exit of the hemostat on the medial side may be troublesome, and the lateral two-thirds of the muscle is first incised and then the hemostat is repassed. Muscle bleeders are clamped and tied. Using a periosteal elevator, the flexor pronator muscles are stripped distally. Motor branches to the flexor pronator mass may need to be neurolyzed to prevent undue tension on them during the muscle elevation.

The tourniquet is released. The field must be dry before the ulnar nerve is translocated (Fig.

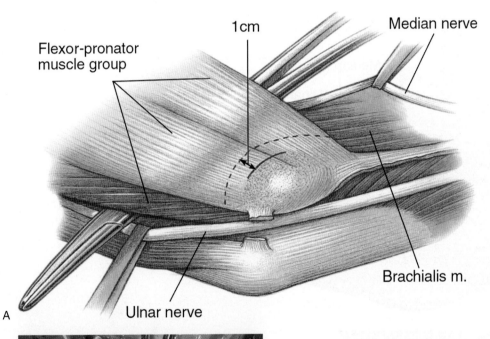

A

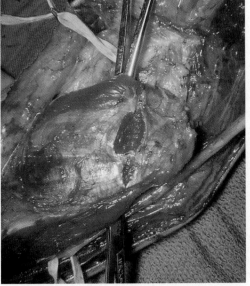

B

Figure 16-9. The tonsillar hemostat is deep to the flexor pronator group of muscles. It is usually inserted from the lateral side. Care is given to avoiding the collateral vessels on the anteromedial aspect of the elbow joint. It is superficial to the brachialis fascia. The adjacent rubber band is about the median nerve. The ulnar nerve is medial (**A,B**).

16-10) and the flexor pronator group of muscles is repaired either in its original or in an elongated (e.g., Z-lengthened) position. Multiple 2-0 interrupted Maxon sutures are utilized. The fascia of the medial longitudinal incision in the flexor pronator muscles is closed with 3-0 chromic sutures (Fig. 16-11). The skin is closed with interrupted nylon sutures or staples.

On occasion, microsurgical epineurotomy may be necessary to address focal scarring (Fig. 16-12). The perineurium is rarely released.

Following anterior transposition of the ulnar nerve, the elbow should be flexed and extended passively to ensure that any site of compression has been eliminated and that any dislocation of the nerve or triceps has been corrected. A dislocating medial triceps can be treated by excision or lateral transposition of the offending portion of triceps (Fig. 16-13).

Revision Surgery

Patients may present with persistent or recurrent ulnar nerve symptoms, often admixed with elbow pain, sometimes with snapping. Failed ulnar nerve surgery is typically due to either

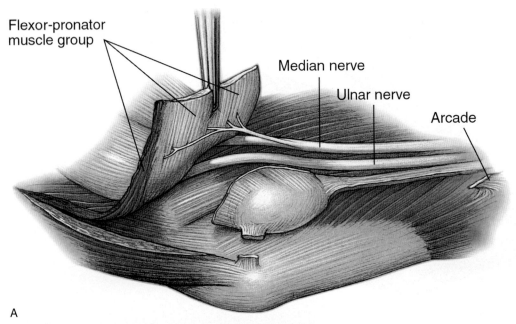

A

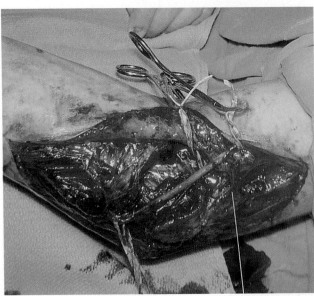

B

Figure 16-10. The tourniquet has been released. The ulnar nerve has been transferred deep to the flexor pronator group of muscles (**A**) adjacent to the median nerve (in rubber band) (**B**).

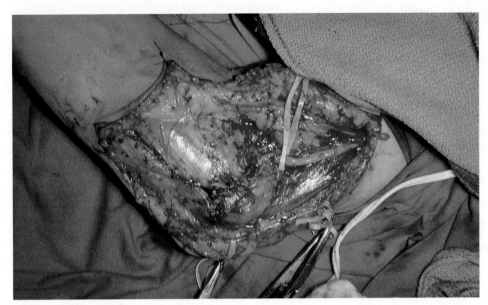

Figure 16-11. The flexor pronator group of muscle has been repaired. The ulnar nerve has been translocated submuscularly.

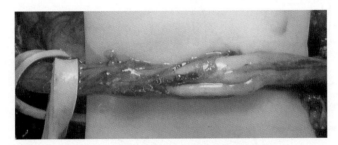

Figure 16-12. Epineurotomy of the nerve is necessary in some secondary cases.

misdiagnosis or compression from incomplete decompression of the original pathology or from secondary compression due to kinking at a nonreleased proximal or distal structure, scarring within a surgical bed or constriction by an overly tight sling. Neuromas from cutaneous nerves may result in new pain or dysethesias. Recurrent ulnar nerve dislocation may result from a ruptured sling or suture, and persistent snapping may become manifest after transposition due to unrecognized dislocation of the medial triceps.

Selection of patients who would best benefit from revision surgery is extremely difficult. Based on our experiences, we are more cognizant of the potential for kinking of the ulnar nerve when just a small incision is made and the nerve is pulled anteriorly. It can angulate very easily. Kinking of the ulnar nerve typically occurs several centimeters proximal or distal to the medial epicondyle. For example, the translocated nerve may be entrapped in a dense tendinous path, especially if the distal aponeurotic arch has not been released (Fig. 16-14). Other factors that may sway us include patients who underwent previous *in situ* decompression without relief, or intramuscular transposition with transient relief. Conversely, factors that would discourage secondary surgery include procedures performed by experienced surgeons or operative notes that sounded technically sufficient, or patients with a bizarre array of somatic complaints. In addition, patients presenting with evidence of chronic, severe neurologic findings or muscle fibrosis would not benefit from revision. In these patients, one can estimate how many motor fibers are left in the hand with the pinch dynamometer. If the strength of pinch on the dynamometer is less than 1 kg, motor fibers

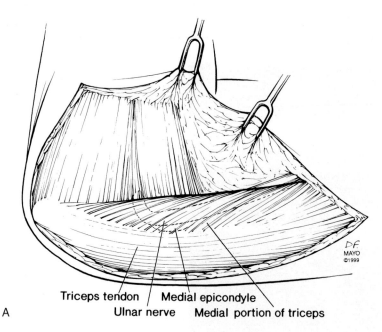

A

Triceps tendon | Medial epicondyle
Ulnar nerve | Medial portion of triceps

Figure 16-13. A: Snapping of a portion of the medial triceps and dislocation of the ulnar nerve needs to be considered in patients undergoing ulnar nerve surgery. Patients should be examined for snapping triceps preoperatively and intraoperatively. **B:** The offending dislocating portion of the triceps can be excised or transposed laterally. *(continued)*

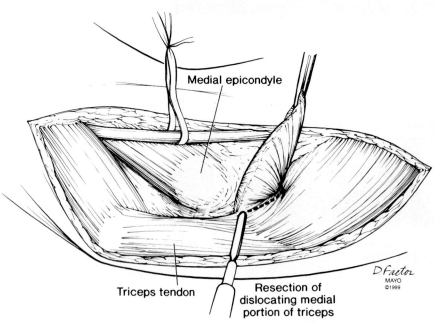

Medial epicondyle

Triceps tendon | Resection of dislocating medial portion of triceps

B

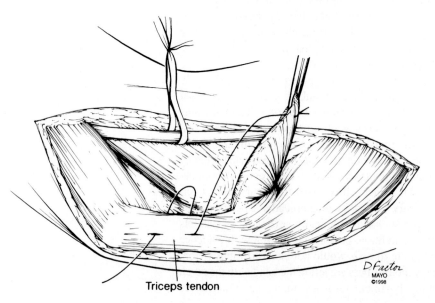

Triceps tendon

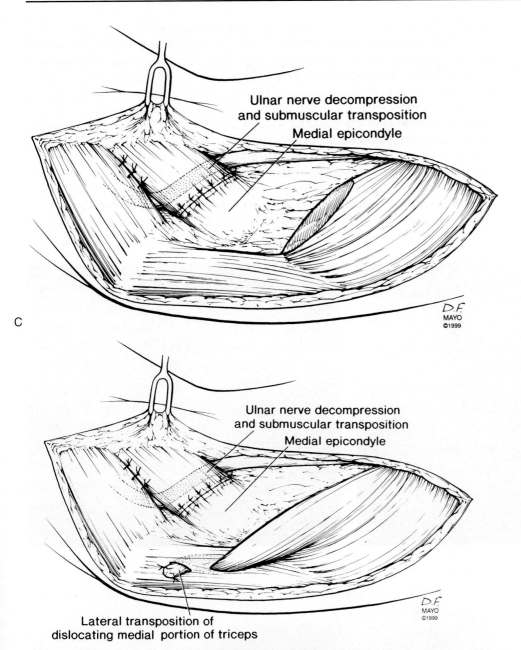

C

Figure 16-13. *Continued.* **C:** Neurolysis and transposition of the ulnar nerve can then be performed. A submuscular transposition was performed in these examples. Snapping of the triceps was eliminated. (From Spinner RJ, O'Driscoll SW, Jupiter JB, et al. Unrecognized dislocation of the medial portion of the triceps: another cause of failed ulnar nerve transposition. *J Neurosurg* 2000;92:52–57, with permission.)

may well be all out and the nerve can be almost nonfunctioning. Electrical conductivity can be on the order of 0 to 17 m/sec across the elbow. If the patient has had a prior anterior translocation and is in this poor state, submuscular transposition may offer little if any chance of success and could increase the symptomatology with an infarcted nerve.

The old scar is incorporated into the new longer scar. A Brunner zigzag type is frequently used in secondary procedures. The incision often extends 10 to 12 cm proximal and distal to the epicondyle. It is particularly important to define normal tissue planes. To identify the ulnar nerve through the region of the earlier surgery most easily, one should isolate the nerve proximally and distally and then trace it through the elbow region. The multiple muscular branches to the flexor carpi ulnaris and the one to the flexor digitorum profundus should be preserved. Of these, the most important is the branch to the flexor digitorum profundus; failure to maintain its continuity results in the inability to flex the distal interphalangeal joint of the little finger. On occasion, the ulnar nerve distally must be identified in the midforearm. The plane between the flexor carpi ulnaris and flexor digitorum superficialis is developed to identify and trace the ulnar nerve proximally to the elbow. Crossing vessels are clamped and tied with fine sutures. The deep fascia over the nerve is released to permit the mobilization. The muscular branches are preserved. The Learmonth procedure has proved to be the most reliable salvage operation.

In addition, these patients often have painful neuromas from the primary surgery. These must be removed, and the ends of the nerves should retract into normal fatty tissue. To prevent recurrent neuromas, gently pull down the involved medial cutaneous nerve of the arm or forearm and double-crush the nerve a centimeter apart. The site of the distal crush is tied with 5-0 nonabsorbent suture and the nerve is severed just distal to the suture. The nerve ends can also be bipolared.

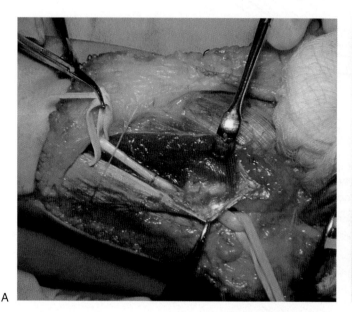

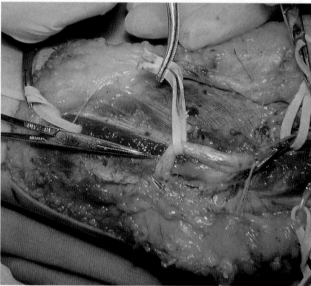

A   B

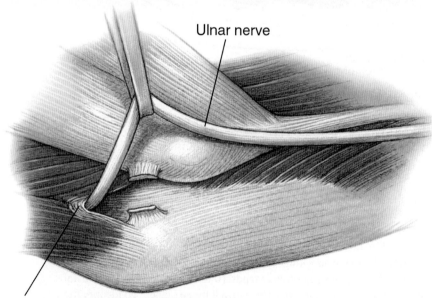

C Flexor carpi ulnaris: inadequate release

Figure 16-14. The ulnar nerve is seen passing below the arcade distal to the medial epicondyle (**A**). If the arcade is not released, then kinking at the level distal to the elbow joint can be produced with a limited anterior ulnar nerve translocation (**B,C**). *(continued)*

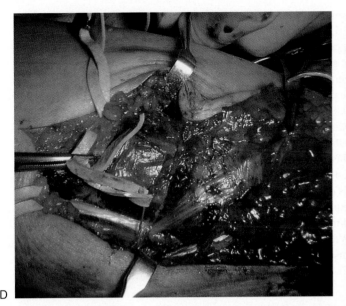

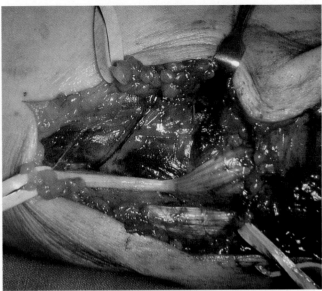

D

E

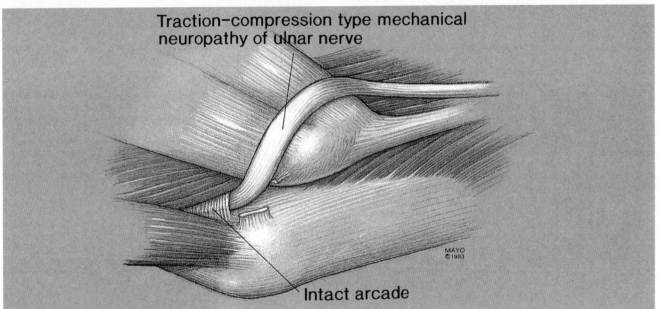

Traction–compression type mechanical neuropathy of ulnar nerve

Intact arcade

MAYO
©1993

F

Figure 16-14. *Continued.* A case in which this was the cause of the resistant ulnar nerve neuritis: A traction-compression type mechanical neuropathy of the ulnar nerve is noted distal to the epicondyle (**D–F**).

In rare cases, the senior author has used interposition of a thin Silastic sheathing on one side of the nerve. Usually there is good fat on the anterior side, while the Silastic membrane is placed on the side that is adjacent to the dense fascial scar. The Silastic is never put circumferentially about the nerve. This procedure is utilized strictly to help with the traction neuritis. It is placed at the level at which the percussion test is positive.

POSTOPERATIVE MANAGEMENT

After both *in situ* decompression and transposition procedures, the extremity is immobilized in a long-arm posterior splint for 5 to 7 days. Full motion is encouraged after the splint is removed in patients who underwent *in situ* decompression. In patients who had transposition and are relatively pain-free, controlled movement is then initiated that balances the need for gliding of the ulnar nerve in its new transposed bed, and adequate time for healing (e.g., submuscular repair or fascial sling). While anterior translocation provides a more lax environment for the nerve (i.e., an approximately 2-cm-shorter course of the nerve), earlier movement is thought to improve nerve gliding with filmier and longer adhesions that have excursions to them. In this group of patients, elbow flexion is permitted. Elbow extension is gradually increased during the subsequent 2 weeks. As numbness in the little finger resolves and the preoperative pain decreases, movement is progressed once or twice a day for a few minutes over the 3-week period. By starting the mobilization in this manner, providing that there are no untoward symptoms, the patient comes out of the dressing and immobilization at 3 weeks and elbow movement is almost, if not fully, complete. One of the authors (RJS) has extended this concept and starts movement immediately after transposition. Physical therapy is required following the Learmonth to help strengthen and mobilize the arm. In cases where there is digital clawing, an ulnar metacarpophalangeal (MP) joint flexion cap orthosis is often required to prevent hyperextension at the MP joint.

With the simpler procedure of release of the cubital tunnel, the patient is frequently back to work by 3 to 4 weeks. With the anterior subcutaneous transposition, 6 to 8 weeks are required, and with the submuscular Learmonth procedure the disability is usually 3 months.

RESULTS

There are several reports regarding the optimum treatment for ulnar decompression that are not conclusive. Because of variable degrees of compression and neural involvement preoperatively, comparison of different studies and techniques has been difficult. Typically, in addition, the results are strongly a function of the surgeon rather than his or her technique. If the procedure is done properly, approximately an 80–90% satisfactory result can be achieved following ulnar nerve decompression.

Patients who have had one or possibly two prior ulnar nerve surgeries are instructed that we are looking for overall 50% improvement. In them the goal of surgery is often to decrease the severity of the pain. Some improvement in sensation and in strength of the hand, as well as range of movement of the fingers, can be achieved. The Learmonth procedure never restores a fully normal arm in secondary or tertiary cases.

COMPLICATIONS

Persistent or recurrent ulnar neuritis and painful neuromas are not uncommon following nerve decompression. In our experience, ulnar nerve symptoms develop from mechanical irritation that persists or is brought about by an improper translocation, usually with a kink or bend in the nerve or the nerve placed in a region that allows intense scarring. The treatment for this is ideally to avoid the circumstance. This can be done by placing the nerve in as straight a line as possible, as has been emphasized in this surgical technique. Cutaneous nerves must be identified and preserved.

ILLUSTRATIVE CASE

This patient had electromyographic (EMG) evidence of motor dysfunction that required an extensive dissection. A submuscular transposition was performed. Here the flexor pronator group was elevated to a large degree to avoid kinking of the nerve (Fig. 16-15).

RADIAL NERVE ENTRAPMENT

The two major branches of the radial nerve at the level of the elbow are the posterior interosseous and the superficial radial nerves. The posterior interosseous nerve basically is motor, whereas the superficial radial is sensory.

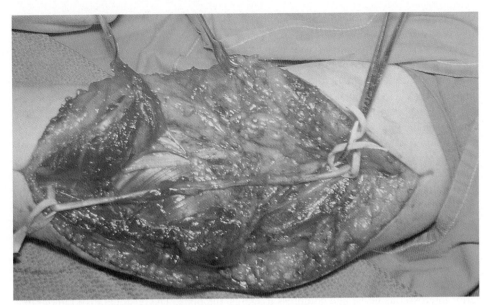

Figure 16-15. Adequate mobilization of the ulnar nerve permitted its straight course during this submuscular translocation.

A small motor branch to the extensor carpi radialis brevis usually arises between these two nerve branches at the division of the radial nerve.

The posterior interosseous nerve forms a cauda equina type arborization pattern 1 cm distal to the distal edge of the supinator muscle.

PREOPERATIVE PLANNING

Identify the etiology and location of the posterior interosseous nerve pathology. The key to localizing the lesion is the classic appearance of the hand. The wrist dorsiflexes in a radial direction, and the fingers do not extend at the MP joints. There is a dropped thumb (Fig. 16-16). Sensation is intact. This is the presentation with a complete lesion. A partial posterior interosseous nerve paralysis presents with weakness or paralysis of some of the digits at MP joints. When the ring and little fingers are initially involved, the term *pseudo-ulnar claw* applies. If there is a dropped wrist, the localization is more proximal in the arm. In contrast to posterior interosseous nerve compression, superficial radial nerve compression would produce isolated sensory disturbance in the dorsoradial aspect of the hand. More commonly, the irritation occurs more distally at the radial styloid or where the nerve passes from beneath the brachioradialis; however, it may occur in the proximal forearm as well.

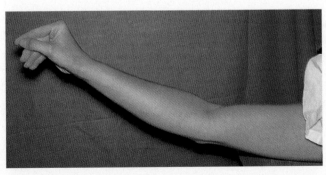
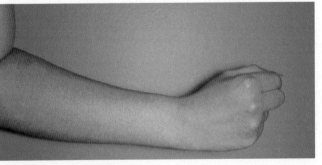

A   B

Figure 16-16. Typical appearance of a hand with a complete posterior interosseous nerve paralysis. The fingers and thumb do not extend at the MCP joints (**A**). The wrist does extend but in a radial direction (**B**).

The site of percussion tenderness can help localize the level of the entrapment to the proximal or distal forearm.

The posterior interosseous nerve is usually entrapped at the proximal end of the supinator muscle (i.e., at the arcade of Frohse). The offending pathology is either the arcade alone or in association with a systematic process like rheumatoid arthritis with synovitis of the elbow joint, a lipoma, a radial bursa, a ganglion, or other soft-tissue tumors. Routine radiographs are of help if they reveal a soft-tissue shadow with the appearance of a lipoma in the region. Changes in the joint suggestive of rheumatoid arthritis in association with a synovitis are often diagnosed with articular changes in the radial head and the adjacent elbow joint. The combination of a posterior radial dislocation of the elbow in a Monteggia fracture with posterior interosseous nerve paralysis is not an infrequent coexistent condition. Similarly, comminuted fractures of the radial head, especially with displacement, can be associated with this specific motoneuron involvement. Fractures and bullet wounds of the proximal third of the radius can be associated with this neural complication. Furthermore, in preoperative planning, computed tomography (CT) and magnetic resonance imaging (MRI) are occasionally helpful in delineating further soft-tissue masses that can be palpable or nonpalpable.

A posterior interosseous nerve paralysis may occur from plating a fracture of the junction of the middle and proximal third of the radius. A six-hole plate may well catch the posterior interosseous nerve and compress it against the bone. The postoperative radiographs reveal the most proximal screw at the level of the bicipital tuberosity. The posterior interosseous nerve passes obliquely directly opposite the bicipital tuberosity, where there is a bare area and entrapment as a complication of plate fixation if diagnosed early can be corrected. Exploration, neurolysis of the posterior interosseous nerve, and replacement of the plate with one that is one hole shorter proximally are usually successful. Similarly, if the posterior interosseous nerve had been identified, a rubber band had been placed about it for retraction at the time of the plating, and paralysis is present after surgery, it is logical to observe this complication without intervention. The lesion may well be neuropractic, because of excess traction on the nerve at the time of the plating. The paralysis may recover spontaneously. In a similar fashion, if one wants to remove a long six-hole plate with three holes proximal to the fracture level, it is wise to identify the posterior interosseous nerve proximally in normal soft tissues. It is then traced through the plated area before removal of the screws and plate. We have treated several patients who have had a posterior interosseous nerve paralysis following plate removal in this area, if the nerve had not been identified before removal of the hardware.

If the posterior interosseous nerve lesion is spontaneous, the lesion most often is at the arcade of Frohse. Electromyographic (EMG) studies will reveal fibrillations in the supinator muscle. If, however, the pathology is at the level of the distal end of the supinator, innervation of the supinator will not be altered. There is a fibrotic band within the muscle that has been described with spontaneous compression directly under the supinator muscle. Here EMG changes within this muscle are most often found.

SURGERY

We use two major approaches for posterior interosseous nerve decompression: the posterior (Thompson) and the anterior (Henry) approaches. If the arcade of Frohse is to be exposed, this is done anteriorly. If the distal third of the supinator is involved, then the exposure can be done either from a posterior approach or with a combination of the anterior and posterior approaches. If there has been prior surgery in the region, then the combined approach must be utilized to gain control of both the proximal and distal portions of the posterior interosseous nerve.

Posterior Approach

To expose the posterior interosseous nerve from the posterior approach, the patient is supine. The arm is draped free and is placed on an arm board, and the forearm is pronated (Fig. 16-17).

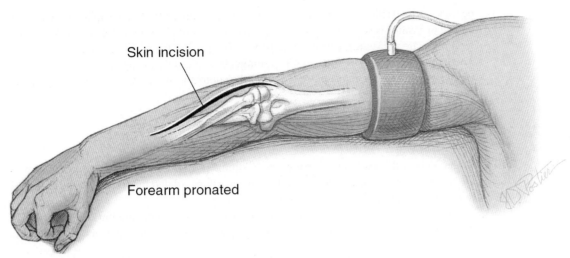

Figure 16-17. To expose the posterior interosseous nerve the arm is draped free and placed on an arm board. The Thompson incision is used to expose the proximal forearm. The incision passes in a line from the wrist to the center of the lateral epicondyle.

The basic Thompson approach is extended proximally onto the arm. In this approach the skin incision is linear in line with the midportion of the wrist and the lateral epicondyle (Fig. 16-17). The incision in the proximal half of the line is extended further proximally onto the lateral ridge of the epicondyle. The posterior cutaneous nerve of the forearm is identified and preserved. The plane between the extensor carpi radialis brevis and extensor digitorum communis is developed from the level of the outcropping muscles in the midforearm proximally (Fig. 16-18). The supinator muscle is seen on the deep plane at the level of the epicondyle. To expose the arcade of Frohse, the following variation in the exposure can be applied: Detach the extensor carpi radialis from its origin at the distal humerus and strip the distal half of the extensor carpi radialis longus. By flexing the elbow and rotating the forearm, the direction and course of the posterior interosseous nerve deep to the superficial head of the supinator is determined by digital palpation. This is done by gently running the index finger over the supinator in a radial-to-ulnar direction. The course of the

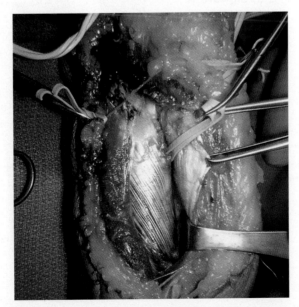

Figure 16-18. The plane between the extensor carpi radialis brevis and the extensor digitorum communis is entered and developed in a distal-to-proximal direction.

nerve is defined (Fig. 16-19). It is followed to the proximal edge of the supinator, where the arcade of Frohse is seen. The posterior interosseous nerve is in fat at this level. At this region there are adjacent recurrent vessels; vessels crossing the nerve are clamped and tied. The nerve can be exposed through its entire course through this approach. The arcade of Frohse is released, as is the entire length of the supinator muscle to its distal end (Fig. 16-20).

Anterior Approach

Under a general anesthesia the patient is in supine position. For exposure of the posterior interosseous nerve, the arm is draped free on an arm board and the forearm is supinated. A tourniquet at 250 mm Hg is utilized.

For exposure of the proximal half of the nerve through the supinator muscle, a curvilinear incision or a chevron incision is made; both of these come lateral to the antecubital crease,

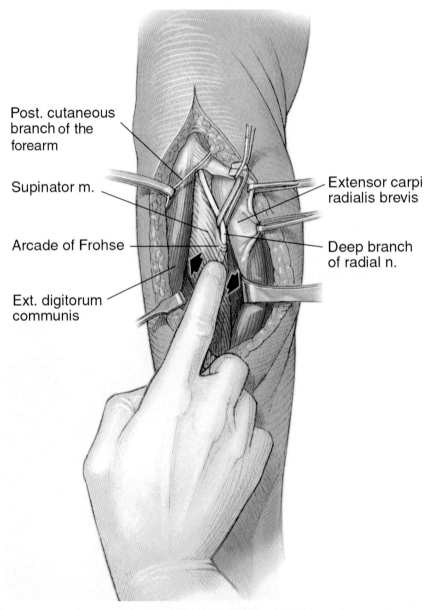

Post. cutaneous branch of the forearm

Supinator m.

Arcade of Frohse

Ext. digitorum communis

Extensor carpi radialis brevis

Deep branch of radial n.

Figure 16-19. The posterior interosseous nerve is identified by palpation. Running the index finger over the supinator muscle in a radial to ulnar direction identifies the location and course of the nerve deep to the muscle.

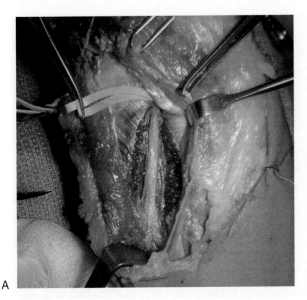

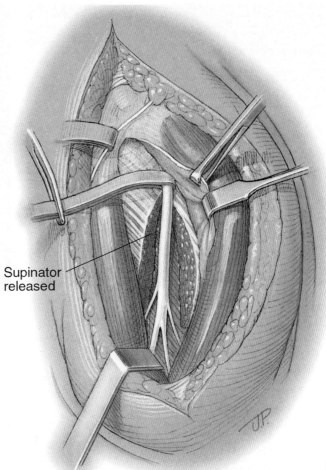

Supinator
released

Figure 16-20. The supinator muscle may be released, exposing the full course of the nerve (**A,B**).

A

B

then down the anterior aspect of the proximal third of the forearm. The lateral antebrachial
cutaneous nerve and its branches will be found just superficial to the antebrachial fascia at
the elbow; rubber bands are placed about it to maintain its identity and to retract a bit.

The radial nerve is identified before its division at the elbow in the interval between the
brachioradialis and the brachialis. A rubber band is placed about it (Fig. 16-21A). The
nerve is then traced distally to its major branches at the elbow level. At the elbow level the
posterior interosseous nerve and the motor branches to the extensor carpi radialis brevis and
the superficial radial nerve are identified. There can be difficulty in identifying the radial
nerve proximally because on occasion there is a fusion between the brachialis and the brachioradialis muscle. Another key to this approach is to identify and protect the superficial
branch of the radial nerve, which is vulnerable to excessive traction. In this instance the superficial radial nerve is identified in the fascia of the brachioradialis on its posterior surface.
It is traced proximally to the main radial trunk and then the other two branches are identified and the dissection is traced distally. Difficulty can occur if one does not stay in the in-
ternervous plane or if there is partial or complete fusion between the brachialis and brachioradialis. The appropriate cleavage plane is identified by tracing the superficial radial
nerve proximally. There is an anterior and posterior leash of vessels about the superficial
radial nerve. These branches of the radial artery are clamped and tied.

The posterior interosseous nerve is traced to the level of the supinator muscle. There are
numerous recurrent branches in this area of the radial recurrent system. These are clamped
and tied (Fig. 16-21B). The posterior interosseous nerve is traced through the proximal half
of the supinator; a hemostat is passed deep to the arcade and the supinator muscle, and superficial to the posterior interosseous nerve. The arcade is cut by sharp dissection with scissors, and the supinator muscle is split. It will be noted that there are numerous branches from

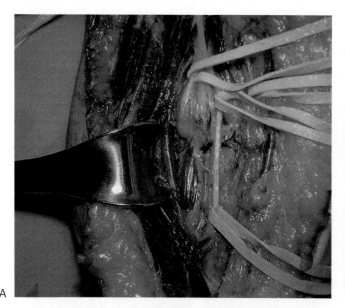
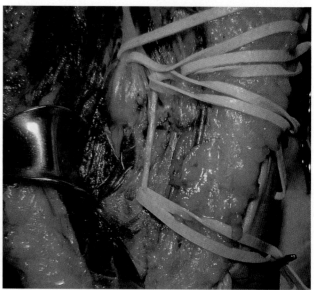

A

C

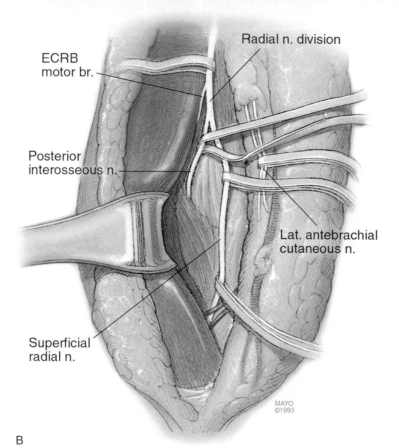

ECRB
motor br.

Radial n. division

Posterior
interosseous n.

Lat. antebrachial
cutaneous n.

Superficial
radial n.

MAYO
©1993

B

Figure 16-21. In the anterior approach, the radial nerve is identified between the brachialis and brachioradialis muscles. The region of the arcade of Frohse is exposed (**A**). The rubber bands are about the lateral antebrachial cutaneous and superficial radial nerves. The posterior interosseous nerve and the motor branch to the extensor carpi radialis brevis are seen. Note the radial recurrent vessels. Some of the key crossing vessels are seen tied (**B**). The arcade of Frohse has been released. See how flattened the nerve is under the arcade (**C**).

the posterior interosseous nerve to the supinator muscle (Fig. 16-21C). With this approach good exposure of the posterior interosseous nerve in this area is obtained. Once the nerve is freed and fully identified, any compressive source such as a ganglion or tumor can be removed. Similarly, if there has been a comminuted fracture of the radial head, once the posterior interosseous nerve has been identified and protected, the radial head can be removed from this anterior approach. Likewise, in those patients with rheumatoid arthritis, a synovectomy can be performed. It should be noted that the motor branch to the extensor carpi radialis brevis is in the field and should be protected with a rubber band as a gentle retractor.

It is important to release the tourniquet before closing the skin incision to ensure hemostasis.

POSTOPERATIVE MANAGEMENT

The patient is placed in a plaster splint, immobilizing the elbow at 90 degrees, the forearm at midposition, and the wrist in neutral. The plaster extends to the proximal interphalangeal (PIP) joints and allows for stabilization of the MP joints in extension for a short period. Postoperatively, active exercises of the PIP and distal interphalangeal (DIP) joints are encouraged. A protective dynamic splint can be utilized afterward in the recovery phase, if necessary. The thumb is sometimes splinted in extension in a static splint at night until there is restoration of full extension of the thumb, as flexion contracture of the DIP joint can develop.

RESULTS

When there is motor paralysis after surgery, galvanic stimulation to the paralyzed muscles is utilized, and the paralysis usually will subside or show improvement gradually over a 3-month period. The last muscle to recover most commonly is the extensor pollicis longus. When this nerve has been compressed or irritated because of a discrete mechanism, decompression is virtually 100% successful. Less predictable are those instances in which the exploratory decompression was performed in association with symptoms of lateral epicondylitis. In general, as the indications for the exploration are less discrete, so also is the likelihood of realizing a satisfactory result.

COMPLICATIONS

The major complications in the operative room result from failure to obtain adequate hemostasis. The tourniquet should be released before closing the skin. It is conceivable to have a Volkmann's type process develop if good hemostasis has not been achieved. This is an important concept, as hematomas cause more inflammation. The fibrosis that can occur in this instance can jeopardize the neural recovery.

Injuries to the superficial radial nerve with exposure or closure are a distinct possibility with posterior interosseous nerve decompression, and great attention to detail is necessary to avoid this complication.

Another problem that is directly related to the postoperative splinting program is due to extension contractures of the MP and interphalangeal joints. This is especially true if outriggers are utilized and the outrigggers extend to the tips of the fingers. If such splints are used, the loop should extend just under the proximal phalanx, leaving the interphalangeal joints free. It is extension of the MP joint that is lost in a posterior interosseous nerve paralysis in the digits. The patient should be allowed to flex his fingers a few times a day with the outriggers completely removed.

ILLUSTRATIVE CASE

A patient with a partial posterior interosseous nerve palsy presented with a "pseudo-ulnar claw" hand of several months' duration (Fig. 16-22A). Radiographs revealed a lucency consistent with a lipoma present in this vicinity of the radial head (Fig. 16-22B). Exploration was performed through an anterior approach and confirmed compression of the posterior interosseous nerve at the arcade of Frohse by a lipoma (Fig. 16-22C). The tumor was resected (Fig. 16-22D). The patient obtained complete recovery in 2 months (Fig. 16-22E).

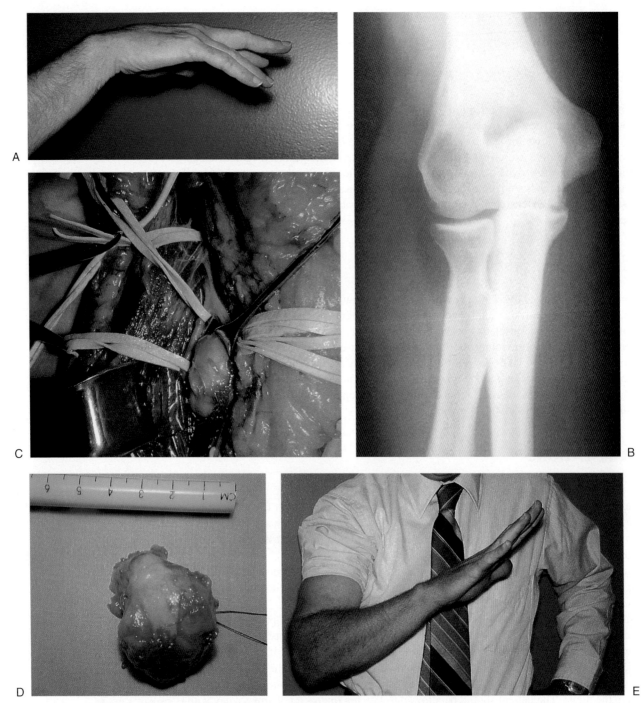

Figure 16-22. A: The "pseudo-ulnar claw" hand representative of a partial posterior interosseous nerve paralysis. It is not a true claw hand seen with low ulnar nerve palsy because there is no hyperextension at the metacarpophalangeal joint of the ring and little fingers; rather, there is a drop in these digits at this joint. **B:** Radiographs revealed a soft-tissue lucency adjacent to the radial head typical of a lipoma. **C:** The lipoma was exposed through the anterior approach. Traction sutures were placed in it to facilitate its delivery of the tumor. The epineurium of the radial nerve was incised longitudinally. This allowed for more room to extricate the tumor safely. **D:** Specimen lipoma. **E:** Recovery occurred gradually over a 6-week period.

RECOMMENDED READINGS

1. Amadio PC, Beckenbaugh RD. Entrapment of the ulnar nerve by the deep flexor pronator aponeurosis. *J Hand Surg* 1986;11A:83–87.
2. Childress HM. Recurrent ulnar-nerve dislocation at the elbow. *Clin Orthop* 1975;108:168–173.
3. Dellon AL. Review of treatment results for ulnar nerve entrapment at the elbow. *J Hand Surg* 1989;14A:688–700.
4. Dellon AL, Mackinnon SE. Injury to the medial antebrachial cutaneous nerve during cubital tunnel surgery. *J Hand Surg* 1985;10B:33–36.
5. Gabel GT, Amadio PC. Reoperation for failed decompression of the ulnar nerve in the region of the elbow. *J Bone Joint Surg* 1990;72:213–219.
6. Inserra S, and Spinner M. An anatomic factor significant in transposition of the ulnar nerve. *J Hand Surg* 1986;11A:80–82.
7. Learmonth JR. Technique for transplanting the ulnar nerve. *Surg Gynecol Obstet* 1942;75:792–793.
8. Leffert RD. Anterior submuscular transposition of the ulnar nerves by the Learmonth technique. *J Hand Surg* 1982;7:147–155.
9. Lundberg G. Editorial. Surgical treatment for ulnar nerve entrapment at the elbow. *J Hand Surg* 1992;17B:245–247.
10. O'Driscoll SW, Horii E, Carmichael SW, et al. The cubital tunnel and ulnar neuropathy. *J Bone Joint Surg* 1991;73B:613–617.
11. Osborne G. The surgical treatment of tardy ulnar neuritis. *J Bone Joint Surg* 1957;39B:782.
12. Rolfsen L. Snapping triceps tendon with ulnar neuritis. *Acta Orthop Scand* 1970;41:74–76.
13. Spinner M, Kaplan EB. The relationship of the ulnar nerve to the medial intermuscular septum in the arm and its clinical significance. *Hand* 1976;8:238–242.
14. Spinner RJ, O'Driscoll SW, Jupiter JB, et al. Unrecognized dislocation of the medial portion of the triceps: another cause of failed ulnar nerve transposition. *J Neurosurg* 2000;92:52–57.
15. Vanderpool DW, Chalmers J, Lamb DW, et al. Peripheral compression lesions of the ulnar nerve. *J Bone Joint Surg* 1968;50B:792–803.

PART IV

Reconstruction

17

Resurfacing Elbow Replacement Arthroplasty

Ian A. Trail, David Stanley, and John K. Stanley

There are many procedures for the management of the destroyed elbow, depending on diagnosis, age, and activity level of the patient, as well as the condition of the bone and ligaments. This chapter reports the indications, planning, surgical technique, and results of resurfacing elbow arthroplasty. Although many resurfacing elbow prostheses are available, this chapter describes only two designs particularly popular in Europe and Asia (4–7), specifically the Souter and the Kudo.

INDICATIONS/CONTRAINDICATIONS

The indications for the use of resurfacing elbow arthroplasty prostheses are those with rheumatoid arthritis who have failed nonoperative measures having intractable pain, limited elbow joint motion, and radiographic evidence of elbow joint destruction. There must be sufficient bone stock to seat and anchor the humeral component on the capitellum and trochlea, and the ulnar component in the trochlear notch of the ulna with bone cement. Low-demand older patients with osteoarthritis or posttraumatic degeneration of the elbow joint are also appropriate indications if the bone stock is adequate, the ligaments and capsule are competent, and the joint is not grossly malaligned.

Contraindications for this type of device include insufficient bone stock to seat the prosthesis, history of sepsis, high-demand young patients, and an absent or attenuated olecranon. These implants are also not usually effective for revision.

PREOPERATIVE PLANNING

With regard to individual patients, there are three criteria. First, the patient must have sufficient bone stock to support the implant; that is, both epicondyles and epicondylar ridges of the humerus must be present. Second, erosion of the olecranon should not preclude ad-

I.A. Trail, m.d., f.r.c.s.: Hand and Limb Department, Wrightington Hospital, Lancashire, England.
D. Stanley, M.D., B.SC., F.R.C.S.: The AMI Thornbury Hospital, Sheffield, England.
J.K. Stanley, M.Ch.ORTH.: University of Manchester, Manchester, England.

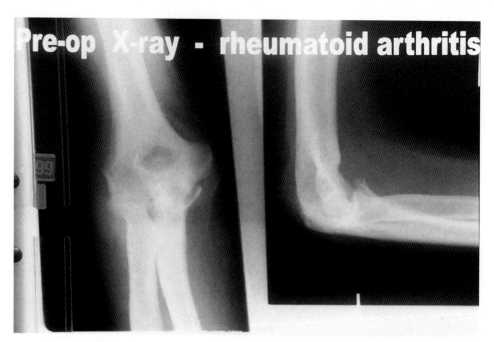

Figure 17-1. Rheumatoid involvement of a 58-year-old female with considerable destruction and alteration of the architecture. There is adequate bone, and the ligaments appear to be intact, allowing consideration of resurfacing implantation.

equate support and fixation of the olecranon component. Finally, the elbow must be stable before surgery. As would be expected, this type of unlinked arthroplasty relies completely on the soft tissues, particularly the collateral ligaments for postoperative stability. It is therefore essential that these be intact and in a satisfactory state before insertion, although the degree of integrity that is required varies according to individual surgeon judgment.

It is also important that the patient have a thorough knowledge of the restrictions imposed and the care required after arthroplasty has been undertaken. More specifically, the elbow should be treated with respect, and repeated heavy lifting, or indeed periods on crutches, or walking sticks, should be avoided. Hence if hip or knee replacement is contemplated, these procedures should precede elbow replacement. Although the Souter is typically not considered in unstable conditions, the Kudo total elbow replacement has been offered for some patients who have either painful stiffness of the elbow or painful instability. Painful stiffness is defined as elbow pain with less than 100 degrees of flexion. This invariably makes it difficult for patients to bring their hand to their face.

Painful instability occurs if, despite adequate passive range of movement, the elbow cannot be actively moved while carrying any weight.

Radiologic Assessment

Patients for whom the Kudo or Souter total elbow replacement is appropriate usually lie between grades III and V of the Larsen et al. classification (8) (Fig. 17-1). Professor Kudo has also on occasion used the implant for mutilans deformity in rheumatoid arthritis (7). In this group of patients, bone grafting is necessary at the time of insertion of the implant.

Before surgery, templates are available such that the appropriate sizing of the humeral and other components can be assessed. The final determination is of course made at the time of surgery.

THE SOUTER-STRATHCLYDE DEVICE (*Ian Trail*)

The Souter-Strathclyde device employs the bone of the medial and lateral supracondylar columns for stable fixation. Currently, both humeral and ulnar components employ stems (Fig. 17-2).

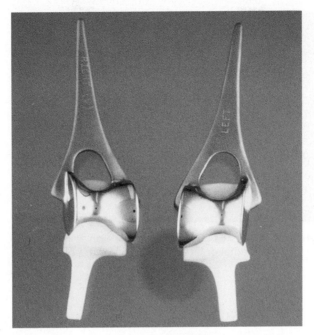

Figure 17-2. The current Souter implant involves an intramedullary stem on the humeral component and a smaller stem on the ulnar component.

SURGERY

The operation is always undertaken under general anesthetic. The patient is brought into the operating room in the lateral decubitus with the arm suspended over a support, which allows free flexion and extension as well as pro-supination of the forearm (Fig. 17-3). A high tourniquet is applied and the operation proceeds under strict asepsis using body exhaust suits and antibiotic cover.

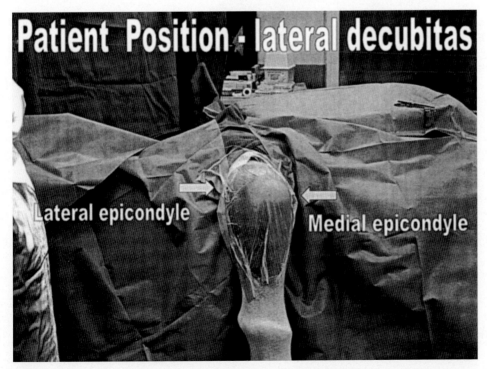

Figure 17-3. The patient prepped and draped in the prone or lateral decubitus position.

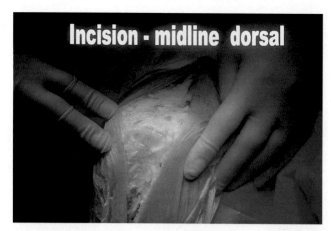

Figure 17-4. A straight posterior incision is preferred coursing just medial or lateral to the tip of the olecranon.

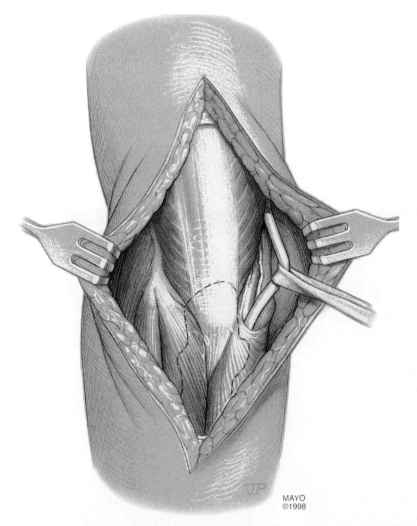

Figure 17-5. The ulnar nerve is identified and tagged but is not routinely translocated.

A dorsal longitudinal skin incision is made avoiding the tip of the olecranon (Fig. 17-4). The incision is taken down to the plane of the triceps and deep fascia. The skin flaps are then reflected out to both epicondyles and a self-retaining retractor is inserted. The ulnar nerve is then identified proximally and tagged (Fig. 17-5).

The nerve is completely decompressed down through the cubital tunnel into the forearm, releasing Osborne's band. Note that the nerve is not transposed, as our results have shown increased postoperative morbidity of the ulnar nerve following transposition.

A reverse triceps flap based on the tip of the olecranon is then developed (Fig. 17-6). It is important to leave 5-mm strips of triceps tendon laterally and medially to allow resuture at the end of the procedure. The triceps muscle is then split in the midline and reflected again medially and laterally out to the epicondylar ridges and epicondyles. The dorsal fat pad is identified and preserved.

The initial incision in the triceps tendon is developed distally on the radial side down along the lateral border of the olecranon at a distance of approximately half a centimeter from that bone. Again this remaining flap allows resuture at the end of the procedure. The incision is taken down to the level of the neck of the radial head, which is isolated by sharp dissection. The head is removed proximal to the annular ligament by an oscillating saw.

On the medial side, the triceps incision again processes distally, this time, however, over a much shorter distance to the dorsal edge of the medial collateral ligament. It is the author's view with this particular prosthesis that the anterior part of the medial collateral lig-

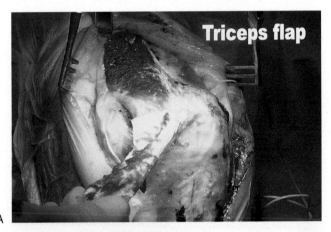

Figure 17-6. A,B: The authors prefer the Van Gorder "turndown procedure" of a sleeve of fascia. The triceps is then split to expose the distal humerus and ulna.

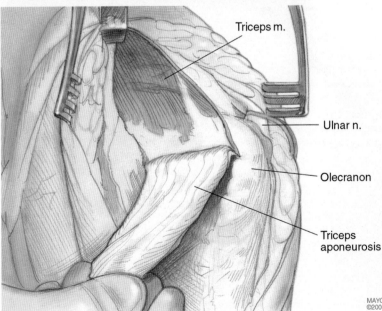

A

B

ament should *never* be compromised. Once this dissection has been undertaken and the tip of the olecranon has been removed with an oscillating saw, it should be possible to dislocate the elbow (Fig. 17-7). If this is not the case, then sometimes a coronoid osteotomy and possibly an anterior capsular release can facilitate the dislocation.

With the elbow dislocated and the forearm rotated toward the patient's head, the humerus is prepared for insertion of the humeral component. First, part of the articular surface of the trochlea is removed, together with the trochlear notch, and a small reamer is passed up the intramedullary canal (Fig. 17-8). Using a power bur, the cancellous bone contained within both epicondylar ridges and epicondyles is removed. This is the most tedious portion of the procedure (Fig. 17-9). An alignment jig and a cutting block allow an appropriate amount of humerus to be removed to accept the body of the humeral component. A trial component is then inserted (Fig. 17-10). At this stage it is extremely important not only to have the implant aligned correctly in both the anterior-posterior (AP) and lateral planes, but also to insert the implant to the correct depth and rotation. The former is achieved by the use of cutting jigs and the latter by using the patient's normal anatomy as a guide. More specifically, the articulating surface of the implant matches and is at the same level as the capitellum.

Attention is then turned to the ulna, which is cleared of soft tissue. A hole is made in the base of the coronoid to gain access to the ulnar intramedullary canal, and a trough from the coronoid through the olecranon is developed (Fig. 17-11). An intramedullary rod and cut-

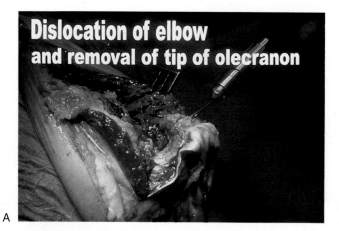

Dislocation of elbow and removal of tip of olecranon

A

Figure 17-7. A,B: The tip of the olecranon is removed and a complete synovectomy is carried out as necessary.

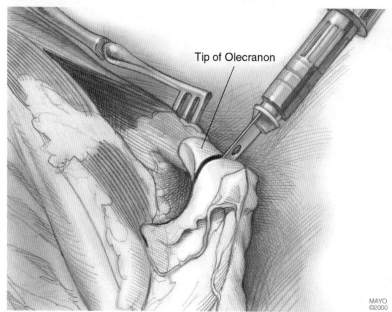

Tip of Olecranon

MAYO
©2000

B

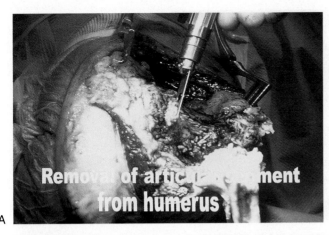

A

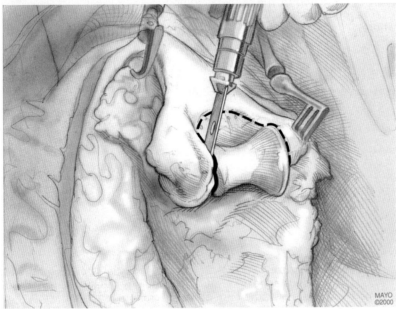

B

Figure 17-8. A,B: The trochlear portion of the distal humerus is removed with an oscillating saw and the medullary canal of the humerus is identified.

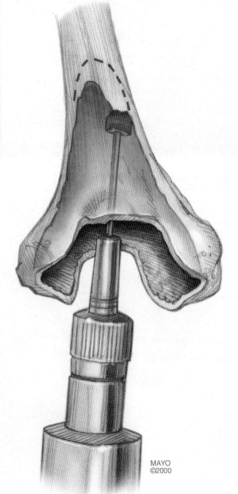

Figure 17-9. A bur is used to excavate bone from both the medial and the lateral supracondylar ridge to accommodate the wings of the device.

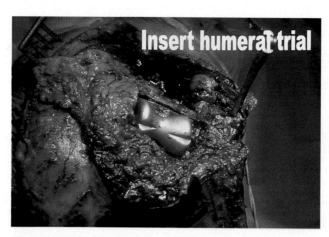

Figure 17-10. A trial reduction of the humeral component. Particular care should be taken to ensure proper rotational orientation.

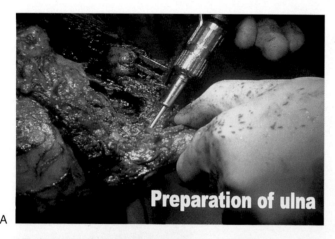

A

Figure 17-11. A,B: The triceps fascial sleeve is grasped to secure the ulna, and the medullary canal is identified with a bur at the base of the olecranon.

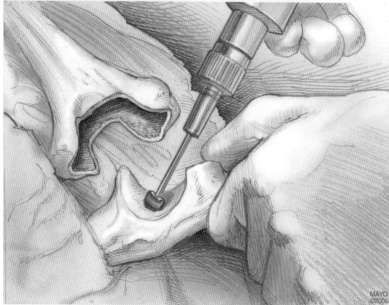

B

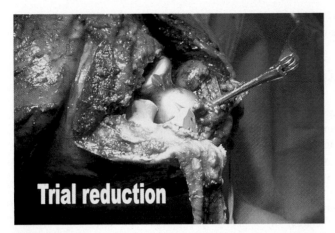

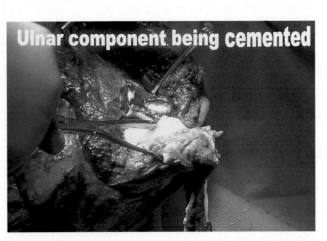

Figure 17-12. A trial reduction of both the humeral and ulnar components. Axial rotation as well as varus/valgus alignment are extremely important to ensure proper stability and function.

Figure 17-13. The components may be cemented simultaneously with special devices used to hold the device securely while the cement hardens.

ting jig are applied and the articulated surface is removed using an oscillating saw. A power bur is used for final modifications. It is important that the ulnar component be inserted to the correct depth within the olecranon and that it be totally supported by bone. In addition, alignment in both the AP and lateral planes should be checked. At this time a trial reduction is undertaken (Fig. 17-12) to assess the stability of the reduction in all positions and ensure unrestricted flexion and extension. The intramedullary canals are then prepared first by the use of hydrogen peroxide, then by saline; then they are dried. Bone blocks are prepared and inserted up the humeral canal for use as cement restrictors. Then, using a gun, the cement is inserted under pressure and the components are inserted (Fig. 17-13). Clamps are available, particularly for the ulnar component, to hold the component in place while the cement sets. Once this has occurred the arthroplasty is reduced.

Subsequent to reduction the authors emphasize meticulous repair of the soft tissues (Fig. 17-14). The incisions on the lateral and medial borders of the olecranon and the triceps muscle are closed to the tip of the olecranon. A deep drain is then inserted and the triceps fascial tongue is reattached, again using a strong suture. It is at this point that any preoperative flexion contracture can be addressed by allowing the tongue to slide distally. A sec-

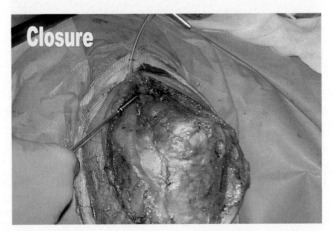

Figure 17-14. A careful closure of the triceps sleeve and fascial tongue is important, and a drain is routinely placed deep to the triceps reflection.

ond, more superficial drain is then inserted and the skin is closed. A plaster back-slap is applied with the elbow at 90 degrees and the forearm in neutral rotation.

POSTOPERATIVE MANAGEMENT

After 2 days the drains are removed and the wound is inspected. A radiograph is taken to confirm alignment of the components and the integrity of the implant. If they are satisfactory, early active mobilization is begun. Almost invariably in the first instance, this is done in conjunction with a therapist. At the same time the patient is given a resting splint at 90 degrees. After 6 weeks this splint is used only at night. Full active movement, including light weights, is allowed at 3 months. Finally, if there is concern about the integrity of the soft-tissue repair, then the author often immobilizes the elbow at 90 degrees flexion and in neutral forearm rotation for 3 weeks.

THE KUDO TOTAL ELBOW REPLACEMENT (*David Stanley*)

The original Kudo elbow arthroplasty was first used in 1972. This consisted of a humeral component made of stainless steel, which in appearance was basically a cylinder and went over the distal humeral articular surface. The implant was a surface fit and had no intramedullary system. The ulnar component was made of high-density polyethylene with a short intramedullary stem. Its articulating surface was reciprocal to that of the humeral component.

Unfortunately, although the early results with the use of this implant were encouraging (5), in the longer term, subsistence of the humeral component was seen (4) and this complication led Professor Kudo to perform a number of revisions to the design of his total elbow arthroplasty.

The humeral component was modified so that the articular surface became saddle-shaped, rather than cylindrical. The ulna articulation was also modified to allow for the redesign of the humeral component.

In 1983, an intramedullary stem was added to the humeral component and the humeral articular surface was designed with 5 degrees of valgus angulation and 20 degrees of anterior flexion. The current implant is made from a cobalt-chromium alloy (Fig. 17-15).

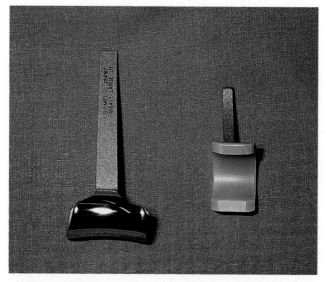

Figure 17-15. The current Kudo design involves stemmed humeral and ulnar components and a nonconstrained articulation.

SURGERY

Either the patient can be placed in the semilateral position with the arm across the chest and with the posterior aspect of the elbow facing superiorly or the patient can be put in the full lateral position with the upper arm horizontal and the forearm hanging vertically (Fig. 17-16). This is the operative position of the author. A nonsterile tourniquet is applied and a straight midline skin incision is made centered at the tip of the olecranon.

The ulnar nerve should then be identified and protected. The exact surgical exposure used depends on the surgeon's preference, but triceps splitting or reflecting techniques are effective (1,2,14) (Fig. 17-17).

The radial head should be excised, and the ulnar collateral ligament, including the tight anterior band, is released from the humerus, enabling dislocation of the elbow joint. This gives adequate access to both the distal humerus and the proximal ulna.

The distal humerus is first prepared by removing a portion of the articulation with a dual osteotome (Fig. 17-18). A rasp enlarges the canal (Fig. 17-19). A special rasp is used to prepare the humeral canal, with care being taken to ensure proper alignment in varus/valgus and axial rotation (Fig. 17-20). The ulna is prepared by isolating the olecranon, removing the tip of the olecranon (Fig. 17-21),and identifying the canal (Fig. 17-22). A special circular rasp is used to create a circular bed for the olecranon component (Fig. 17-23).

Once a satisfactory trial reduction has been achieved, the appropriate implants are secured. Although Kudo has recently advocated an uncemented technique, the author always cements both devices (Fig. 17-24).

The extensor mechanism is then repaired, as determined by the initial surgical approach. The wound is closed over suction drainage to reduce the risk of postoperative hematoma formation (Fig. 17-25). A plaster slab is applied, maintaining the arm in as much extension

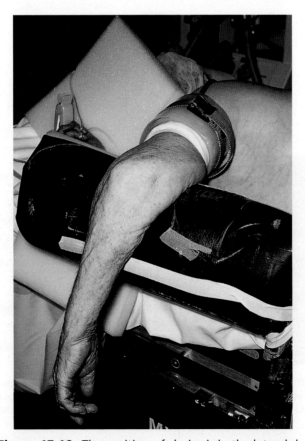

Figure 17-16. The position of choice is in the lateral decubitus position with the arm brought across a padded bolster.

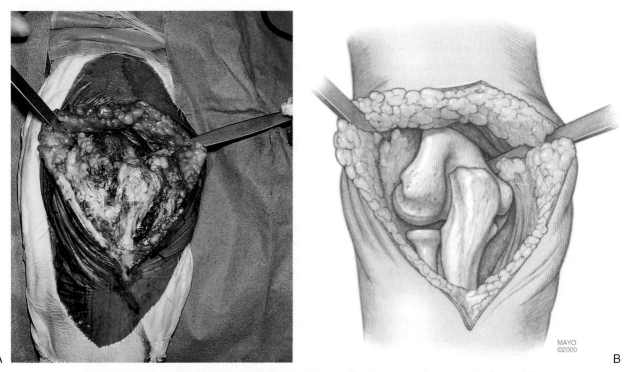

Figure 17-17. A,B: A triceps splitting incision reflecting the triceps medially and laterally and from the subcutaneous border of the ulna is the most commonly used exposure.

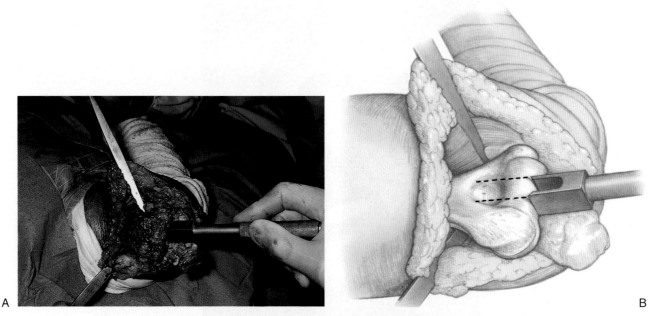

Figure 17-18. A,B: After the distal humerus has been exposed the lateral collateral ligament is released and the ulna is rotated and dislocated, the midportion of the trochlea is removed with a box osteotome in line with the olecranon fossa.

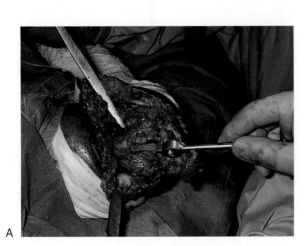
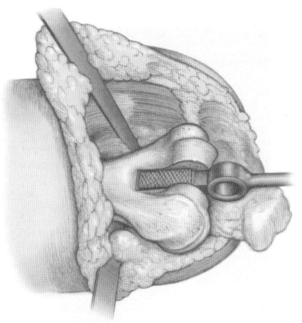

Figure 17-19. A,B: A bone rasp is used to enlarge the humeral canal.

A

B

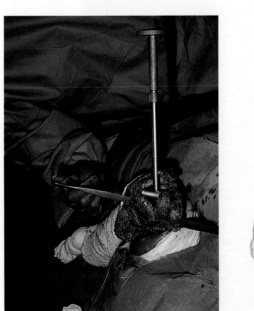
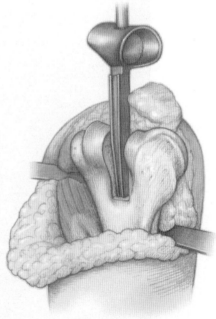

A

B

Figure 17-20. A,B: A specially designed spacer is used to further demonstrate the amount of bone to be removed and to orient and align the humeral component in a varus/valgus and from a rotatory perspective.

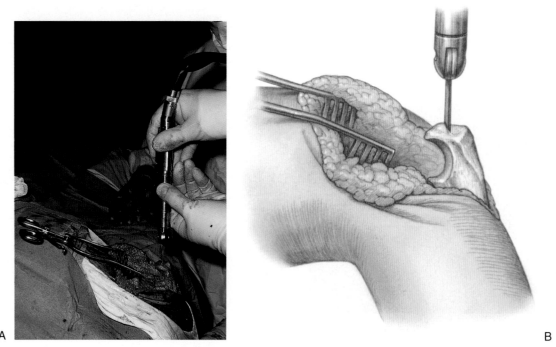

A   B

Figure 17-21. **A,B:** The tip of the olecranon is removed with an oscillating saw.

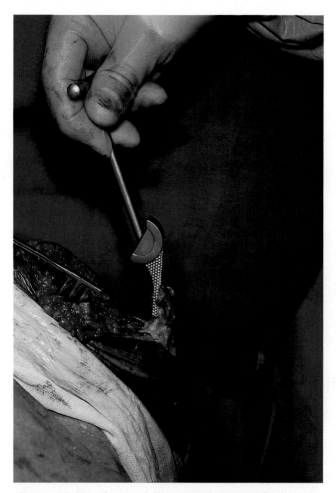

Figure 17-22. The medullary canal is identified at the base of the coronoid and entered with a rasp.

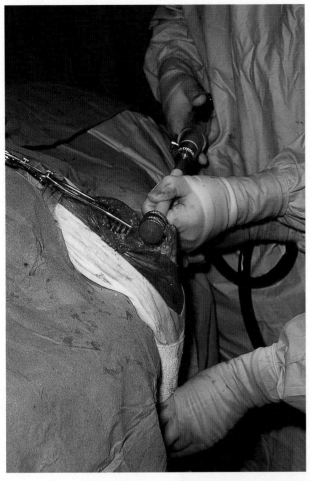

A

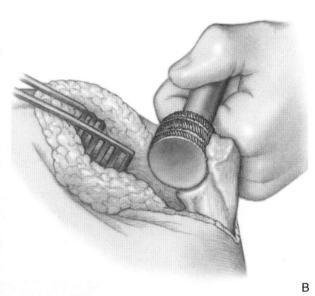

B

Figure 17-23. A,B: A specially designed circular reamer is used to contour the bone of the olecranon to conform to the ulnar component and appropriately fit the ulna.

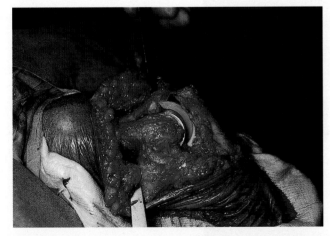

Figure 17-24. Both humeral and ulnar components are secured with methylmethacrylate.

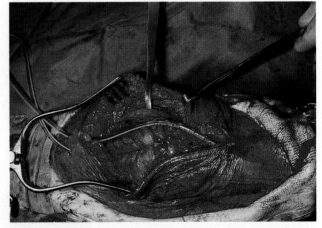

Figure 17-25. After closure of the triceps a drain is placed in the subcutaneous tissue to minimize the likelihood of hematoma formation and problems of wound healing.

as possible. The plaster slab is removed after 48 hours, and the patient is permitted to begin mobilization of the elbow.

RESULTS

Resurfacing devices have been shown to give good or excellent results in up to 90% of patients, provided that the indications for surgery were appropriate. Pain relief is frequently significantly improved (6), as is the patient's ability to undertake activities of daily living. An average increase in flexion postoperatively of 25 to 130 degrees has been reported (4,6,12,17). No improvement in extension might be expected. However, with the Souter device the flexion contracture is felt to lessen the likelihood of dislocation (11,17). Improvement in rotation movements has also been noted, with a mean of about 100 degrees, greater pronation and supination arc. In 1989, Souter published his experience with 250 cases, reporting pain relief in 92% and an improvement in flexion from 127 to 135 degrees but no gain in extension.

COMPLICATIONS

The complication that distinguishes unlinked surface replacement implants from linked devices is the incidence of dislocation. The rate varies from 3% to 15% (3,4,11,13,17). In our experience of 86 Kudo elbow arthroplasties inserted since 1992, three have dislocated (Stanley, unpublished). The first dislocation occurred early in Stanley's clinical experience. In hindsight it was not an appropriate joint to insert into the patient. The gross instability was present preoperatively. Of the other two dislocations, one required soft-tissue tensioning and the other required revision, owing to a poorly positioned ulna component.

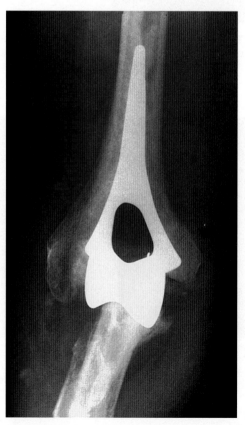

Figure 17-26. The Souter-Strathclyde resurfacing device.

A report from Pöll and associates reviewed the results of 33 patients with the Souter implant followed for a mean of 4 years (11). Five (15%) were revised—three for dislocation, one for loosening, and one for infection. The mean arc of flexion was 31 to 138 degrees. A similar experience was reported by Chiu and co-workers. Of 20 replacements followed a mean of 43 months, only one had instability and one required revision (3). The complication rate was 45%, and the loss of extension averaged 7 degrees, but the flexion arc increased a mean of 14 degrees. More recent reports have revealed radiographic loosening rates of up to 30% and instability in 15% (10,15).

At Wrightington at 12 years, 87% survival free of revision was recorded after 186 Souter procedures. The causes of failure, which accounted for 75% of all revisions, included infection and instability, and aseptic loosening of the humeral component (17).

ILLUSTRATIVE CASES

A 54-year-old female had marked pain, and motion was 30 to 115 degrees as a result of rheumatoid arthritis, but acceptable bone stock was present (Fig. 17-1). She continues to do well 5 years after replacement with the Souter implant (Fig. 17-26).

A 61-year-old female has marked functional limitation caused by rheumatoid arthritis with severe joint dislocation (Fig. 17-27). A successful outcome persists 7 years after replacement with the Kudo implant (Fig. 17-28).

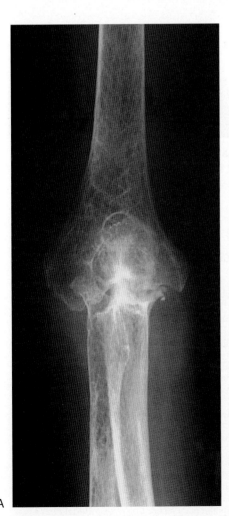
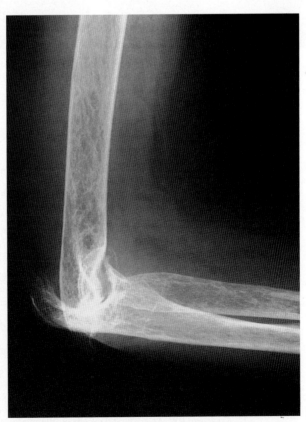

A

B

Figure 17-27. A,B: Patient with significant bone deterioration but adequate stock and collateral ligaments for the minimally constrained Kudo implant.

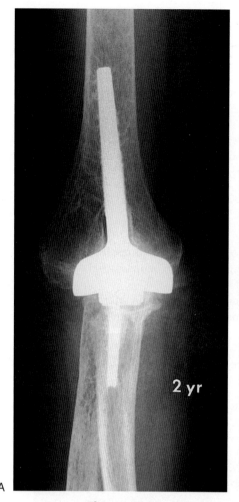
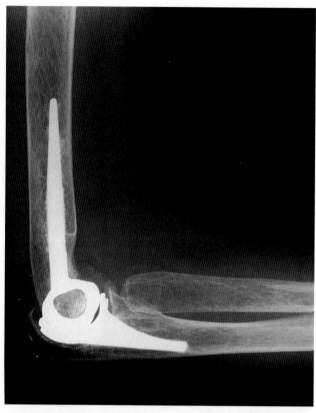

Figure 17-28. A,B: Two years after implantation with methylmethacrylate, the patient has functional motion and no pain, and there is no evidence of implant loosening.

RECOMMENDED READINGS

1. Bryan RS, Morrey BF. Extensive posterior exposure of the elbow: a triceps-sparing approach. *Clin Orthop* 1982;166:188.
2. Campbell WC. Incision for exposure of the elbow joint. *Am J Surg* 1932;15:65.
3. Chiu KY, Luk KDK, Pan WK. Souter-Strathclyde elbow replacement for severe rheumatoid arthritis. *J Orthop Rheum* 1996;9:194.
4. Kudo H, Iwano K. Total elbow arthroplasty with a nonconstrained surface replacement prosthesis in patients who have rheumatoid arthritis. *J Bone Joint Surg* 1990;72A:355.
5. Kudo H, Iwano K, Watanabe S. Total replacement of the rheumatoid elbow with a hingeless prosthesis. *J Bone Joint Surg* 1980;62A:277.
6. Kudo H, Iwano K, Nishino J. Cementless or hybrid total elbow arthroplasty with titanium-alloy implants: a study of interim clinical results and specific complications. *J Arthroplasty* 1994;9:269.
7. Kudo H. Nonconstrained elbow arthroplasty for mutilans deformity in rheumatoid arthritis. *J Bone Joint Surg* 1998;80B:234.
8. Larsen A, Dale K, Eek M. Radiographic evaluation of rheumatoid arthritis and related conditions by standard reference films. *Acta Radiol Diagn* 1977;18:481.
9. Lowe LW, Miller AJ, Alum RL, et al. The development of an unconstrained elbow arthroplasty. *J Bone Joint Surg* 1984;66B:243.
10. Lyall HA, Cohen B, Clatworthy M, et al. Results of the Souter-Strathclyde total elbow arthroplasty in patients with rheumatoid arthritis: a preliminary report. *J Arthroplasty* 1994;9:279–284.
11. Pöll RG, Rozing PM. Use of the Souter-Strathclyde total elbow prosthesis in patients who have rheumatoid arthritis. *J Bone Joint Surg* 1991;73A:1227.
12. Prictchard RW. Anatomic surface elbow arthroplasty: a preliminary report. *Clin Orthop* 1981;179:223.
13. Roper BA, Tuke M, O'Riordan SM, et al. A new unconstrained elbow. *J Bone Joint Surg* 1986;68B:566.

14. Shahane SA, Stanley D. A posterior approach to the elbow joint. *J Bone Joint Surg* 1999;81B:1020–1022.

15. Sjoden GO, Lundberg A, Blomgren GA. Late results of the Souter-Strathclyde total elbow prosthesis in rheumatoid arthritis: 6/19 implants loose after 5 years. *Acta Orthop Scand* 1995;66:391–394.

16. Souter WA. Surgery for rheumatoid arthritis: 1. Upper limb surgery of the elbow. *Curr Orthop* 1989;3:9–13.

17. Trail D, Nuttall D, Stanley JK. Survivorship and radiological analysis of the standard Souter-Strathclyde total elbow arthroplasty. *J Bone Joint Surg* 1999;81B:80–83.

18

Semiconstrained Total Elbow Replacement

Bernard F. Morrey

The value of and rationale for the semiconstrained joint replacement has been well established since the first edition of this text. A major value is to broaden the indications beyond
rheumatoid arthritis. Improved stability with the anticipation of minimizing stress to the
bone cement interface is realized by the laxity or "play" that occurs at the ulnohumeral articulation (13). Although several designs are available, I will describe in detail the surgical
procedure for the insertion of a Mayo modified Coonrad total elbow arthroplasty (Coonrad-Morrey), which has been used almost exclusively at our institution since 1981.

INDICATIONS/CONTRAINDICATIONS

The indications for total elbow arthroplasty are similar to those of other joints, the most
common being pain that significantly alters activities of daily living. This is typically seen
in the patient with rheumatoid arthritis or certain traumatic conditions.

The second most frequent indication for joint replacement is dysfunctional instability.
This presentation is seen in the very severe grade IV type of rheumatoid arthritic elbows as
well as with posttraumatic arthrosis resulting from distal humeral nonunion or resection.

A third and the least common indication for elbow joint replacement is that of the ankylosed elbow; this may be seen in several circumstances, including juvenile rheumatoid
arthritis, some forms of adult-onset rheumatoid arthritis, posttraumatic arthritis, and other
inflammatory conditions that involve this joint.

The techniques specific for each of these indications are illustrated and discussed.

Absolute contraindications are two: (a) an active or a subacute infection and (b) neuromuscular deficiency of the elbow joint flexors.

A history of previous infection is a relative contraindication. Replacement may proceed
if the absence of an active infection can be demonstrated.

Severe soft-tissue scarring and poor tissue coverage are relative contraindications. How-

B.F. Morrey, M.D.: Mayo Medical School and Department of Orthopaedics, Mayo Clinic and Mayo
Foundation, Rochester, Minnesota.

ever, such a situation can usually be converted to an acceptable setting with a soft-tissue surgical procedure that is performed before or occasionally concurrent with joint replacement.

Deficiency or absence of the triceps musculature markedly decreases the effectiveness of elbow extension and the ability to work overhead. However, in some instances, active flexion and relief of pain justify joint replacement in this setting.

PREOPERATIVE PLANNING

Routine anteroposterior (AP) and lateral radiographs are all the imaging that is necessary for this procedure. The most important factors in this process are (a) to assess humeral bow and medullary canal size in the lateral projection and (b) to note size and angulation of the ulnar medullary canal in both projections. In patients with juvenile rheumatoid arthritis, the medullary canal may be extremely small. In such cases the special small ulnar implant should be used.

SURGERY

While some use an arm board, I prefer to place the patient in a supine position with a sandbag under the scapula. The arm is draped free and the table is rotated approximately 10 degrees away from the operated extremities to further elevate the elbow and extremity (Fig. 18-1). A general anesthesia is most often used.

Technique: Rheumatoid Arthritis

Any one of a number of approaches may be used. I prefer the Bryan-Morrey approach (1) (see Chapter 1). A straight incision is made just medial to the tip of the olecranon between the medial epicondyle. The incision extends approximately 5 cm distal and 7 cm proximal to the tip of the olecranon (Fig. 18-2). As the subcutaneous tissue to the medial aspect of

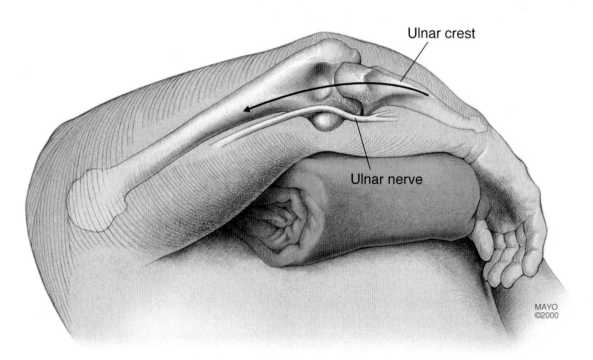

Figure 18-1. The patient is placed supine on the operating table. The arm is draped free and brought across the chest.

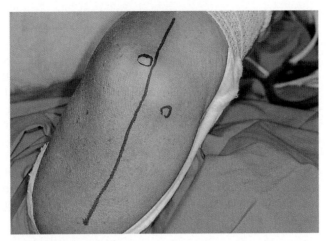

Figure 18-2. A straight incision is made between the medial epicondyle and the tip of the olecranon.

the triceps is released, exposing the medial margin of the triceps and the ulnar nerve, I always identify and translocate the ulnar nerve that has not been previously moved. The nerve is isolated at the medial margin of the triceps proximally. The dissection is carried distally to the cubital tunnel retinaculum, which is split, and carried further distally to the first motor branch to the flexor carpi ulnaris (Fig. 18-3). If there are adhesions to the cap-

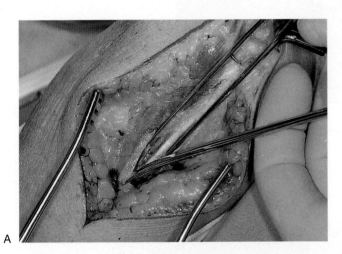

Figure 18-3. A,B: The ulnar nerve is identified at the medial margins of the triceps.

A

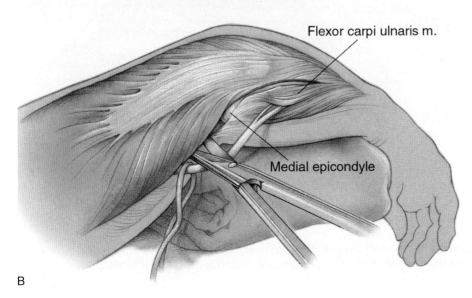

Flexor carpi ulnaris m.

Medial epicondyle

B

sule, as sometimes occurs with rheumatoid arthritis or scarring from a traumatic cause, the use of loops may be effective. Bipolar cautery is used.

The intramuscular septum is identified and released (Fig. 18-4), and a subcutaneous pocket is developed distally over the flexor pronator fascia and proximally anterior to the triceps. An incision is then made just to the medial aspect of the crest of the ulna, which releases the forearm fascia and the periosteum over the ulna (Fig. 18-5). The medial aspect of the triceps is then elevated from the posterior aspect of the humerus and from the posterior capsule. Retractors exist proximally and distally to the triceps insertion. The discrete insertion of the triceps by way of Sharpey's fibers to the tip of the olecranon is identified and released by a sharp dissection, allowing a flap of tissue to be raised, including the triceps, forearm fascia, and ulnar periosteum. As the extensor mechanism is further reflected laterally, the anconeus is identified to the lateral aspect of the proximal ulna. This is elevated from its bed (Fig. 18-6). Continued release of the extensor mechanism from the lat-

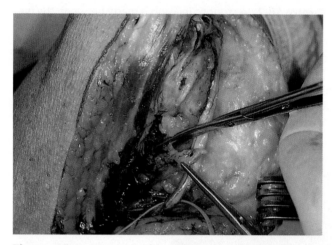

Figure 18-4. Intermuscular septum is removed. A deep subcutaneous pocket is created to receive the ulnar nerve.

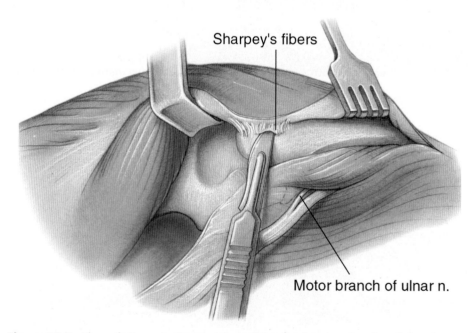

Figure 18-5. The soft tissue is elevated from the subcutaneous border of the ulna and the medial margin of the triceps from the posterior aspect of the humerus.

eral epicondyle allows complete exposure of the posterior aspect of the joint. The lateral and medial collateral ligaments are then released from its humeral attachment and the elbow is fully flexed, providing excellent exposure of the distal humerus and proximal ulna (Fig. 18-7). The ulnar nerve is carefully protected during this release.

To adequately expose the humerus, the tip of the olecranon is removed (Fig. 18-8), the humerus is externally rotated, and the forearm is fully flexed (Fig. 18-9). The midportion

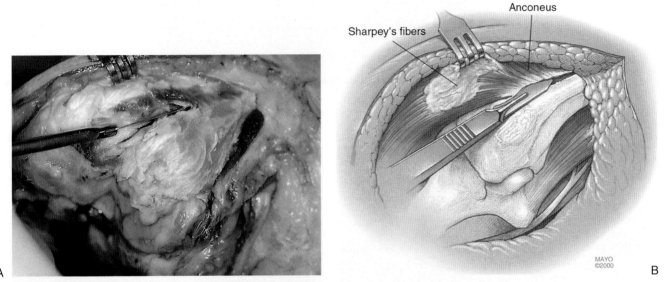

A   B

Figure 18-6. A,B: The anconeus is released and maintains the continuity of the extensor mechanism.

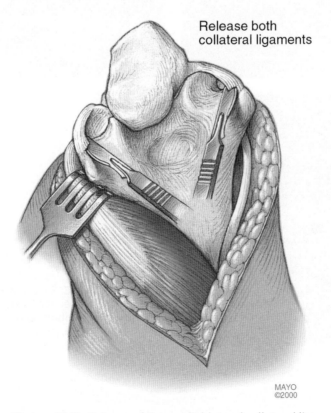

Figure 18-7. Release of the medial-lateral collateral ligaments.

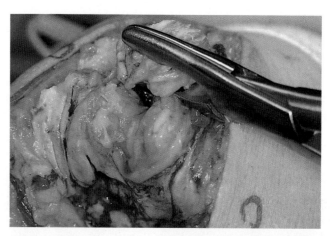

Figure 18-8. The tip of the olecranon is removed with a rongeur or oscillating saw if the bone is dense.

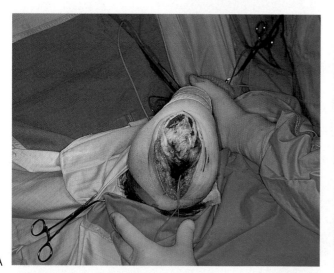

A

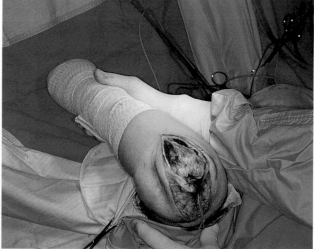

B

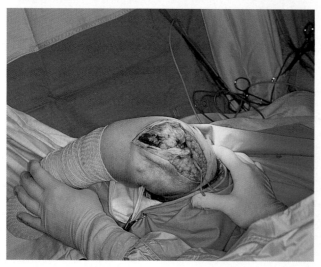

C

Figure 18-9. A-C: External rotation of the humerus is termed "the maneuver." Externally rotating the humerus and flexing the elbow allows ready access to the entire humerus and ulna, especially after the ligaments are released.

of the trochlea is removed with a rongeur or a saw, depending upon the quality of the bone (Fig. 18-10). The medial and lateral columns are identified, and the roof of the olecranon is entered using either a bur or a rongeur, again depending on the bone quality (Fig. 18-11). The medullary canal of the humerus is then identified with a long twist reamer, which also serves as the alignment stem. The humeral canal is typically very spacious, allowing easy access of this instrument (Fig. 18-12).

Placement of the alignment stem down the full length in the humeral canal accurately centers the distal cut. The handle is removed and a cutting block is attached, which allows accurate dimensions and a template for removal of the articular surface of the distal humerus (Fig. 18-13). The side arm, which rests on the capitellum, is interchangeable and the same device can be used for the left or right elbow. The flat of the template is oriented to the plane of the posterior columns to ensure accurate rotatory alignment (Fig. 18-14).

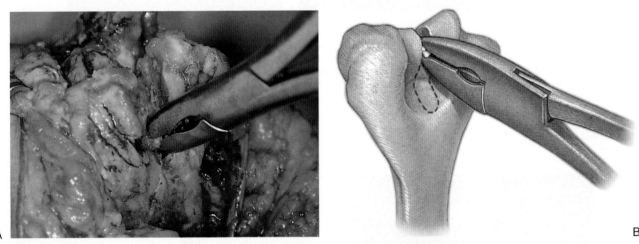

A   B

Figure 18-10. A,B: A rongeur for soft bone or oscillating saw for more sclerotic bone is used to remove the midportion of the trochlea.

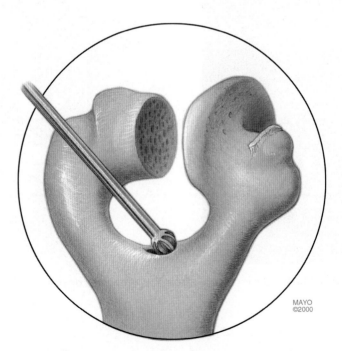

MAYO
©2000

Figure 18-11. The roof of the olecranon is entered with a rongeur or bur and expanded to receive the twist reamer.

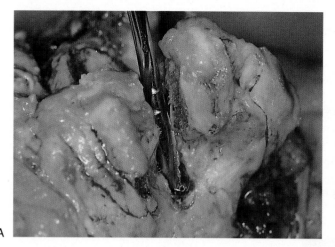

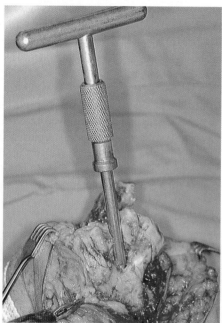

Figure 18-12. The canal is entered with a twist reamer (**A**) that serves as an alignment guide with a removable handle (**B**).

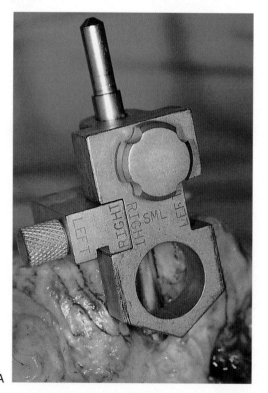

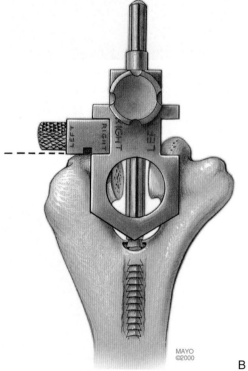

Figure 18-13. A,B: The handle is removed from the alignment device and the humeral cutting jig is in place.

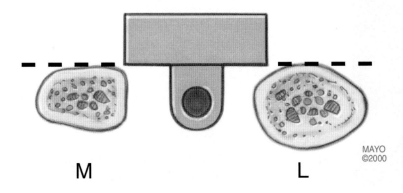

M L

Figure 18-14. The humeral cutting block is oriented coplanar with the plane of the posterior aspect of the medial and lateral humeral columns.

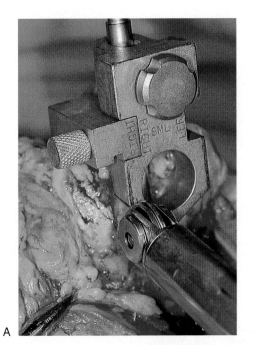

A

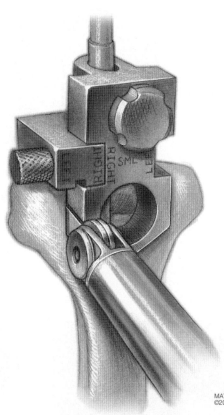

B

Figure 18-15. A,B: Accurate removal of bone with the oscillating saw.

With an oscillating saw the trochlea is removed (Fig. 18-15). We prefer not to cut tightly on the cutting template so as to avoid too narrow a resection that could place excessive force on the medial or lateral column with the introduction of the component. For the transverse cut, the oscillating saw blade is not angled from posterior to anterior but rather is oriented obliquely to lessen the likelihood of a cross-hatch at the junction of the column and the olecranon fossa that can serve as a stress-riser, allowing the column to fracture (Fig. 18-16). A small, thin rasp is initially used to again identify the canal and ensure that the rasp is centered on the completed cut of the humerus. The appropriate rasp is then used, depending upon the size of the canal (standard or small) (Fig. 18-17). The most typically employed is the 4-inch in the rheumatoid elbow, as there may be shoulder pathology.

In most traumatic problems, the 6-inch stem is used. The brachialis muscle is released from the anterior cortex of the humerus with a curved elevator to accommodate the flange (Fig. 18-18). The articulation of the trial humeral component is placed within the resected trochlea. If there has been adequate bone removed to accommodate the width of the implant articulation, it is then inserted down the canal (Fig. 18-19).

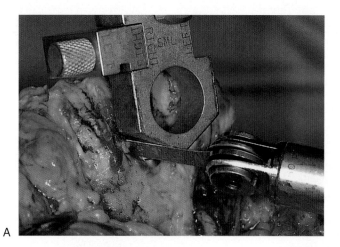

A

Figure 18-16. A,B: By placing the oscillating saw at an oblique angle one can avoid cross-hatching the supra-condylar columns.

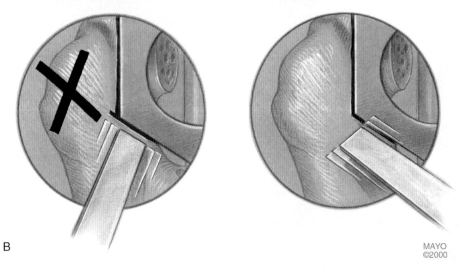

B

MAYO
©2000

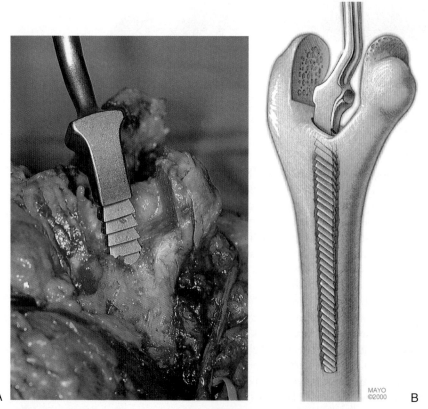

A

B

MAYO
©2000

Figure 18-17. A,B: The humeral canal is rasped to the appropriate size.

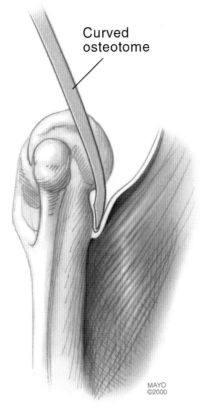

Curved
osteotome

MAYO
©2000

Figure 18-18. The anterior capsule and brachialis muscle insertion are released from the anterior humeral cortex with a curved osteotome.

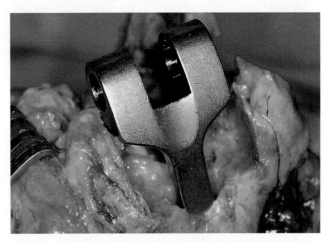

Figure 18-19. Trial reduction of the humeral component.

The medullary canal of the ulna is easily identified since the proximal ulna has been denuded. The canal is most easily entered with a high-speed bur placed approximately at a 45-degree angle to the olecranon at the base of the coronoid (Fig. 18-20). The orientation of the canal is established with a small awl (Fig. 18-21). To ensure longitudinal access down the ulna the olecranon is notched in line with the awl (Fig. 18-22). A pilot rasp is used with a twisting motion to further identify and enlarge the canal (Fig. 18-23). Next, the appropriate-sized ulnar rasp is inserted initially with a twisting motion. Complete seating often requires the use of a mallet (Fig. 18-24), and care is taken to ensure that rotation is at a right

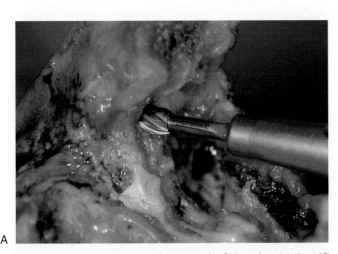

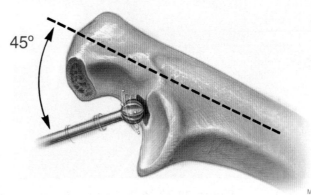

45°

MAYO
©2000

A   B

Figure 18-20. A,B: Medullary canal of the ulna is identified with a high-speed bur. If the bone is soft, a rongeur can be used.

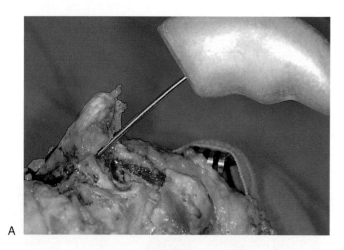

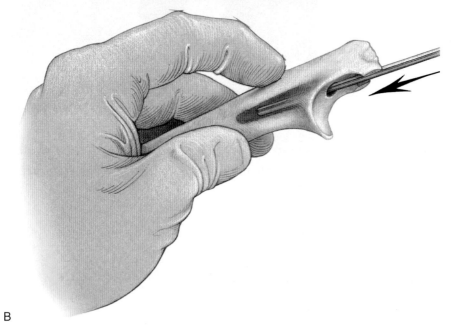

A

Figure 18-21. A,B: An awl identifies the medullary canal.

B

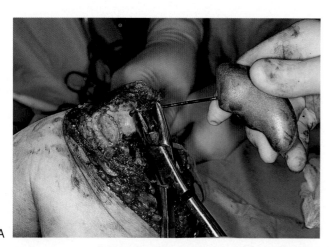

A

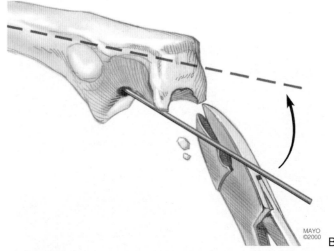

B

Figure 18-22. A,B: To assist in proper alignment the olecranon is notched with a rongeur in line with the awl.

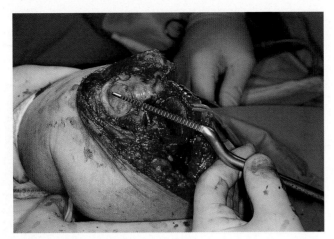

Figure 18-23. The canal is enlarged with a pilot rasp using a twisting maneuver.

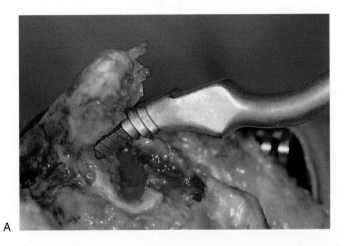

Figure 18-24. A,B: The appropriate-sized rasp is introduced down the canal. Occasionally, the orifice must be opened with a bur. This stage often requires the use of a mallet to adequately seat the rasp.

A

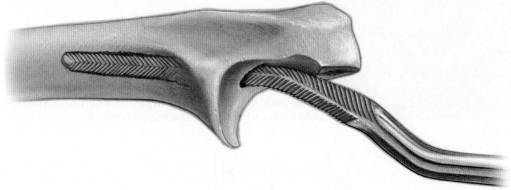

B

angle with the flat portion of the olecranon implanted (Fig. 18-25). In small bones the "trial rasp" is used. If the canal allows, the larger rasp is inserted.

After the ulnar canal has been prepared, the trial ulnar component is inserted down the canal. The depth of the insertion should be such that the center of the olecranon component is coincident with the center of curvature of the greater sigmoid fossa that is halfway between the tip of the olecranon and the coronoid (Fig. 18-26). It is wise then to insert the humeral component and perform a trial reduction to ensure that there is no residual flexion contracture to identify impingement and to ensure that the humeral component can readily be articulated with the ulnar component (Fig. 18-27).

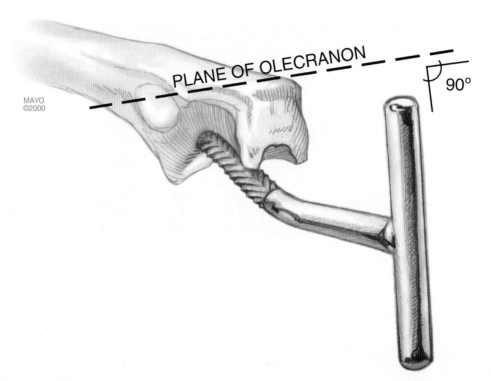

Figure 18-25. Proper orientation of the rasp is with the handle perpendicular to the flat of the proximal ulna.

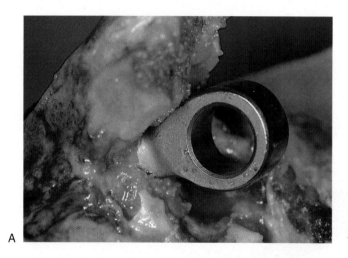

A

Figure 18-26. A,B: A trial reduction of the ulna ensures axial rotation, and proper depth of insertion replicates the center of the normal articular contour.

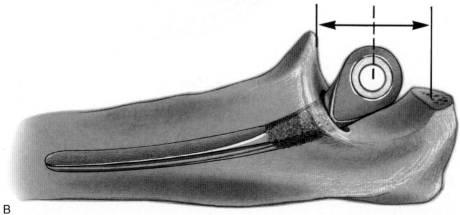

B

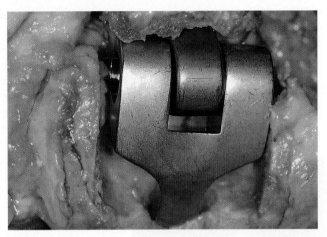

Figure 18-27. A trial reduction of both components ensures that the flexion contracture has been released and an adequate arc of motion has been attained.

Medullary canals of both the bones are cleansed with a pulsating lavage system and dried. For those less experienced with the procedure it is safest to cement the implants separately. If this is done, the ulnar component is first cemented using an injection system that is cut to the length of the ulnar component (Fig. 18-28). The ulnar component is inserted into the cemented medullary canal and impacted into proper position as noted earlier.

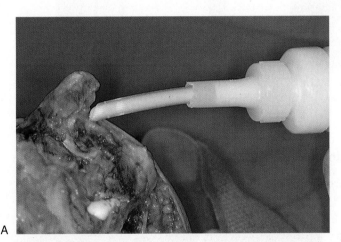

A

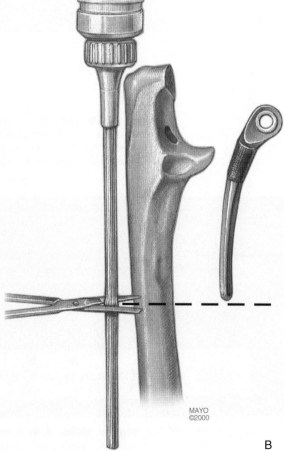

B

MAYO
©2000

Figure 18-28. A,B: An injection system is used to reliably and reproducibly introduce cement down the medullary canal of the ulna.

A cement restrictor is under development. If concern exists about cement extending too far down the canal, cancellous bone chips from the trochlea may be used. Otherwise, no attempt is made to plug the canal and the injector nozzle is cut to the proper length and placed down the medullary canal to deliver the cement to the appropriate depth (Fig. 18-29).

A bone graft is prepared from the excised trochlea measuring approximately 2 × 2 cm and 2 to 4 mm in thickness. This is placed at the anterior aspect of the humerus just proximal to the cut in the distal humerus (Fig. 18-30). The humeral component is then inserted down the canal to the point at which articulation with the ulna is possible. The previously

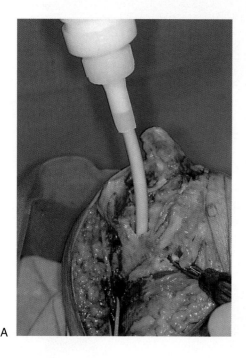

Figure 18-29. A,B: The length of the injector system is determined by the anticipated length of the appropriate-sized humeral component to be used.

MAYO
©2000

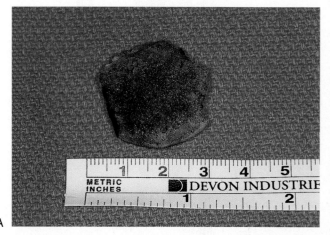

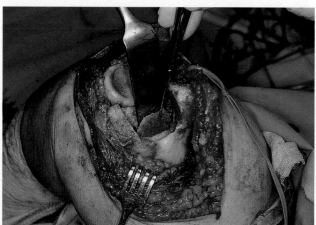

Figure 18-30. A,B: A bone graft is placed behind the anterior cortex of the distal humerus against which the flange of the implant articulates.

placed bone graft engages the flange at the time of implant coupling (Fig. 18-31). The ulnar component is then articulated by placing a pin across the humerus through the ulna and is secured with the "pin-in-pin" axis system (Fig. 18-32).

Note: In some instances there is a slight bow to the humerus and a small canal. These circumstances are recognized with the trial reductions, and a slight bow measuring approximately 5 degrees is placed in the distal one-third of the humeral component with the plate binder. This allows accommodation of the anterior bow of the humerus (Fig. 18-33).

After the prosthesis has been coupled, the ulna is placed in a 90-degree angle and the humeral component is impacted down the medullary canal (Fig. 18-34). The humeral component is usually inserted such that the distal aspect of the component is at the level of or slightly proximal (1 or 2 mm) to the contour of the distal capitellum. The actual depth of insertion is governed by the depth at which the flange articulates with the roof of the olecranon. The bone graft is anterior to the distal humeral cortex and posterior to the flange at

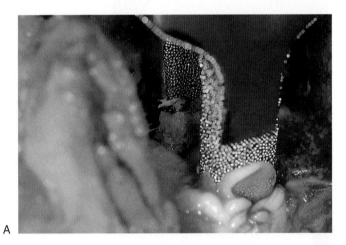

A

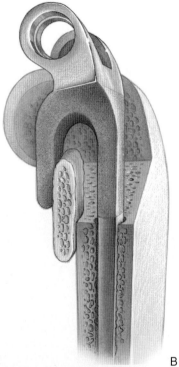

B

Figure 18-31. A,B: After the ulnar component has been rigidly fixed, the bone graft is partially elevated and the humeral component is inserted to the point where the graft is captured by the flange, and this allows the juxtaposition and articulation of the ulna with the humeral component.

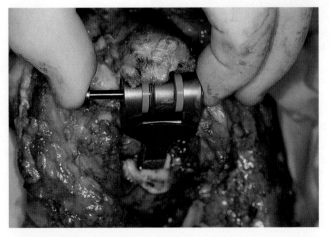

Figure 18-32. The pin-within-the-pin articulating mechanism couples the device.

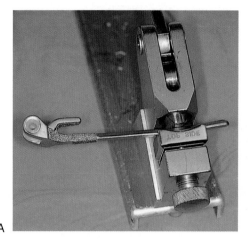

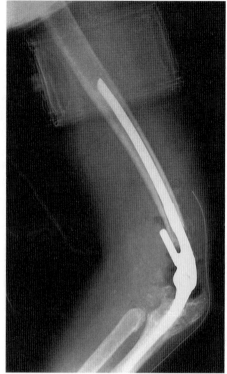

Figure 18-33. A,B: In those instances in which there is a small canal and an anterior bow of the humerus the humeral component is slightly bent with a plate bender.

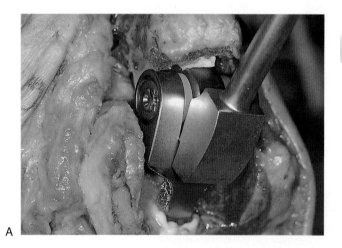

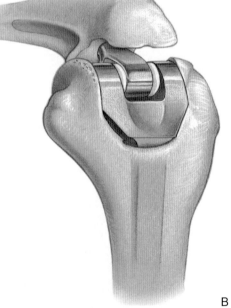

Figure 18-34. A,B: The humeral component is placed to the proper depth by impaction with the elbow at 90 degrees of flexion.

this point. After the prosthesis has been inserted, the tourniquet is deflated and hemostasis is obtained.

The elbow is placed through a range of motion to ensure full extension and flexion. Usually, an arc of 0 to 140 degrees is obtainable at the time of surgery. The radial head need not be removed for proper functioning of the device but should be excised if the pathology dictates this. The proximal ulna is prepared for reattachment of the triceps by placing drill holes obliquely both medially and laterally in a cruciate fashion (Fig. 18-35A,B). A third transverse hole is placed across the proximal ulna (Fig. 18-35C). A heavy nonabsorbable (No. 5) suture is then brought through the distal medial hole with a Keith needle. The elbow is placed in 90 degrees of flexion and the triceps is reduced over the tip of the olecranon. The suture is then inserted in the triceps at this point and a criss-cross stitch is placed in the triceps tendon (Fig. 18-36). The suture then penetrates from the tendon medially and is directed obliquely through the second hole to emerge on the lateral aspect of the ulna. The suture is then brought through the forearm and ulnar periosteum in such a way as to meet the initial suture on the medial aspect of the ulna and is tied off the subcutaneous border (Fig. 18-36). A transverse suture is then placed across the ulna and through the tendon to further stabilize the attachment.

The wound is closed in layers, with particular care taken to move the ulnar nerve into the subcutaneous pocket. Stitches are placed in the subcutaneous tissue to the soft tissue at the medial column (Fig. 18-37). This keeps the ulnar nerve from subluxing into the articulation. A drain is optional and the remainder is closed in layers with absorbable sutures on the deep structures and stainless steel staples on the skin (Fig. 18-38). In patients with rheumatoid arthritis a 3-0 monofilament running suture is used if the skin is thin or atrophic.

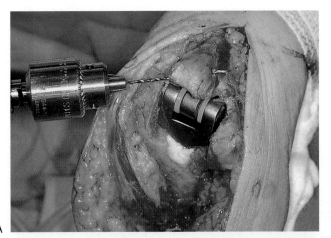

A

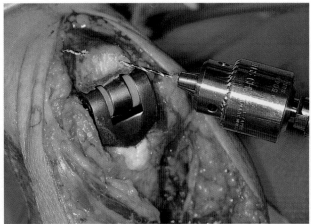

B

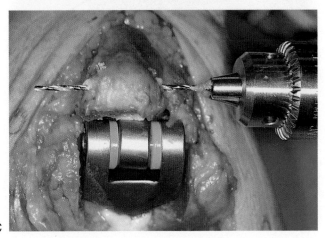

C

Figure 18-35. Cruciate (**A,B**) and transverse (**C**) drill holes are placed in the proximal ulna.

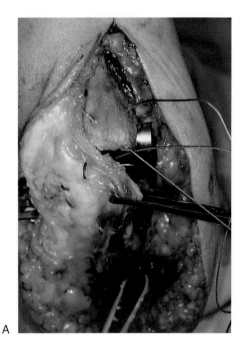

A

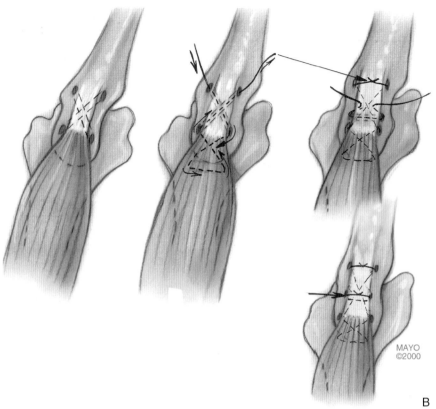

MAYO
©2000

B

Figure 18-36. A,B: The sutures have been placed through the ulna and in a criss-cross fashion in the tendon. The elbow is at 90 degrees of flexion when these sutures are tied.

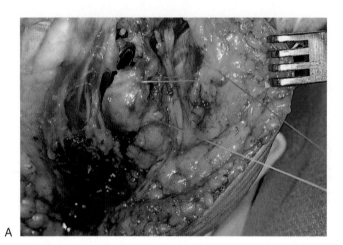

A

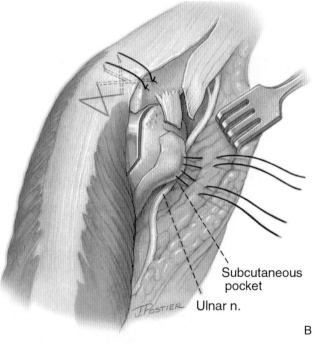

Subcutaneous pocket

Ulnar n.

B

Figure 18-37. A,B: The ulnar nerve is carefully brought into the subcutaneous pocket and secured with a 3-0 absorbable suture placed in the subcutaneous tissue to the medial epicondylar region.

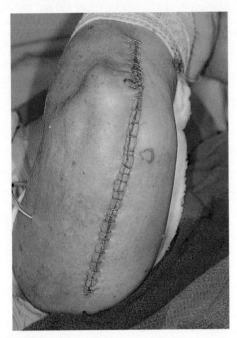

Figure 18-38. Skin closure is routine. In this instance, dermal staples were used.

POSTOPERATIVE MANAGEMENT

The arm is wrapped in full extension. If there has been a significant flexion contracture, an anterior splint is used. The arm is elevated overnight and for the second day. If drains are used they are removed the following day. The patient is then allowed to move the elbow as tolerated. A light-weight dressing is used during this period of time. A collar and cuff is helpful to keep the patient comfortable. No formal physical therapy is required or employed. Occupational therapy may be helpful for very debilitated patients, but we have not found this necessary in recent years.

The patient is advised before surgery that limitations after the procedure are not to lift 1 to 2 pounds on a repetitive basis or more than 5 to 10 pounds in a single event. Occasionally, if a flexion contracture of greater than 40 degrees is observed by the fifth postoperative day, then a turnbuckle splint is used to try to resolve this. This splint is typically used for 8 to 12 weeks.

Technical Notes

- The current design employs a universal articulation allowing interchange among all three sizes of the humeral and ulnar components.
- The implant comes in three humeral lengths: 10, 15, 20 cm; and three cross-sectional dimensions—extra-small, small, and standard (Fig. 18-39). Three stem lengths are available: 10 cm for rheumatoid arthritis to allow shoulder replacement if needed; 15 cm for post-trauma and revision; and 20 cm for revision and special problems with distal bone loss.
- The ulnar component is available in three diameters with an extra-long device available for revisions (Fig. 18-39).
- The polyethylene bushings are removable and interchangeable should these wear over time and require replacement.

Technique: Trauma With Absence of Distal Humerus

Indications include acute distal humeral fracture, humeral nonunion, gross instability (2,7,10,15,16).

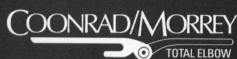

Humeral Stems

4"

6"

8"

| X-Small | Small | Regular |

Ulnar Stems

STANDARD

LONG

| X-Small | Small | Regular |

Figure 18-39. Three lengths and three dimensions of the humeral components and two lengths and three sizes of ulnar components are available.

Several unique technical considerations exist to treat the patient with a grossly unstable elbow due to a distal humeral nonunion or prior resection.

We leave the triceps attached as the absent distal humerus allows ready access to the humeral canal by translating the distal segment to the lateral margin of the triceps muscle. For acute fracture or for nonunion, we first excise all fragments while leaving the triceps left attached to the olecranon (Fig. 18-40) (2,7).

The resected distal humerus is translated laterally and is readily accessible for preparation (Fig. 18-41). The most difficult technique is exposure of the ulna shaft with the triceps attached. The ulna is prepared from the medial margin protecting the ulnar nerve. The essential step is a partial (25% to 50%) Mayo type subperiosteal reflection of the triceps attachment allowing subluxation of the triceps and greater rotation of the ulna (Fig. 18-42). The actual execution of the replacement is relatively easy, as the absent distal humerus eliminates obstruction to coupling the device. Because of the extent of the usual dissection, we recommend release of the tourniquet to secure hemostasis before closure. Closure includes the reattachment of the flexor and extensor muscle mass, as able, to the margins of the triceps with a No. 0 suture.

Postoperative management is as outlined earlier. No concern exists regarding tissue healing, so motion is immediately allowed, as tolerated.

Technique: The Fused, Ankylosed Joint (6,16)

For the fused, ankylosed joint, reflection of the triceps from the olecranon is essential. An aggressive transection of the fused joint or release of joint adhesions is coupled with a very aggressive release of the anterior capsule *and* release of the collateral ligaments *and* release

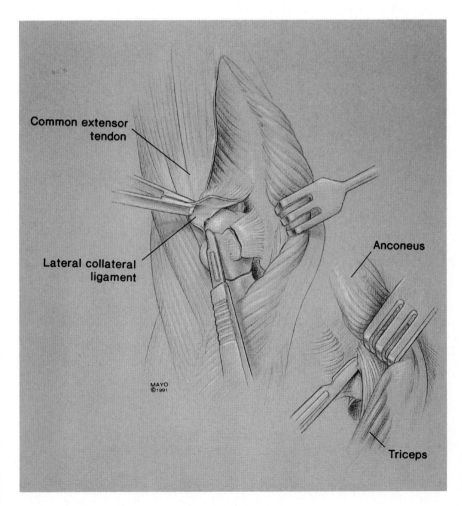

Figure 18-40. The distal humeral nonunion or acute fracture is excised, leaving the triceps attached.

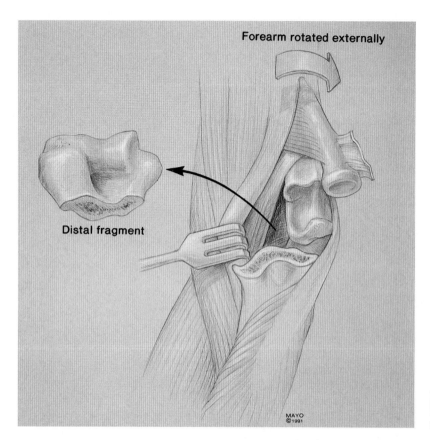

Figure 18-41. Exposure of the distal humerus at the lateral margin of the triceps.

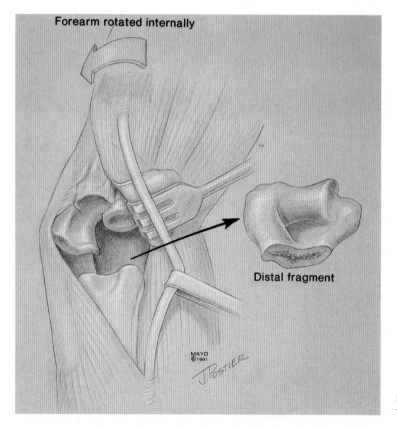

Figure 18-42. Exposure of the distal humerus at the medial aspect of the triceps.

of the flexor/extensor attachments to the humerus (Fig. 18-43). Additional steps to improve extension include the more proximal palcement of the humeral component (Fig. 18-44). If this is limited by fear of fracture or thinness of the medial column, the epicondyle may be excised. Increasing the depth of the insertion of the ulnar component is limited by the coronoid, and too excessive distal placement results in a prominence of the olecranon. After the implant has been coupled the last special consideration is that of the triceps attachment. If

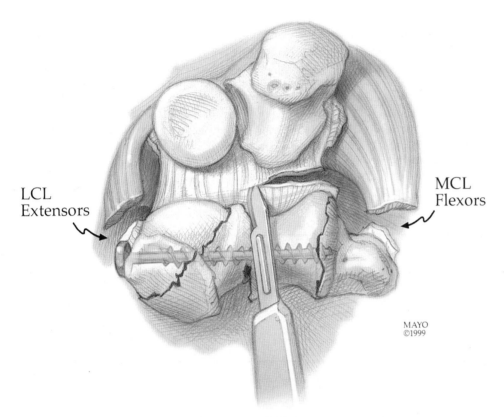

LCL
Extensors

MCL
Flexors

MAYO
©1999

Figure 18-43. Aggressive soft-tissue release includes the capsule, collateral ligaments, and flexor/extensor muscle origins.

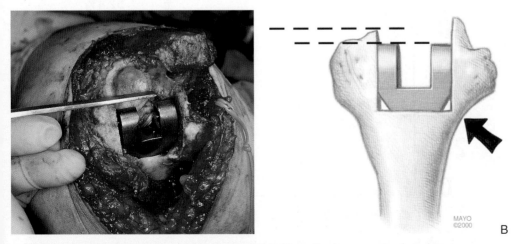

MAYO
©2000

B

Figure 18-44. A,B: In those with fixed contracture, the humerus is placed more proximally. The integrity of the medial column limits the depth of insertion. However, clinical experience indicates that medial epicondyle integrity is not essential for the implant to function in an effective manner.

the triceps is compliant, reattachment may not be a problem and will not limit flexion. If, however, the anatomic reattachment is not possible without markedly restricting flexion, we perform an anconeus slide procedure and reattach the anconeus-triceps complex to the olecranon in 90 to 110 degrees of flexion as appropriate to allow functional flexion without excessive weakening of the extension force of the mechanism.

RESULTS

This semiconstrained implant was first used in the latter part of 1981 and has been used almost exclusively by the author since then with few modifications. This implant, Coonrad-Morrey, has been used in more than 800 patients in our Mayo practice. The most common indications have been rheumatoid arthritis (39%), posttraumatic arthritis (30%), and revision total elbow replacement surgery (24%). The results for the spectrum of indications are summarized in Table 18-1. The outcome for rheumatoid arthritis is particularly gratifying as the survival now rivals that of hip replacement, with 93% survival at 12.5 years (3,9) (Fig. 18-45). Others also report good early results with the semiconstrained concept (4,14).

TABLE 18-1. *Mayo Experience with Semiconstrained Elbow Replacement for a Spectrum of Conditions*

Diagnosis	Procedures	Surveillance	Outcome satisfactory	
			MEPS	Subjective
Rheumatoid (3)	78	12.5	88	92
Traumatic arthritis (16)	41	6.5	86	91
Humeral nonunion (7)	39	4.5	88	91
Acute fracture (2)	21	5.0	87	92
Resection (15)	19	6.0	86	84
Ankylosis (6)	14	5.3	66	78

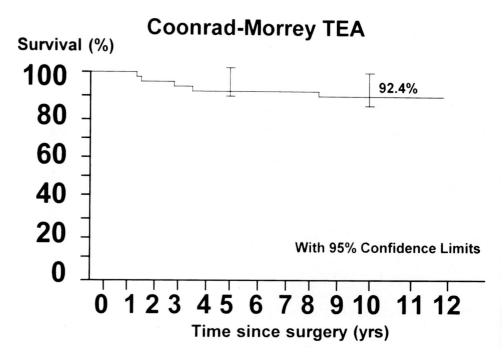

Figure 18-45. Kaplan-Meier survival curve free of revision of a group of 78 patients with rheumatoid arthritis followed a mean of 12.5 years.

TABLE 18-2. *Type and frequency of complications after semiconstrained TEA*

Type	Frequency (%)
Fractured epicondyle	5
Infection	3
Lysis/revision	2
Mechanical failure	
Loosening (5–10 yr follow-up)	2
Component fracture	1.5
Nerve injury (partial, permanent)	1
Wound healing	1.5
Triceps deficiency	2

Abbreviation: TEA, total elbow arthroplasty.

COMPLICATIONS

The complications following elbow arthroplasty are generally considered prohibitive (5,11) (Table 18-1). It is now well known that semiconstrained implants have a lower incidence of loosening than the earlier, more rigidly constrained articulated devices (4,9,12,14). Our experience with loosening was almost nonexistent (9) until recently. In the last 5 years an increased incidence in ulnar osteolysis has prompted the change from a polymethylacrylate (PMMA) precoat to a plasma spray surface finish for the ulnar component. The treatment for loose or unstable implants is treated by revision/reimplantation, if possible, and is discussed in Chapter 19.

Mechanical failure is an uncommon problem with most elbow replacements. We have observed 10 fractured components: eight of the ulna and two of the humeral component over the last 10 years (1.3%). In all but two instances, the patient had sustained a significant injury or was using the elbow in an aggressive manner such as lifting 100-pound bags of feed. Reimplantation has been successful in all to date (16).

Injury to the ulnar nerve is a well-recognized complication of total elbow arthroplasty, cited in the literature as a complication with a 2% to 26% incidence (8) averaging about 5% (2,11). Our personal experience is an incidence of 0.5% of patients with motor deficiency and fewer than 3% with permanent paresthesias. In our opinion, this complication is lessened by exposing and protecting the ulnar nerve.

Triceps deficiency has required a second operation in 1.3%. Reattachment is successful in 50% either with the same technique as used for the primary procedure or with an anconeus rotational reconstruction (see Chapter 11). Notable weakness of the triceps was observed in fewer than 10% of patients.

Although wound healing was a major problem in the early experience with total elbow arthroplasty, in our personal experience the incidence is currently just over 1%. In the last 10 years there have been five significant wound problems from among 300 procedures.

In patients with very thin bones, such as those with rheumatoid arthritis, fracture of the medial supracondylar column is not uncommon and is not considered a significant event. This has occurred in approximately 5% of our patients. If the column is extremely thin, we simply excise the fragment. Otherwise, the fragment is secured to the implant with a No. 5 Mersilene suture. We do not alter our postoperative course as a result of this occurrence, as no adverse effects have been appreciated as a result of this to date.

ILLUSTRATIVE CASES

A 57-year-old with severe grade IV rheumatoid arthritis of the elbow (Fig. 18-46) was treated with semiconstrained total elbow replacement. The Mayo Modified Coonrad implant was selected for stability and because of the favorable long-term results (Fig. 18-47). At 5 years the patient is pain free, has an arc of motion of 25 to 135 degrees, and shows no evidence of loosening (Fig. 18-48).

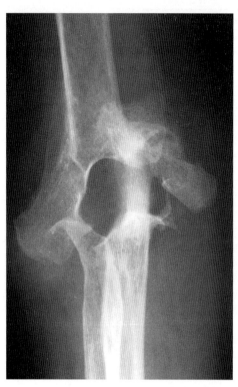

Figure 18-46. Severe rheumatoid arthritis with grade IV radiographic changes (severe architectural distribution).

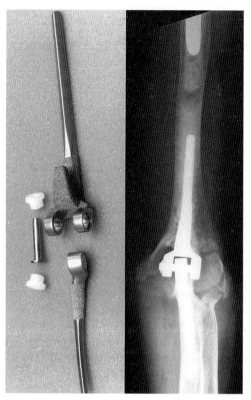

Figure 18-47. After replacement with a Mayo modified Coonrad implant (**A**), a stable cement interface is observed (**B**).

A 72-year-old female has a distal humeral nonunion (Fig. 18-49A). Four years after replacement she has a fully functional elbow and feels it is "normal" (Fig. 18-49B).

At age 28 a posttraumatic fusion with a one-bone forearm and neural deficit was offered (Fig. 18-50). At 16 years after surgery she has flexion from 40 to 100 degrees and no pain (Fig. 18-50B).

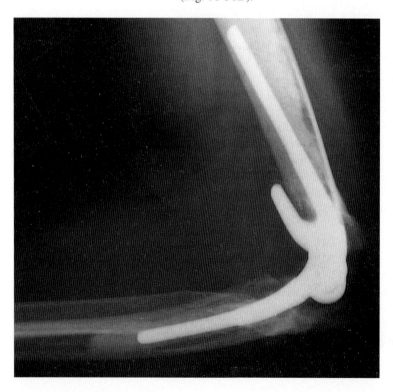

Figure 18-48. At 5 years no loosening has occurred, the bone graft has matured, and virtually normal function has been restored.

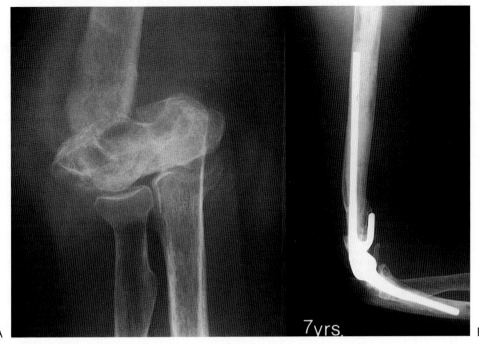

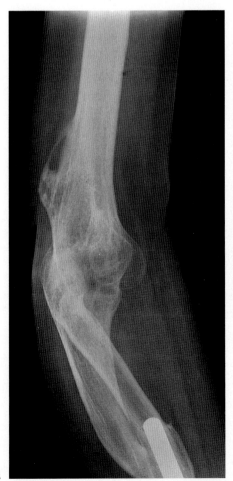

A

Figure 18-49. Patient with distal humeral nonunion of 2 years' duration (**A**). Excellent function persists 4 years after replacement (**B**).

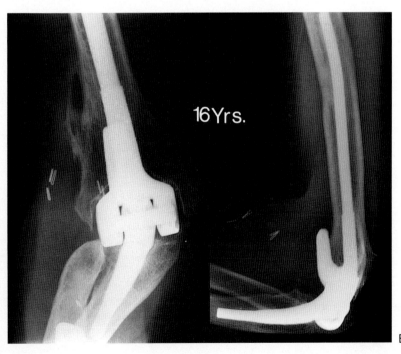

Figure 18-50. Severe deformity, spontaneously fused elbow, and one-bone forearm (**A**). Patient continues to function well 16 years after replacement (**B**).

RECOMMENDED READINGS

1. Bryan RS, Morrey BF. Extensive posterior exposure of the elbow. A triceps-sparing approach. *Clin Orthop* 1982;166:188.
2. Cobb TK, Morrey BF. Total elbow arthroplasty as primary treatment for distal humeral fracture in elderly patients. *J Bone Joint Surg* 1997;79A:826–832.
3. Gill DRJ, Morrey BF. The Coonrad-Morrey total elbow arthroplasty in patients who have rheumatoid arthritis: a ten to fifteen year follow-up study. *J Bone Joint Surg* 1998;80A:1327–1335.
4. Gschwend N, Loehr J, Ivosevic-Radovanovic D, et al. Semiconstrained elbow prostheses with special reference to the GSB III prosthesis. *Clin Orthop* 1988;232:104.
5. Gschwend N, Simmen BR, Matejovsky Z. Late complications in elbow arthroplasty. *J Shoulder Elbow Surg* 1996;5:86.
6. Mansat P, Morrey BF, Adams RA. Semiconstrained elbow replacement for gross ankylosis of the elbow. *J Bone Joint Surg* 2000;82A:1261–1268.
7. Morrey BF, Adams RA. Semiconstrained joint replacement arthroplasty for distal humeral nonunion. *J Bone Joint Surg* 1995;77B:67–72.
8. Morrey BF. Complications of total elbow arthroplasty. In: Morrey BF, ed. *The elbow and its disorders,* 3rd ed. Philadelphia: WB Saunders; 2000.
9. Morrey BF, Adams RA. Semiconstrained elbow replacement for rheumatoid arthritis. *J Bone Joint Surg* 1992;74A:479.
10. Morrey BF, Adams RA, Bryan RS. Total replacement for post-traumatic arthritis of the elbow. *J Bone Joint Surg* 1991;73B:607.
11. Morrey BF, Bryan RS. Complications after total elbow arthroplasty. *Clin Orthop* 1982;170:202.
12. Morrey BF, Bryan RS, Dobyns JH, et al. Total elbow arthroplasty: a five-year experience at the Mayo Clinic. *J Bone Joint Surg* 1981;63A:1050.
13. O'Driscoll S, An K, Morrey BF. The kinematics of elbow semiconstrained joint replacement. *J Bone Joint Surg* 1992;74B:297.
14. Pritchard RW. Long-term follow-up study: semiconstrained elbow prosthesis. *Orthopedics* 1981;4:151.
15. Ramsey ML, Adams RA, Morrey BF. Instability of the elbow treated with semi-constrained total elbow arthroplasty. *J Bone Joint Surg* 1999;81A:38–47.
16. Schneeberger AG, Adams R, Morrey BF. Semiconstrained total elbow replacement for the treatment of post-traumatic arthritis and dysfunction. *J Bone Joint Surg* 1997;79A:1211–1222.

19

Revision of Total Elbow Arthroplasty

Bernard F. Morrey

There are several considerations when undertaking the salvage of a failed elbow prosthesis (2,6,9,10,11,14). Of these, reimplantation with a semiconstrained device provides the most predictable result and is clearly the treatment of choice in the authors' experience. The results of this option are, however, dependent upon technique and implant design (3,4,13).

INDICATIONS/CONTRAINDICATIONS

In the following situations, revision is indicated:

1. A painful loose elbow prosthesis should be revised.
2. Those with a painless but radiographically loose total elbow arthroplasty of either the humeral or ulnar component should be followed carefully. Many of these patients may not have pain, but progressive resorption due to particulate debris or mechanical resorption can be extreme, may weaken the bone, and may predispose the bone to fracture. Intervention and revision are obviously indicated before this occurs.
3. Evidence of joint sepsis demands immediate surgical attention. Resection is recommended if the organism is gram negative, the organism is antibiotic resistant, and/or the process is chronic. Debridement may be offered for the acute infection with a less virulent organism (15).
4. Periprosthetic fracture with a loose implant.
5. Gross instability of the articulation.
6. Progressive ulnar neuropathy due to changes associated with failure of the previous surgery justifies reoperation to correct both conditions.

Contraindications to revision arthroplasty are as follows:

1. A loose implant but with minimal pain and no evidence of progression and no radiographic evidence of osseous resorption. Care must be taken, however, to follow pa-

B.F. Morrey, M.D.: Mayo Medical School and Department of Orthopaedics, Mayo Clinic and Mayo Foundation, Rochester, Minnesota.

tients with loose implants carefully to ensure that progression is not occurring. If a patient is lost to follow-up, significant resorption can occur, leading to pathologic fracture and making revision very difficult.

2. Acute or subacute sepsis is an absolute contraindication to reimplantation. Reoperation for debridement and resection is the treatment of choice (15).

3. Chronic, severe, debilitating comorbidity may be reason not to revise the loose implant.

PREOPERATIVE PLANNING

No special imaging techniques are used or are useful. However, from a technical perspective it is important to be aware of the location of the tip of the implant referable to the intramedullary canal and cortex, as this predicts cortex penetration and possible fracture. Simple anterior-posterior and lateral views of the humerus and ulna, usually attainable on the same film, are adequate to provide this information. The precaution is to visualize sufficient proximal and distal bone in both planes.

The Implant Device

Unlike many revision conditions (3), complicated custom implants have not been necessary to replace the humeral component in our practice. Since 1981, the implant used at the Mayo Clinic is the Coonrad-Morrey (Zimmer, Warsaw, ID) with an anterior flange that allows fixation to the anterior osseous cortex. When the bone graft matures, the flange decreases the likelihood of posterior forces and rotatory torque from loosening the device. A larger flanged device is now available for the specific purpose of providing greater humeral fixation in the patient with compromised distal humeral bone. The longer flange also allows greater flexibility when revising those with more significant distal humeral bone deficiency. This technique may be used with strut grafting in conditions that warrant it and is discussed later.

The articulation is semiconstrained, allowing 7 to 10 degrees of laxity. The device is available in 100-, 150-, and 200-cm lengths with small and standard humeral component options. An extra-small 100-cm implant is also now available (Fig. 19-1). The 200-cm implant has been of sufficient length for every condition encountered to date.

On the ulnar side there is also a need for flexibility. Extremely small canals require an extra-small implant. The small-diameter implant is also available in an extended length to bypass olecranon fractures, areas of avascular change, or lytic segments caused by loosening or wear (Fig. 19-2). Careful assessment of the radiographs before the surgery to determine the need for any of the special devices is critical, so these are available to the surgeon if needed.

Bone Graft

In addition to the implant, the second consideration of preoperative planning is the availability of adequate bone graft. In the primary procedure there is sufficient local bone to place behind the flange. However, in revision procedures this is not the case. There are three types of bone graft that may be needed in the revision procedure:

1. *A 1.5- × 2-cm corticocancellous graft.* This is sufficient to place behind the flange if reimplantation is possible with a standard flanged device and if the bone quality allows.

2. *Cancellous impaction.* As used at the hip (5,13) for lytic defects, autologous cancellous bone is used in an impaction mode. The volume required necessitates access to allograft material.

3. *Strut graft.* For periprosthetic fracture and extreme bone deficiency, allograft struts are used. These features of the reconstruction are discussed with the patient before surgery as appropriate.

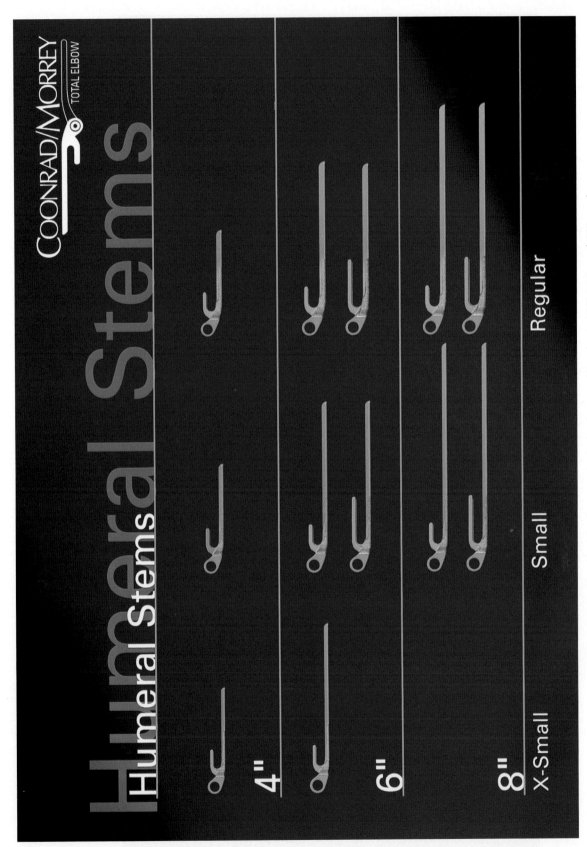

Figure 19-1. The standard system includes humeral implants 100, 150, and 200 cm in length with small and standard sizes available. Extended flanges are available in 150- and 200-cm lengths.

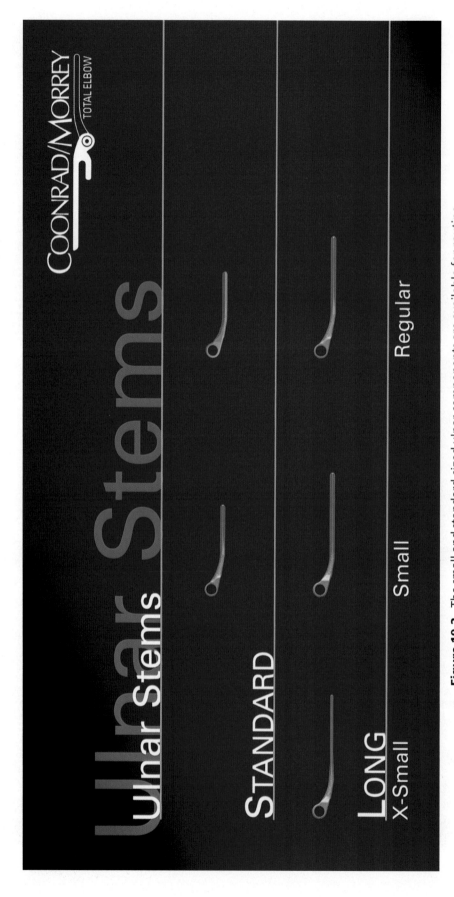

Figure 19-2. The small and standard-sized ulnar components are available for routine ulnar component revisions. If the previous implant has been associated with a fracture or the tip of the implant must be bypassed, several longer components are available.

Cement Delivery Systems

A third consideration is an adequate cement delivery system. If a long-stem device is to be used, an injection system to deliver the cement throughout the course of the 200-cm device is required. In most circumstances the cement must be mixed rapidly and injected in the less viscous stage to attain adequate flow through the nozzle into the humeral canal. If a cancellous impaction technique is performed, the availability of the appropriately sized tubes and nozzles is required (see later).

Ulnar Nerve

In patients who have had previous injury or surgical procedures or those with neurologic deficiencies, anticipation of a nerve exploration requires the availability of a nerve stimulator and magnification. A careful history and physical examination to ascertain whether it has been transferred in the past and the current status of the ulnar nerve is essential before the revision. Specifically, palpation should try to elicit whether the problem is proximal at or distal to the joint.

Cement Extraction

If the implant has broken, the revision will require removal of cement, which may still be rigidly fixed. The availability of a long-stemmed high-speed bone bur and an ultrasonic cement removal system have been extremely helpful. It is important to either expose the radial nerve and protect this nerve during the removal of humeral cement or at least to palpate and protect against laceration or injury during surgery.

Component Removal

In those implants that are well fixed, note the design of the articulation or contact the manufacturer for determination of the method by which the implant may be removed. In some designs a specific instrument is required to disarticulate the device.

A special note should be made as to whether or not both components have failed. If one component is solidly fixed, consideration of whether or not the well-fixed component can be left intact is appropriate. This is often determined at surgery, but the availability of the matching humeral or ulnar component must be assessed before the procedure.

SURGERY

Since the first edition of this text, the issue of revision surgery has become more clearly understood, if no less easily managed. There are three basic revision strategies that are applied as a function of the specific pathology (Table 19-1). In this chapter we will detail revision management by removal/reimplantation, the salient features of strut graft management, and impaction cancellous grafting.

Technique: Removal/Reimplantation

The patient is placed in the supine position and the arm is draped free and brought across the chest (Fig. 19-3). We usually use a sterile Esmarch tourniquet to ensure the maximum proximal exposure of the arm should this become necessary. The incision is carried proximally as far as needed or as far as the drape and tourniquet allow. The dissection is carried down to the triceps. In reoperations we prefer to grasp the skin to ensure that the medial and lateral subcutaneous flaps are as thick as possible and to avoid a "button-hole" in the skin. The ulnar nerve is identified at the medial aspect of the triceps as far proximal as necessary (Fig. 19-4). Even if the nerve has been moved we do identify the structure proximally and ensure ourselves of the position and location of the translocated nerve. If it has not been

TABLE 19-1. *Complication After 40 Revision Procedures*

Neuropathy	2
Radial nerve	1
Ulnar nerve	1
Wound	2
Triceps	1
Fractured implant	1
Infection	0
Loose	0
Total	6 (15%)

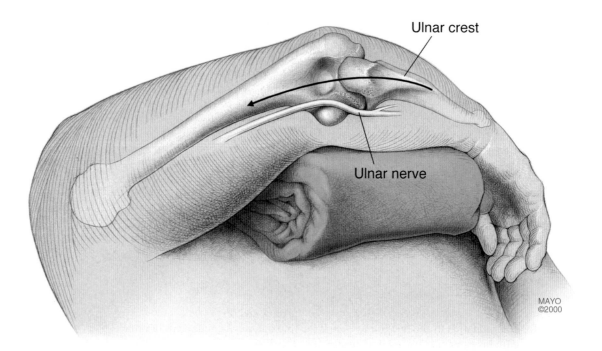

Figure 19-3. As for primary cases the patient is placed in the supine position with the arm draped free and brought across the chest. The tip of the olecranon and medial epicondyle are marked.

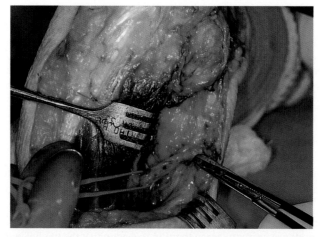

Figure 19-4. The medial aspect of the triceps is identified and the ulnar nerve is isolated. This may be rather easy or it can be extremely difficult, depending upon the previous surgery.

translocated we isolate the nerve and dissect it free to its first motor branch. Sometimes this can be rather difficult. If dense scarring or deformity is present, magnification loops and possibly a nerve stimulator are used.

Because exposure of the shaft of the ulna is required for most ulnar revisions, we reflect the triceps from the tip of the olecranon in continuity with the forearm fascia as for a primary procedure (Fig. 19-5) (1). After the triceps has been adequately removed to expose the ulnar and the medial and lateral aspect of the humerus, in virtually every instance of ulnar revision we perform an extensive subperiosteal exposure of the ulna past the tip of the implant to be revised. The anterior condylar bone is removed if this is required for disarticulation of the components. This is the case for the Coonrad-Morrey implant (Fig. 19-6). The device is disarticulated, and if the ulna is being revised, the component is usually loose and easily removed (Fig. 19-7). Exposure of the subcutaneous border of the ulna allows palpation of the very thin cortex, which helps minimize the likelihood of penetration or fracture at the time of preparation for the revision (Fig. 19-8). Meticulous cleansing of the medullary canal is required. If a foreign-body reaction has occurred, osteolysis is common. The debris-contain-

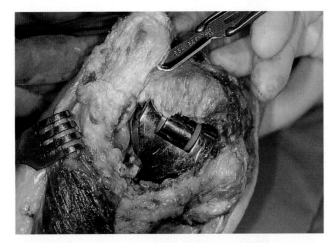

Figure 19-5. The extensor mechanism is again reflected from the tip of the olecranon. The remnants of previous nonabsorbable suture are noted. The mechanism is reflected past the lateral column for adequate exposure.

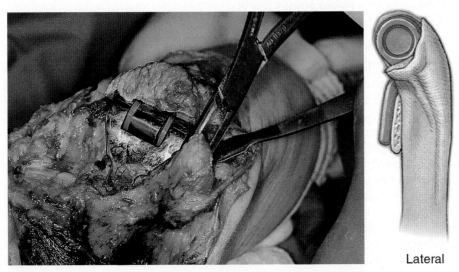

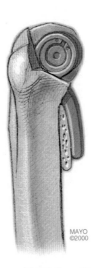

A   Lateral   Medial   B

Figure 19-6. The medial and lateral epicondyle may be left intact (**A**). If a Coonrad-Morrey implant is being revised a small amount of bone removed from the anterior aspect of the trochlea or capitellum is all that is necessary to allow disarticulation of the device (**B**).

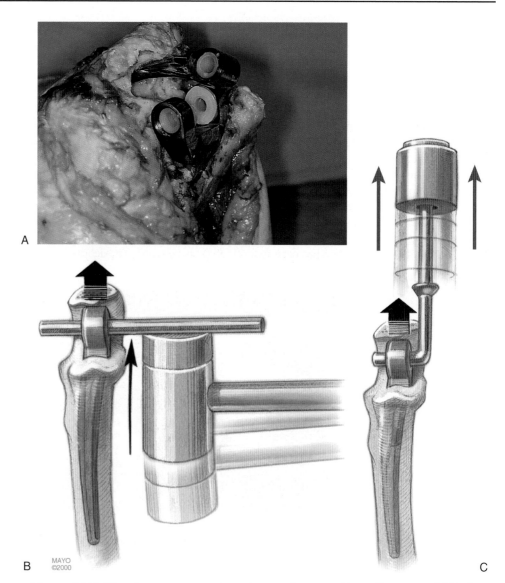

Figure 19-7. The ulnar component may be very loose and is easily removed (**A**). If not, a straight impacter is placed across the articulation and the implant is disengaged with direct blows (**B**), or a modified femoral component system is used (**C**).

ing membrane is thoroughly removed (Fig. 19-9). The cement is removed with an osteotome. The ultrasound probe may also be used to cleanse the canal; if the cement remains well fixed, it is left intact and the canal is expanded to allow the reinsertion of another component. This expansion is typically done with a simple long-stemmed bone bur (Fig. 19-10).

The medullary canal can also be cleaned and prepared with a flexible reamer. Special 4.5- to 7-mm cannulated flexible reamers are available for this purpose (Fig. 19-11). If the canal has undergone extensive thinning or if there is concern about the likelihood of penetration of the canal, a radiograph taken with the instrument down the medullary canal may be obtained to ensure containment within the canal. Penetration allows extravasation of the cement, causes loss of effective compression, increases the possibility of stress fracture, and may cause mechanical or thermal damage to the nerve (Fig. 19-12). If moderate osseous compromise has occurred, the longer-stemmed component is used to bypass the poor-quality bone of the proximal ulna. If the bone is of insufficient quality to "hold" the cement, an impaction grafting technique is done (see later). After a trial insertion the canal is filled with cement and the implant is inserted to the correct depth (Fig. 19-13). The depth of insertion is as recommended for the primary implant; that is, the center of rotation is in the middle of the greater sigmoid notch. The triceps is then reattached, as with a primary procedure. Cru-

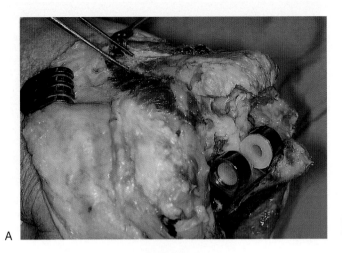

A

Figure 19-8. A,B: The proximal subcutaneous border of the ulna is identified to avoid cortical penetration.

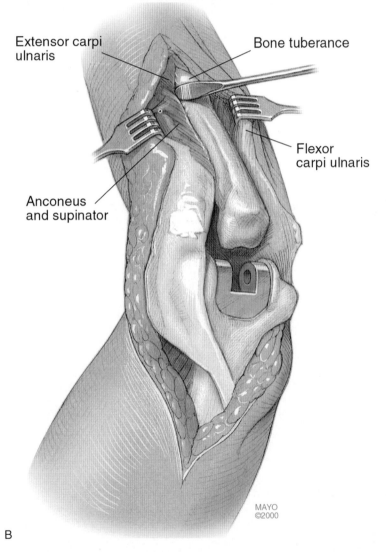

Extensor carpi ulnaris

Bone tuberance

Flexor carpi ulnaris

Anconeus and supinator

MAYO
©2000

B

ciate drill holes and a transverse drill hole are placed in the proximal ulna (Fig. 19-14). Non-absorbable suture is used to reattach the triceps. The needle enters the ulna from distal to proximal, starting on the side of the reflection, in this instance, from the medial side. The triceps is brought to its anatomic position, and the first suture passes into the tendon (Fig. 19-15). The suture then crisscrosses in the triceps tendon and is brought back through the opposite cruciate drill hole. A transverse suture is then placed across the triceps to further secure the repair. This is tied with the elbow in 90 degrees of flexion (Fig. 19-16).

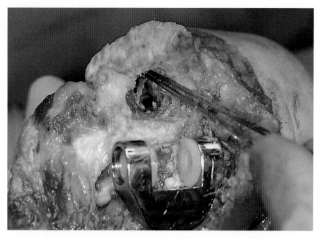

Figure 19-9. Any debris or soft tissue and membrane is identified and carefully removed. Loose cement is removed with an osteotome.

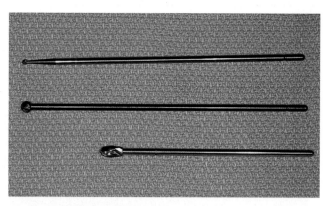

Figure 19-10. A small, 2-mm head on an extended bone bur shaft is effective to remove cement from an intact implant. A larger 5-mm "olive" is effective to expand the canal.

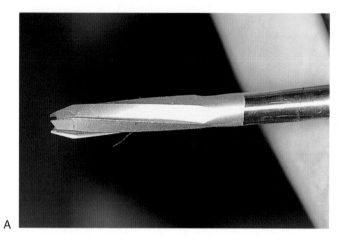

A

Figure 19-11. A flexible 4.5- to 7-mm intramedullary reamer (**A**) is used to bypass defects and to safely prepare the medullary canal (**B**).

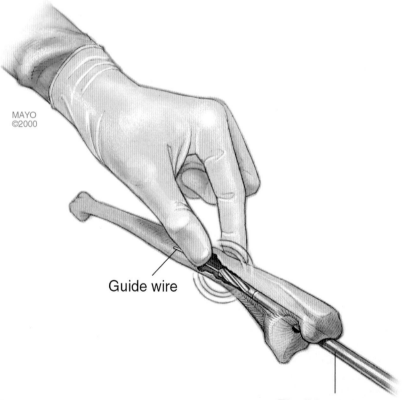

MAYO
©2000

Guide wire

Flexible reamer

B

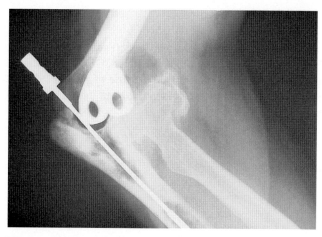

Figure 19-12. A lateral and an anteroposterior (AP) radiograph are obtained to ensure that the medullary canal has been safely identified and the cortex has not been violated.

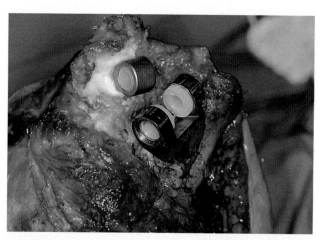

Figure 19-13. The implant has been inserted to the optimum depth, leaving the center of rotation of the ulnar component at the level of the center of rotation of the proximal ulna.

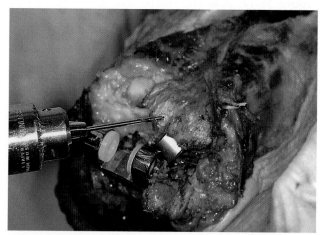

Figure 19-14. Cruciate drill holes are placed in the proximal ulna to reattach the triceps.

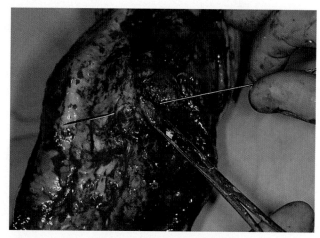

Figure 19-15. Triceps reattachment begins from the side of reflection. Thus the first move is medially across the olecranon and into the triceps tendon.

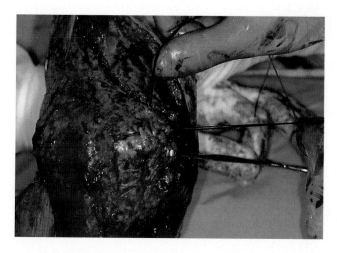

Figure 19-16. The transverse suture is also inserted and these sutures are tied with the elbow in 90 degrees of flexion.

HUMERAL COMPONENT REVISION

If only the humeral component is to be revised, the triceps may be left attached to the ulna. The extensor mechanism is identified and Kocher's interval is entered. Often the anconeus will not be evident or will have been replaced by scar tissue because of previous dissections. In any event, the lateral column of the humerus is identified and the triceps is elevated from its posterior aspect.

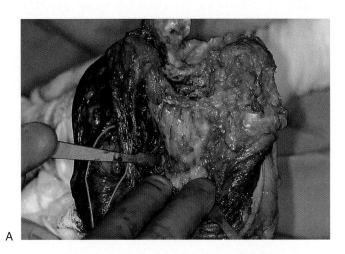

A

Figure 19-17. A,B: The medial and lateral shaft of the distal humerus is identified and palpated to ensure proper orientation of the cement removal instruments.

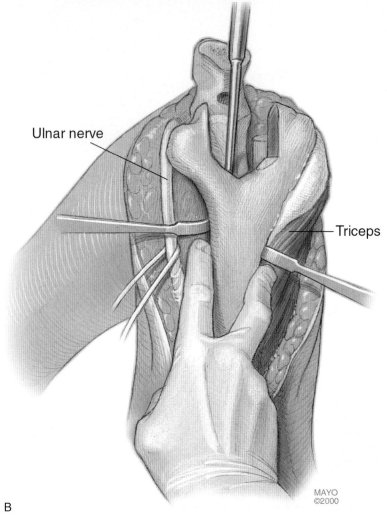

Ulnar nerve

Triceps

MAYO
©2000

B

The ulnar nerve is observed and protected as the medial triceps margin is elevated from the humerus and the pseudocapsule is entered. The articulation is then identified and the components are separated. This allows the ulna to displace from the humerus. We then "buttonhole" the humerus across the medial or lateral margin of the triceps. Usually, the distal humerus emerges from the lateral aspect of the triceps protecting the ulnar nerve. Sufficient release of soft tissue allows the humeral component to be adequately exposed.

If grossly loose, the device is easily removed. If this is not the case, a modest effort to disimpact the component is carried out. If the implant remains well fixed, a long-stemmed, small bone bur or similar device may be required to free the cement from the distal humerus. Some form of disimpaction device is necessary to remove the well-fixed implant. For loose implants this is not an issue.

If the cement is well fixed, the retrieval requires attention to the humeral shaft at the level of the spiral groove (Fig. 19-17). A limited exposure allows visualization and/or palpation of the radial nerve during humeral cement removal (Figs. 19-18 and 19-19).

Once the implant has been removed the cement is meticulously removed as well. We use small osteotomes, a high-speed bone bur (Fig. 19-10), and an ultrasonic cement remover as necessary (Fig. 19-20). Great care should be used to avoid penetration of the cortex, especially in the vicinity of the radial nerve. We are perfectly content to leave a well-fixed bone

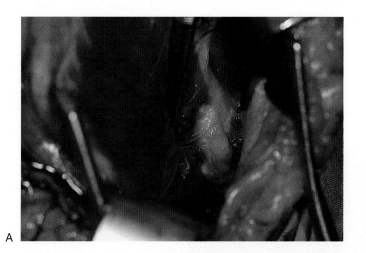

A

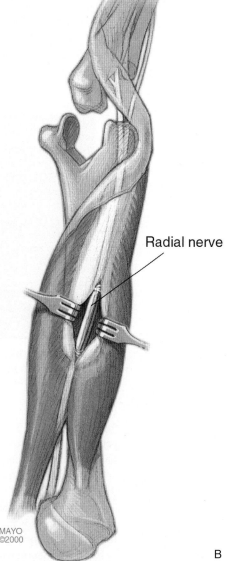

Radial nerve

Figure 19-18. A,B: The skin incision is extended proximally if cement removal in the midshaft is anticipated. The radial nerve is exposed and is protected.

MAYO
©2000

B

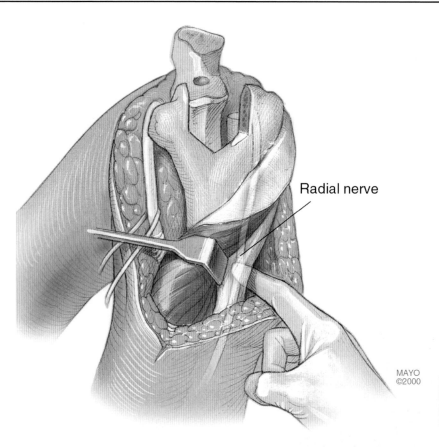

Radial nerve

MAYO
©2000

Figure 19-19. In some instances it is acceptable to expose and just palpate the nerve during cement removal.

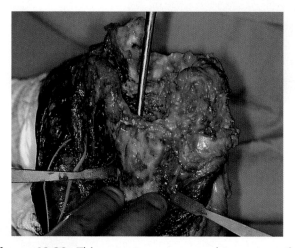

Figure 19-20. Thin osteotomes are used to remove the cement in most instances. An ultrasonic device is the safest way to remove the cement that remains well fixed to the bone.

cement interface intact and simply create an adequate space to receive the new implant. The basic technique of cement removal is similar to that used for femoral cement removal.

In patients with fracture, the plan is to bypass the fracture with a long-stem implant. In this setting a cortical strut graft is also used as discussed later.

After the cement has been removed and the humerus has been adequately prepared, the ulnar component is identified; if it is intact, the humeral component is matched to it. If it is loose this component must also be revised according to the technique described earlier.

Before cementing the new components we always remove the tourniquet and obtain hemostasis, after which the tourniquet is reapplied. We drain only those in which the bleeding has not been well controlled. If both components are being revised, the ulnar component is first inserted and the cement is allowed to harden. The humeral canal is then filled with the injection system to deliver the cement to the desired level of the medullary canal. In most instances the 15-cm or occasionally the 20-cm humeral stem will be used. If possible, a canal plug of cancellous bone should be used to improve bone/cement intrusion. If it has been released, the triceps is reattached with nonabsorbable sutures in a crisscross fashion described earlier.

The closure is done in layers. The fascia is closed with an absorbable 0 suture. The deep structures around the ulnar nerve are brought anterior to the medial epicondyle to isolate the nerve in a subcutaneous pocket. The remainder of the closure is routine. If flexion contracture or wound healing is a concern, we place the patient in full extension with an anterior splint.

POSTOPERATIVE MANAGEMENT

The arm is elevated for 24 hours. The patient uses the extremity as tolerated if there are no wound problems. Discharge from the hospital occurs at about 3 to 5 days with instructions to use the extremity as dictated by functional demands. Rechecking at 3 weeks allows removal of the stitches and inspection of the wound. If all is going well, the patient may increase activity as tolerated. No formal physical rehabilitation is needed or prescribed. The postoperative recommendation is for the patient not to lift more than 4 or 5 kg as a single event or more than 1 kg on a repetitive basis. Whether at the humerus or ulna the basic technique is the same.

Technical Points

There are several important features to recognize with regard to any revision procedure, particularly at the elbow:

1. The ulnar nerve must be identified as the initial step in the exposure.
2. The shaft of the component to be revised, either the humerus or the ulna, is exposed in the region of osseous deficiency or potential neural injury. For the humerus this requires exposure of the radial nerve. For the ulna this requires exposure to the level of the tip of the implant, to the fracture, or to the pathology of concern.
3. Trial reduction is essential to ensure adequate soft-tissue release and to be certain that the articulation can be completed without difficulty.
4. If an extensive dissection has been carried out, the tourniquet should be released and hemostasis obtained before cementation.
5. If a fracture has occurred or if osseous integration is required, then a period of immobilization is appropriate. Rigid immobilization for 3 weeks is typically used. Flexion-extension splints may then be used if needed.
6. Be sure that an adequate array of implants and options are available in unpredictable cases.

Strut Graft For periprosthetic fracture or in some instances when it is desirable to augment the length of the humerus, cortical strut allografts are employed (Fig. 19-21). The brachialis is safely elevated subperiosteally for the entire length of the anterior humerus as needed and the strut graft is slid in place. Because the host bone is usually of poor quality, a second graft is used to keep the wire from cutting through the host cortex. For bone deficiency the posterior strut is extended distally to compensate for bone loss (Fig. 19-22). For instances where struts are used, the radial nerve is exposed and protected during the placement of the wire or during passage of the strut itself. We avoid cables and usually employ 18-gauge wire for fixation of the struts. At least three wires are necessary for fractures and at least two for simple augmentation.

Note: When stems are used to augment lost distal humeral bone, the long flange of the device should attain the depth of insertion to overlap the host bone for at least 2 cm (Fig. 19-23).

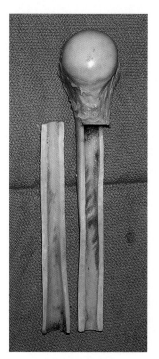

Figure 19-21. A cortical strut allograft is harvested from a humeral allograft. The proximal portion of this graft can be harvested if cancellous bone is needed.

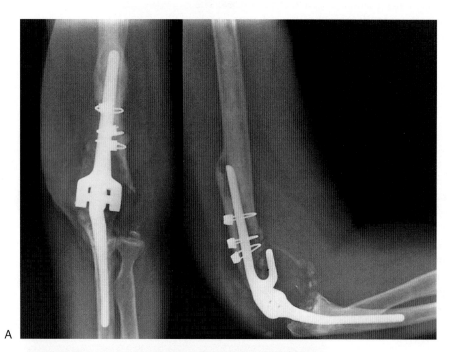

A

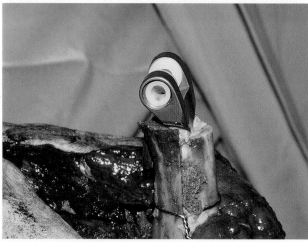

B

Figure 19-22. In instances of complete distal humeral deficiency (**A**), a posterior strut is added (**B**).

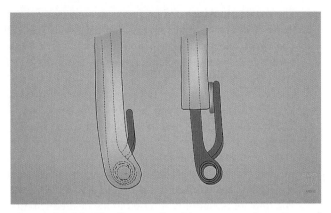

Figure 19-23. The flange should engage at least 2 cm of native bone.

Cancellous Impaction Grafting Cancellous impaction grafting for expansive or osteolytic lesions of the distal humerus or proximal ulna is carried out as follows (Fig. 19-24).

1. All endosteal soft tissue is carefully removed and the canal is plugged with a Silastic device or with cancellous bone.

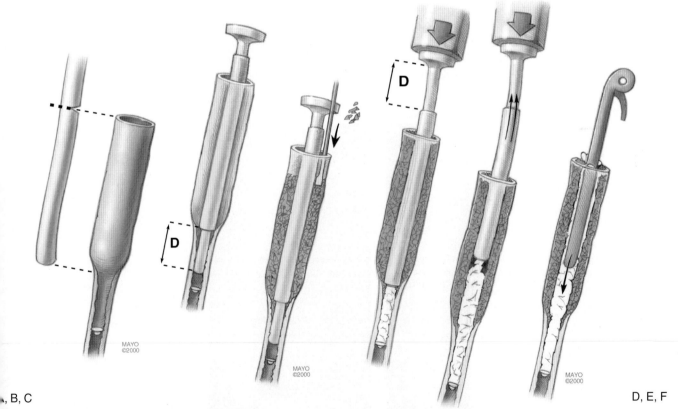

, B, C   D, E, F

Figure 19-24. A: The outer tube or nozzle for impaction grafting is cut to the length that corresponds to the extent of the lytic process. **B:** The elbow injector tube is then inserted through the outer tube extending distally for a distance *D* required to securely fix the component into normal host bone. **C:** Cancellous bone graft is tightly packed around the outer tube. **D:** The cement is then mixed in the canister of the elbow injector system and inserted on the inner nozzle. Cement is injected through the nozzle while withdrawing to the level of the outer tube. **E:** At this point both tubes are simultaneously withdrawn while injecting cement into the void created by the impacted graft sleeve. **F:** The implant is carefully inserted to the desired length. The implant is left undisturbed until the cement is fully cured.

2. The nozzle of tubing used for femoral cementation is cut to the length that corresponds to the extent of the lytic process (Fig. 19-24A). This is the outside tube.

3. The elbow injector tube is then inserted within the femoral tube extending distally into normal host bone to the depth necessary to fix the selected length of the ulnar component (Fig. 19-24B).

4. Cancellous bone graft or graft substitute is tightly packed around the outer tube (Fig. 19-24C). Take care to keep the tubes from being bent.

5. The cement is then mixed in the canister of the smaller elbow injector system and inserted on the nozzle *in situ*. Cement is injected through the nozzle while withdrawing to the level of the outer tube (Fig. 19-24D).

6. At this point both inner and outer tubes are simultaneously withdrawn while injecting cement into the void created by the larger tube (Fig. 19-24E).

7. The implant is carefully inserted to the desired length (Fig. 19-24F) and is left undisturbed until the cement is fully cured.

RESULTS

There is relatively little information in the peer review literature with regard to revision of total elbow arthroplasty. Posttraumatic conditions accounted for the greatest incidence of failures in the early experience with elbow replacement (8). Our experience with 40 cases done over the last 11 years has been rather gratifying but has been associated with the anticipated problems of revision surgery. The mean arc of motion is 25 to 130 degrees. The ulnar nerve is vulnerable with such procedures, as is the possibility of fracturing one of the epicondyles (see later). Nonetheless the overall results in our experience with 40 procedures is 88% satisfactory, with an average follow-up of 5 years (4). Surprisingly, there has been no revision for mechanical loosening in this sample to date (Fig. 19-25). These results are considerably better than our early experience (10). One case report of cancellous im-

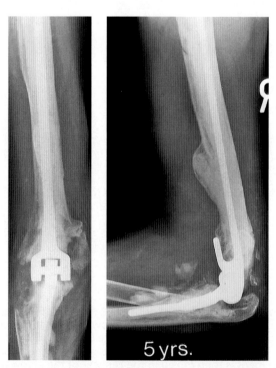

Figure 19-25. A typical 5-year result from simple reimplantation. Note stable bone cement interface and evidence of prior implant, which had eroded into the anterior humeral cortex.

paction grafting has been reported (7). The outcome of 12 of our cases of impaction grafting is currently under review. Preliminary assessment reveals 10 of 12 (88%) are satisfactory between 2 and 6 years after surgery. The results of 14 strut graft augmentations are currently under review. There are no firm data on this experience at this time (12).

COMPLICATIONS

The complications of this procedure are very similar to those of the primary operation but less than those for treatment of the stiff elbow (Table 19-1) (6). Surprisingly, we have only a 20% complication rate over the last 8 years. For reasons not clear and in spite of all of the risk factors, we had no infection in the first review. A subsequent assessment by King et al. also revealed no infections after 41 reimplantation revisions. There has been one (8%) infected after the impaction grafting procedure. If infection occurs with revisions, removal of the implant is usually required. Although the patient is left with a flail elbow, I am not very enthusiastic about another revision procedure at a later date.

Neuropathy has occurred in less than 5%. This is usually due to stretch of the ulnar nerve and is typically a sensory deficiency. I have not reexplored any of these patients. One radial nerve was transected with a Midas Rex in a patient who had extremely thin bone. It is this experience that has prompted the preceding recommendation to always expose the radial nerve if cement is being removed from the midshaft of the humerus. We have had one instance of triceps disruption and two wound-healing problems. To date, there have been no mechanical loosenings requiring revision.

ILLUSTRATIVE CASES

Long-Flange Reimplantation

A 68-year-old man developed loosening of the humeral and ulnar component 3 years after a custom implant was inserted, at which time the ulna was fractured. This device had a rigid hinge with no laxity or freedom at the articulation. The radiograph demonstrated loosening of the ulnar component, but the humeral side looked solidly fixed. Nevertheless the patient had pain with internal and external rotation of the humerus (Fig. 19-26). At the time of revision the humeral component was in fact loose, as was the proximal ulna. A long-flanged humeral component was used (Fig. 19-27). The ulna fracture had not healed, requiring a long ulnar implant with strut grafting. Excellent motion from 20 to 135 degrees and minimal pain were present as found (Fig. 19-28).

Allograft Exchange

A 60-year-old patient with rheumatoid arthritis underwent joint replacement arthroplasty in 1980, but the replacement loosened and was revised in 1988. This implant also loosened, migrating proximally and the tip eroding anterior (Fig. 19-29). With the technique described earlier, an allograft was used to replace the proximal ulna (Fig. 19-30). Bone graft was placed behind the anterior flange and a 150-cm humeral component was inserted down the humeral canal (Fig. 19-31). The patient has excellent motion 1 week after surgery. The radiograph shows a well-fixed implant (Fig. 19-32).

Pathologic Fracture: Strut Graft

A 72-year-old female with three prior procedures sustained a periprosthetic fracture of the humerus and extensive erosion of the posterior distal one-third of the humerus (Fig. 19-33). At surgery the ulnar component was intact. Strut grafts were placed anterior and posterior, both extending past the fracture (Fig. 19-34). At 1 year the implant is solid, the fracture has healed, and the patient has minimal pain (Fig. 19-35A,B).

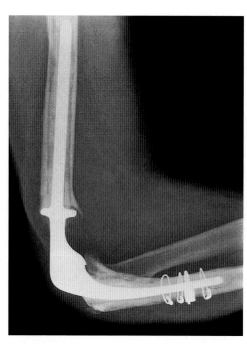

Figure 19-26. The preoperative radiograph showing absence of distal humerus and a prior fracture of ulna treated by cerclage wiring. The ulnar component was loose and the humeral bone deficient.

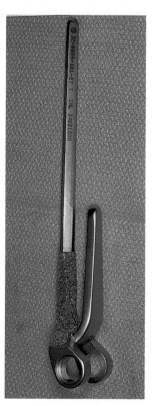

Figure 19-27. A long-flanged implant was used.

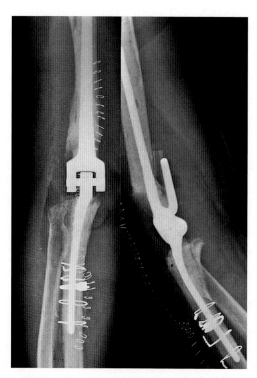

Figure 19-28. The long flange and humeral and ulnar strut grafts were used.

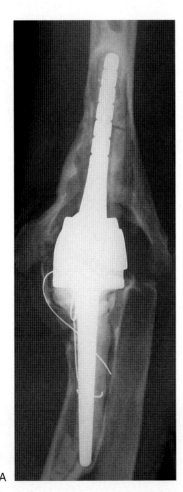

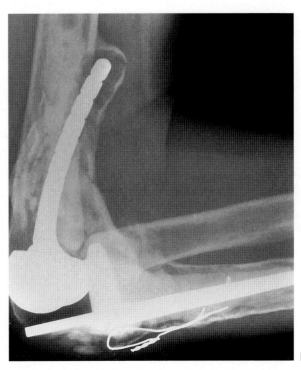

A

B

Figure 19-29. AP (**A**) and lateral radiographs (**B**) of a patient after two failed revision procedures showing the resurfacing implant eroding through the anterior proximal portion of the midhumerus. The lateral view also shows that the proximal ulna is completely eroded and that both the components are loose.

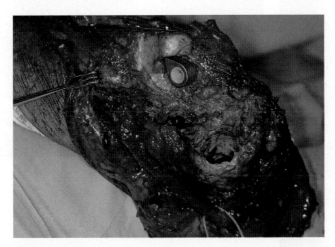

Figure 19-30. An allograft has been used to replace the proximal ulna. The allograft has been secured with a semitubular plate with single cortical screws. The screws are stabilized with cement.

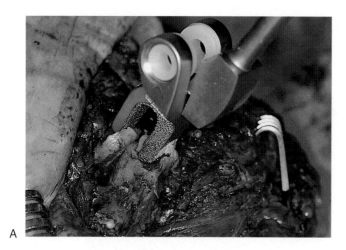

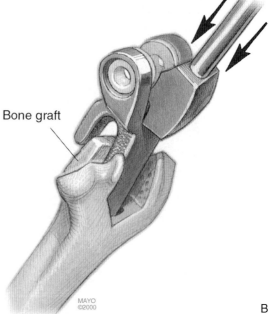

Figure 19-31. A,B: The humeral component is inserted and stabilized with a bone graft behind the flange of the prosthesis.

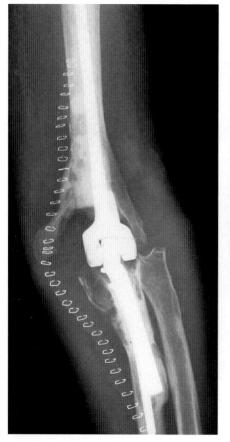

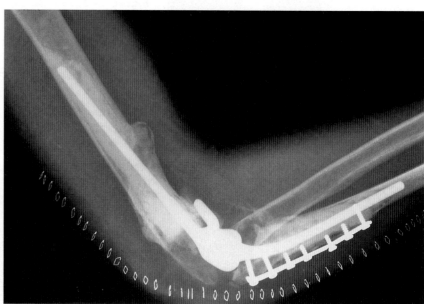

Figure 19-32. A,B: Five days after surgery the patient has very good early motion. The radiograph shows a well-fixed implant with a range of motion between 40 and 110 degrees at 5 days.

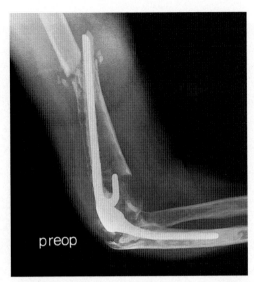

Figure 19-33. A periprosthetic fracture at the mid-humerus associated with grossly loose humeral component and marked distal humeral bone loss.

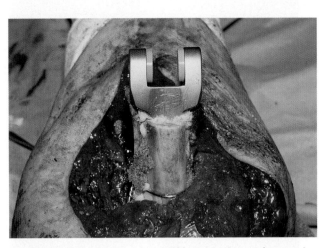

Figure 19-34. This was treated by anterior and posterior strut bone graft extending to the level of the articulation.

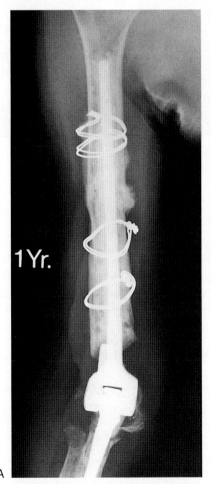

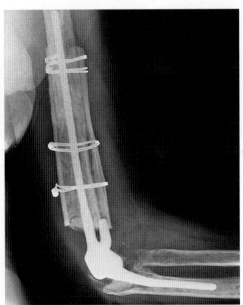

Figure 19-35. A,B: The fracture has healed and the graft has been incorporated at 1 year.

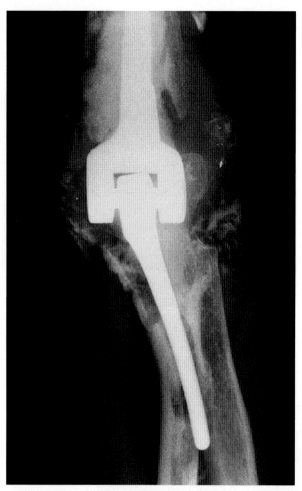

Figure 19-36. Extensive osteolysis of ulnar component 6 years after elbow replacement. The humeral component is also involved in this 58-year-old patient.

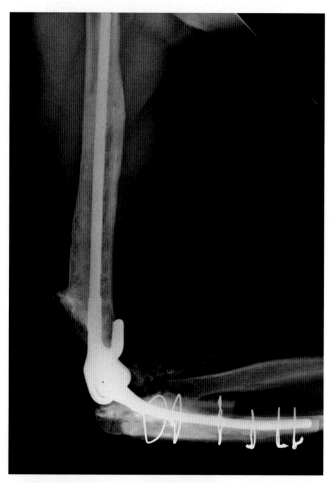

Figure 19-37. An anterior and posterior strut graft was placed along with impaction grafting.

Impaction/Strut Grafting

A 58-year-old man admits to excessive use of his elbow for 6 years. The ulna was grossly loose, with extensive osteolysis (Fig. 19-36). At surgery structural deficiency required anterior and posterior strut grafting as well as impaction grafting of the proximal ulna (Fig. 19-37). At 2 years the reconstruction was stable and pain was minimal.

RECOMMENDED READINGS

1. Bryan RS, Morrey BF. Extensive posterior exposure of the elbow: a triceps-sparing approach. *Clin Orthop* 1982;166:188.
2. Dee R, Ries M. Nonprosthetic elbow reconstruction. In: Morrey BF, ed. *The elbow and its disorders,* 3rd ed. Philadelphia: WB Saunders; 2000.
3. Dent CM, Hoy G, Stanley JK. Revision of failed total elbow arthroplasty. *J Bone Joint Surg* 1995;77B:691–695.
4. Figgie HE, Inglis AE, Ranawat CS, et al. Results of total elbow arthroplasty as a salvage procedure for failed elbow reconstructive operations. *Clin Orthop* 1987;219:185.
5. Gie GA, Linder L, Ling RSM, et al. Impacted cancellous allografts and cement for revision total hip arthroplasty. *J Bone Joint Surg* 1993;75B:14–21.
6. King G, Adams RA, Morrey BF. Revision with a non-custom semiconstrained prosthesis. *J Bone Joint Surg* 1997;79A:394–400.
7. Lee DH. Impaction allograft bone-grafting for revision total elbow arthroplasty. *J Bone Joint Surg* 1999;81A:1008–1012.

8. Loebenberg M, Adams RA, Morrey BF. Impaction grafting in revision total elbow arthroplasty. (In preparation)
9. Mankin HJ, Doppelt S, Tomfort W. Clinical experience with allograft implantation: the first ten years. *Clin Orthop* 1983;174:69.
10. Morrey BF, King GJ. Revision of failed total elbow arthroplasty. In: Morrey BF, ed. *The elbow and its disorders,* 3rd ed. Philadelphia: WB Saunders; 2000.
11. Morrey BF, Bryan RS. Revision total elbow arthroplasty. *J Bone Joint Surg* 1987;69A:523.
12. Sanchez-Sotelo J, Morrey BF. The use of struts for the purpose of revision of total elbow arthroplasty. (In preparation.)
13. Slooff TJ, Huiskes R, van Horn J, et al. Bone grafting in total hip replacement for acetabular protrusion. *Acta Orthop Scand* 1984;55:593–596.
14. Urbaniak JR, Black KE Jr. Cadaveric elbow allografts: a six-year experience. *Clin Orthop* 1985;197:131.
15. Yamaguchi K, Adams RA, Morrey BF. Infection after total elbow arthroplasty. *J Bone Joint Surg* 1998; 80a:481–491.

20

Ulnohumeral Arthroplasty

Bernard F. Morrey

The existence of a degenerative process involving the elbow is becoming increasingly recognized (2,9,14). The process typically limits extension to a minimal or moderate extent. Most symptomatic is impingement pain with terminal extension and, less commonly, terminal flexion with or without ulnar nerve involvement. A debridement procedure termed *ulnohumeral arthroplasty* has proven to be effective and reliable for such conditions, especially if ulnar nerve involvement is an issue.

INDICATIONS/CONTRAINDICATIONS

The patient with primary osteoarthritis is the ideal candidate for ulnohumeral arthroplasty. This process occurs predominantly in males by at least a 5 to 1 ratio (4,11,14). The mean age of onset is approximately 55 years, range 25 (uncommon) to 65. The chief complaint is terminal extension pain; a painful midarc is uncommon. Radiohumeral involvement occurs in approximately 50%, and loose-body formation in approximately 50%. More than half of the individuals will have an occupation or lifestyle associated with repetitive use, such as a carpenter, laborer, or person who requires a wheelchair or crutches for ambulation (11). About one in four will have symptoms of ulnar nerve irritation.

This procedure is particularly indicated in patients presenting with terminal extension pain, radiographic evidence of coronoid or olecranon osteophytes, and ossification of the olecranon foramen. If ulnar nerve symptoms are present, the nerve is inspected.

This procedure is contraindicated in the patient with pain throughout the arc of motion, marked limitation of motion with an arc of less than 30 to 40 degrees, or severe radiohumeral involvement indicating an advanced and generalized process. Isolated symptoms of catching associated with loose bodies are best dealt with by arthroscopy (12,13). If motion loss is the principal concern and the ulnar nerve is not symptomatic, we prefer the column decompression procedure (6) (Chapter 21).

B.F. Morrey, M.D.: Mayo Medical School and Department of Orthopaedics, Mayo Clinic and Mayo Foundation, Rochester, Minnesota.

PREOPERATIVE PLANNING

It is most important to properly select patients for this procedure. This operation is not designed to reliably gain motion but rather to relieve the pain associated with the impingement arthritis, especially in terminal extension. If the impingement is associated with mild osteophyte formation, an arthroscopic debridement has been effective in the hands of the experienced (12,13). However, particular attention should be paid to the presence of ulnar nerve symptoms. This must be addressed at the time of decompression and prompts this rather than the arthroscopic procedure.

Since approximately 50% of the patients will have loose bodies in addition to routine anterior/posterior and lateral radiographs, it is important to assess this before surgery. Careful plain films or CT may be useful to define. The precise size of the osteophytes as well allows identity of any loose bodies. Specific care is taken not to overlook any loose bodies, as these may cause mechanical symptoms later. Other imaging studies such as arthrogram or magnetic resonance imaging (MRI) are worthless.

SURGERY

With the patient supine and a sandbag under the shoulder, general anesthesia is administered and the elbow is brought across the chest.

Technique

A posterior incision courses just medial to the tip of the olecranon. This extends distally about 4 cm and proximally about 6 cm (Fig. 20-1). The subcutaneous tissue is reflected from the medial aspect of the triceps.

The ulnar nerve is identified at the cubital tunnel and carefully inspected. Its possible involvement with an osteophyte or from degenerative changes in the medial epicondylar region should be assessed before surgery (Fig. 20-2). The nerve has been a source of irritation for a growing number of patients, so we have a lower threshold to decompress than we once had. The nerve is carefully inspected. If it appears to be compressed, the cubital tunnel retinaculum is released.

Two approaches to the posterior joint are possible. A simple triceps-splitting technique was originally described and is still used in very muscular individuals (Fig. 20-3). Otherwise, approximately one-third to one-half of the triceps attachment may be elevated from the tip of the olecranon, releasing Sharpey's fibers by sharp dissection (Fig. 20-4). The triceps is elevated from the posterior aspect of the distal humerus by blunt dissection using a periosteal elevator, the capsule is excised, and any loose bodies are removed from the posterior compartment.

The tip of the olecranon is identified (Fig. 20-5). Usually there is a prominent osteophyte present that may extend across the joint and into the medial and lateral aspect posteriorly. The tip of the olecranon with the osteophyte is resected first using an oscillating saw or a 19-mm osteotome to define the exact amount to be resected. A 13-mm osteotome is used to complete the resection (Fig. 20-6) and the olecranon process with its osteophyte is removed (Fig. 20-7). The level should be such that the posterior aspect of the ulna is flush with the midportion of its articulation. The orientation of the osteotome should be parallel to each face of the trochlea rather than directed straight across the olecranon and into the trochlea (Fig. 20-8).

An 18- to 20-mm diameter trephine (Cloward) is then used to remove the ossified olecranon (Fig. 20-9). Often there are osteophytes originating from both the medial and the lateral columns. Proper placement of this foraminectomy is important. The trephine follows the curvature of the trochlea; the osteophyte may be removed in part with an osteotome to allow the trephine to be properly seated. After several turns of the trephine it is removed and the orientation of the foraminectomy is confirmed to be accurately placed (Fig. 20-10). The foraminectomy with the trephine is then completed and the core of bone is removed from the

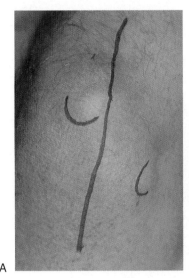

A

Figure 20-1. A,B: A straight skin incision is made just medial to the tip of the olecranon.

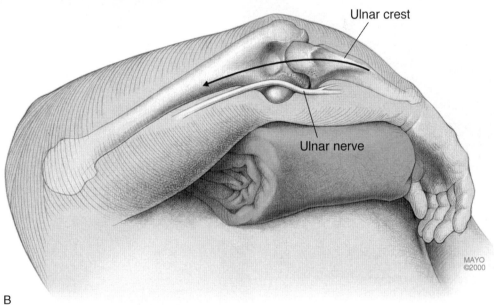

Ulnar crest

Ulnar nerve

MAYO
©2000

B

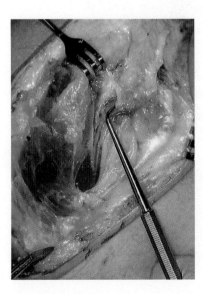

Figure 20-2. The ulnar nerve is identified at the medial margin of the triceps muscle and, if not compressed, is protected in the cubital tunnel (dental probe) but not translocated.

Figure 20-3. A,B: The simplest exposure is that of triceps muscle splitting to expose the posterior joint.

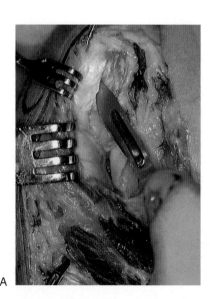

A

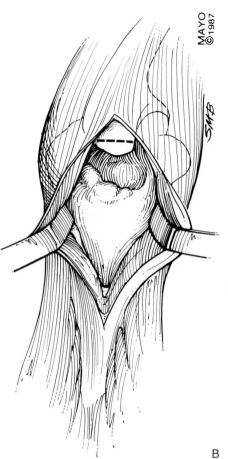

B

Figure 20-4. A,B: The medial aspect of the insertion of the triceps is reflected from the tip of the olecranon. Avoid releasing more than one-half of the Sharpey's fiber insertion.

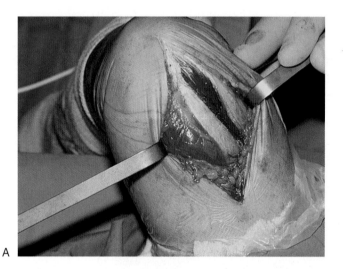

A

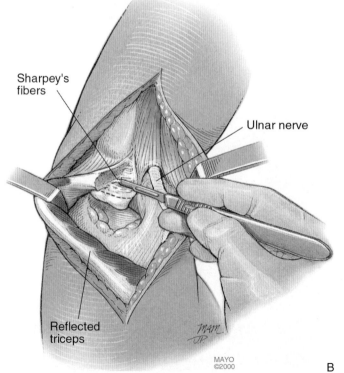

Sharpey's fibers

Ulnar nerve

Reflected triceps

B

Figure 20-5. A,B: The prominent olecranon osteophyte is identified and the line of olecranon process resection is defined.

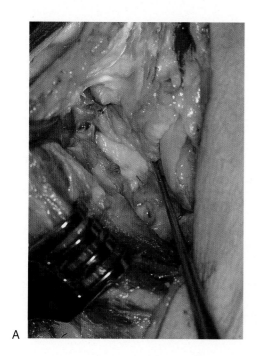

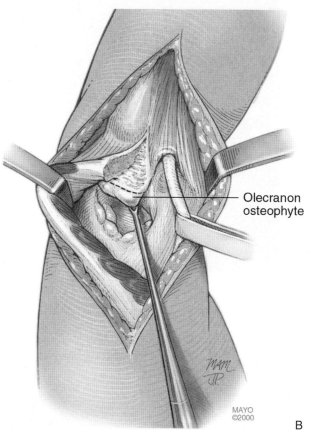

Olecranon osteophyte

MAYO
©2000

A

B

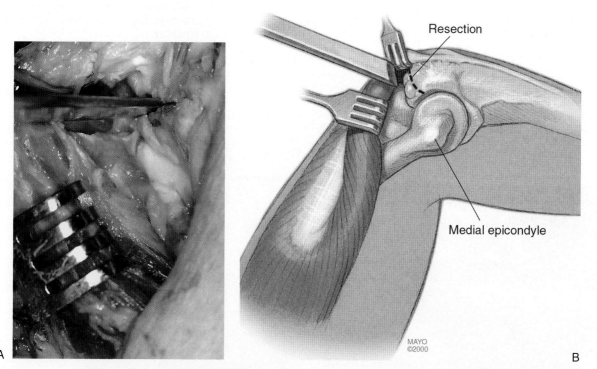

Resection

Medial epicondyle

MAYO
©2000

A

B

Figure 20-6. A,B: The osteophyte and process is removed with an osteotome. The initial cut may be made with an oscillating saw to provide optimum orientation.

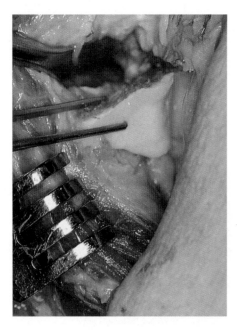

Figure 20-7. Removal of the olecranon process.

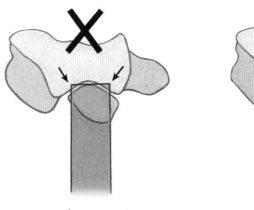

Incorrect   Correct

Figure 20-8. The completion of the osteotomy of the olecranon is with the osteotome parallel to each face of the trochlea. Direct transection will injure the trochlea.

Figure 20-9. A,B: With the triceps reflected laterally a trephine is used to remove the ossified olecranon fossa.

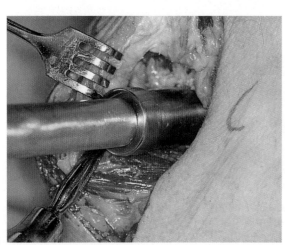

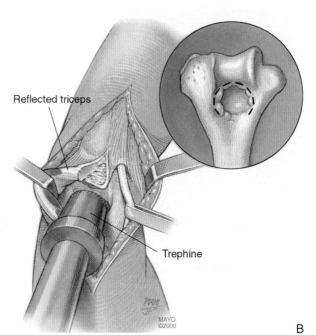

Reflected triceps

Trephine

A   B

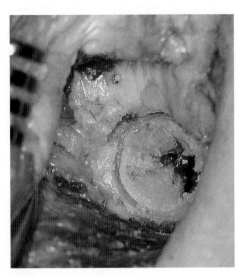

Figure 20-10. The contour of the trephine follows that of the trochlea, and inspection of the initial cut should be made before its completion.

distal humerus. This will frequently include osteophytes from the anterior aspect of the joint (Fig. 20-11). Inspection through the posterior aspect of the elbow into the anterior capsule is then possible. Loose bodies are identified and removed (Fig. 20-12). We then palpate the anterior column and determine whether any particularly tight bands are present that may need to be released. Any loose bodies that may be present or have been identified by a preoperative tomogram are removed and care is taken to be sure that none are left or overlooked.

The next step is the most difficult and involves removing the coronoid osteophyte and a portion of the coronoid process. By fully flexing the elbow the coronoid appears in the orifice created by the trephine. This can only be done with the elbow flexed. This is usually easily accomplished if the triceps has been split (Fig. 20-13A), but if the triceps has been reflected, it must be retracted laterally at the same time as the elbow is being flexed, which

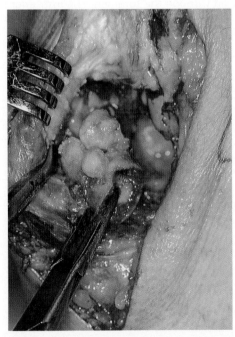

Figure 20-11. The foraminectomized portion of the distal humerus is removed. Note the anterior osteophytes present on this specimen.

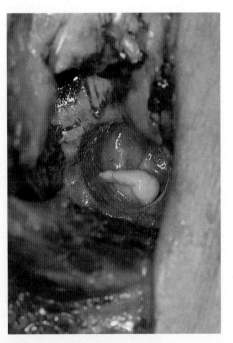

Figure 20-12. Anterior compartment loose bodies then may be identified and removed through the foramen.

is done with difficulty in the heavily muscled patient (Fig. 20-13). A curved 7-mm osteotome follows the distal aspect of the foraminectomized distal humerus. The tip of the olecranon is palpated and with a curvature directed toward the ulna; the coronoid with its osteophyte is resected and removed through the foramen (Fig. 20-14). The anterior aspect of the joint is again palpated with elbow flexion and extension to ensure that this has been adequately resected. A final check for any residual loose bodies or impingement is followed by placing a portion of rolled Gelfoam into the defect to fill the dead space to minimize the chance of hematoma and possibly recalcification (Fig. 20-15).

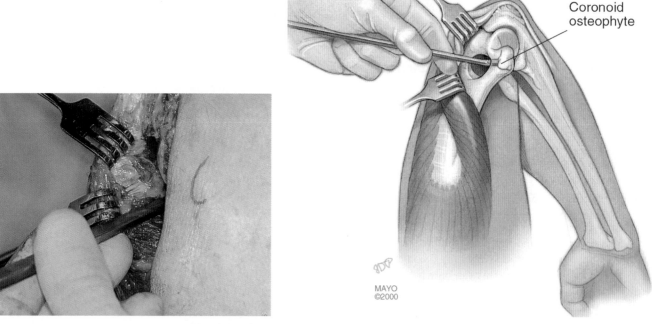

Coronoid osteophyte

MAYO ©2000

A

B

Figure 20-13. A,B: With the triceps reflected laterally and the elbow flexed as much as possible, an osteotome is introduced through the foramen. The instrument follows the distal surface of the foramen, and the coronoid process with its osteophyte is then osteotomized.

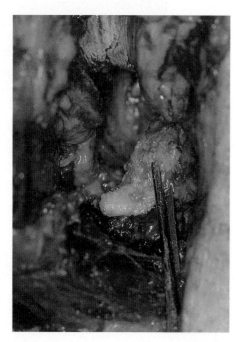

Figure 20-14. The osteophyte and a portion of the coronoid are removed.

The triceps is repaired if split or it resumes its normal position if partially reflected. Reattachment is not necessary since adequate insertion strength persists. The forearm and brachial fascia are brought back to the medial margin of the triceps and secured with absorbable suture (Fig. 20-16). The remainder of the closure is routine and is the choice of the surgeon.

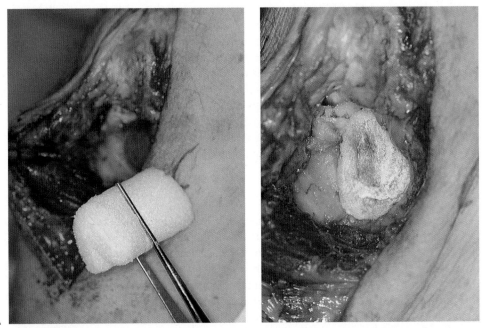

A   B

Figure 20-15. Gelfoam is then rolled in a cylinder-type fashion (**A**) and placed in the foramen (**B**).

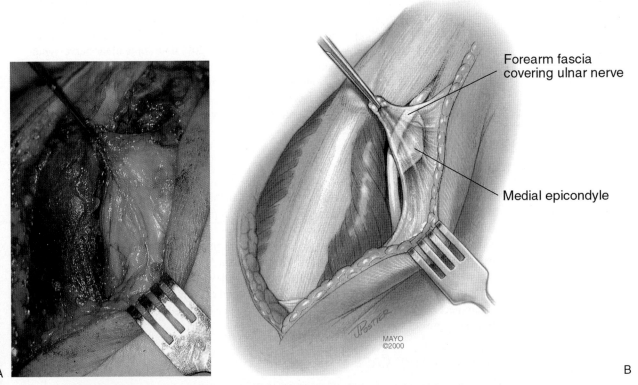

A   B

Figure 20-16. A,B: The triceps is allowed to resume its normal position. Reattachment is not considered necessary unless more than half of the triceps has been reflected. Forearm fascia is brought to the margin of the triceps to prevent any subluxation of the ulnar nerve.

POSTOPERATIVE MANAGEMENT

After surgery these patients are managed similarly to those with ankylosis release (10); that is, after the neurologic assessment has been performed in the recovery room, an axillary block is placed (3). A continuous passive motion (CPM) machine is then used, beginning the day of surgery for approximately 24 to 36 hours, at which time the axillary catheter is discontinued and a portable CPM is provided. The patient is dismissed at day 2 or 3. If significant loss of extension or flexion was observed before surgery and it is felt that this may be improved after the procedure, then flexion and extension braces, again similar to those described for the surgical release of the stiff elbow, are prescribed. Reassessment is made at 3 weeks. At that time the use of the splints is decreased to approximately 2 to 3 hours in the morning and 2 to 3 hours in the evening, with the patient continuing to sleep in the splints. The CPM machine is generally discontinued after the third week as well. The patient is seen again at 6 weeks and at 3 months. It is uncommon to gain or to lose any significant motion after 3 months, but this may still occur up to 6 months or possibly even a year. The exact period of time during which these patients are followed must be individualized.

RESULTS

The basic concept of this procedure was first described by Outerbridge and Kashiwagi in a series of patients in the Japanese literature in 1977 (5). The experience was updated by Minimi et al. in 1996 (8). With longer surveillance, recurrence of both pain and motion loss was observed in about 40%. The original report revealed greater than 90% satisfactory results, but it was recognized that the osteophytes may recur, and the underlying disease process is of course still present. A more recent experience, again from Japan, tends to confirm these findings (7). At the Mayo Clinic the procedure was modified by preserving the triceps, decompressing the ulnar nerve, and using a trephine for decompression. The results of the first 13 patients reveal that approximately 85% were considered satisfactory at an average of 3 years following the surgery. Pain relief is seen in approximately 90%. Improved motion is observed in 80% and averages about 10 to 15 degrees of improved extension and approximately 10 degrees of improved flexion for an overall improvement arc of about 20 to 25 degrees. There has been no instance of instability. The experience is currently being updated (1). Preliminary results reveal that approximately 20% note some ulnar nerve symptoms, which has prompted the current recommendation regarding preoperative ulnar nerve assessment and decompression. Nonetheless, approximately 80% are satisfied a mean of 7 years from surgery. The procedure has been redone in one patient.

As facility increases with arthroscopic debridement, some patients may be effectively decompressed via this modality (12,13).

COMPLICATIONS

We have experienced only one major complication in this patient population, that of a severe ulnar neuropathy. It is felt that a retractor may have compressed this nerve during the surgical procedure. This experience in part prompted the recommended exposure in which the ulnar nerve is identified and protected throughout the surgical procedure. Recurrence of the disease process is a function of time (8). Within the first 5 years, less than 10% symptomatic recurrence has been observed, which is consistent with what is reported in the literature.

With inadequate exposure of the medial and lateral columns, improper placement of the foraminectomy may lead to a column fracture. Hence the need for adequate visualization of the margins of the columns.

ILLUSTRATIVE CASE

A 54-year-old carpenter presented with pain in the elbow. He indicated that he had particular difficulty holding objects overhead for any period of time, and this was limiting his ability to do his job. This process had been noticed approximately 2 years earlier, with the first abnormality noticed being loss of full extension and forearm rotation. He had a radial head excision with only modest impairment limited to forearm rotation. He had little pain through the midarc of flexion and extension. The examination revealed a range of elbow flexion of 30 to 125 degrees, pronation of 70 degrees, and supination of 75 degrees. The ulnar nerve was painless to palpation. Radiographs revealed a prominent osteophyte in the anterior coronoid, less so in the tip of the olecranon (Fig. 20-17). The olecranon foramen was ossified, as was the resected radial head (Fig. 20-18), as demonstrated on the anteroposterior radiograph. Debridement included the olecranon, coronoid, foramen osteophytes, and a loose body (Fig. 20-19). Five years after the surgical procedure the patient has an arc

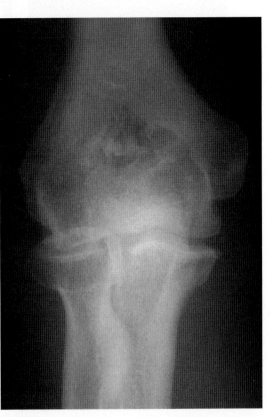

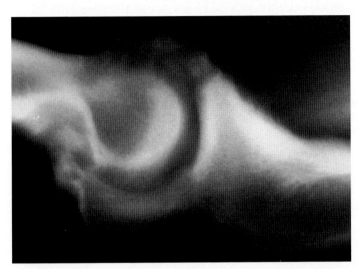

Figure 20-17. A 46-year-old laborer has extensor pain and motion of 40 to 120 degrees. The lateral roentgenograph reveals osteophytes of the olecranon and of the coronoid.

Figure 20-18. The olecranon and coronoid foramen are ossified on the anteroposterior view.

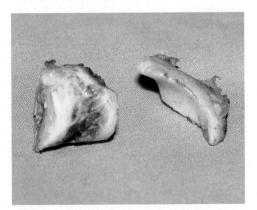

Figure 20-19. The debridement consists of a large olecranon osteophyte and of the foramen resection. The coronoid osteophyte was also removed.

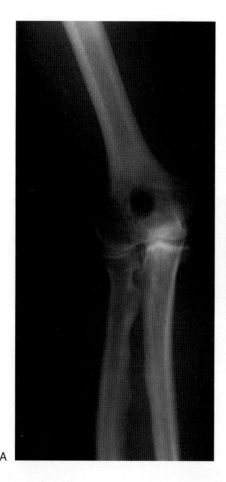

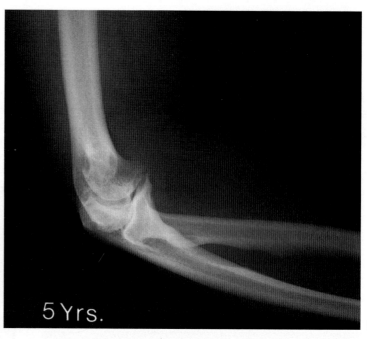

Figure 20-20. A,B: Five years after removal the motion is from 20 to 130 degrees. There is no pain and the foramen osteophytes have not recurred.

of motion of 18 to 130 degrees, and pronation-supination is unchanged. He has essentially no pain and is well pleased with the result (Fig. 20-20).

RECOMMENDED READINGS

1. Antuna S, Morrey BF, O'Driscoll S. Primary osteoarthritis of the elbow treated by ulnohumeral arthroplasty: a long term follow-up study. *J Bone Joint Surg* 2001 (accepted).
2. Doherty M, Preston B. Primary osteoarthritis of the elbow. *Ann Rheum Dis* 1989;48:743.
3. Gaumann DM, Lennon RL, Wodel DJ. Continuous axillary block for postoperative pain management. *Reg Anaesth* 1988;13:77.
4. Kashiwagi D. Intra-articular changes of the osteoarthritic elbow, especially about the fossa olecrani. *Jpn Orthop Assoc* 1978;52:1367.
5. Kashiwagi D. Outerbridge Kashiwagi arthroplasty for osteoarthritis of the elbow in the elbow joint. In: Kashiwagi D, ed. *Proceedings of the International Congress, Kobi, Japan.* Amsterdam: Excerpta Medica; 1986.
6. Mansat P, Morrey BF. The "column procedure," a limited surgical approach for the treatment of stiff elbows. *J Bone Joint Surg* 1998;80A:1603.
7. Minami NM, Ishii S. Outerbridge Kashiwagi arthroplasty for osteoarthritis of the elbow joint. In: Kashiwagi D, ed. *Proceedings of the International Congress, Kobi, Japan.* Amsterdam: Excerpta Medica; 1986.
8. Minami M, Kato S, Kashiwagi D. Outerbridge-Kashiwagi's method for arthroplasty of osteoarthritis of the elbow: 44 elbows followed for 8–16 years. *J Orthop Sci* 1996;1:11.
9. Mintz G, Fraga A. Severe osteoarthritis of the elbow in foundry workers. *Arch Environ Health* 1973;27:78.
10. Morrey BF. Post-traumatic contracture of the elbow: operative treatment including distraction arthroplasty. *J Bone Joint Surg* 1990;72A:601.
11. Morrey BF. Primary arthritis of the elbow treated by ulnohumeral arthroplasty. *J Bone Joint Surg* 1992;74B:409.
12. Ogilvie-Harris DJ, Gordon R, MacKay M. Arthroscopic treatment for posterior impingement in degenerative arthritis of the elbow. *Arthroscopy* 1995;11:437.
13. Redden JF, Stanley D. Arthroscopic fenestration of the olecranon fossa in the treatment of osteoarthritis of the elbow. *Arthroscopy* 1993;9:14.
14. Stanley D, Winson G. A surgical approach to the elbow. *J Bone Joint Surg* 1990;72B:728.

21

Capsular Release for Flexion Contracture: The Column Procedure

Bernard F. Morrey and Pierre Mansat

In some instances of elbow trauma the articular surface has not been badly injured and the loss of motion is limited to extension due primarily to thickening of the anterior capsule. This type of stiffness is termed *extrinsic* and the joint surface is minimally damaged (7). In this circumstance several options are available. The technique described later is used in preference to an anterior exposure. The indications are very similar, and the author has found this technique to be simple and reliable with a low complication rate (6). This exposure is preferable in the author's opinion to a formal anterior approach (3, 8,10) and avoids the more aggressive release needed for intrinsic contracture (7,11). Arthroscopic release of the anterior capsule is discussed in Chapter 2 (5).

INDICATIONS/CONTRAINDICATIONS

Indications include flexion contracture with loss of extension of at least 40 degrees and preservation or minimal changes of the articular surface. Posttraumatic etiology such as dislocation is an ideal indication. If limitation of motion includes loss of flexion, an additional step is needed, but the loss of flexion can usually be effectively treated by anterior capsular release.

This "simple" release cannot be done in instances requiring interposition of the joint. Interposition is used if any of the following three contraindications are present (7): a significant alteration of the articular contour, loss of joint cartilage (50%), or pathology that requires release of one or both collateral ligaments (see Chapter 22).

Additional contraindications include motor deficiency or spasticity, especially involving the flexor muscles and residual impairment from closed head injury.

B.F. Morrey, M.D.: Mayo Medical School and Department of Orthopaedics, Mayo Clinic and Mayo Foundation, Rochester, Minnesota.

P. Mansat, M.D.: Department of Orthopaedics and Traumatology, University Hospital of Toulouse–Purpan, Toulouse, France.

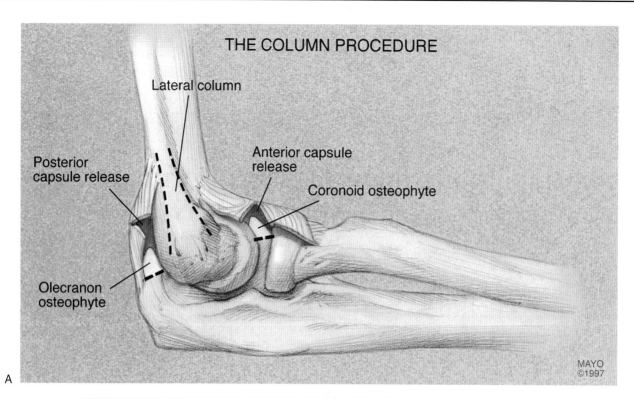

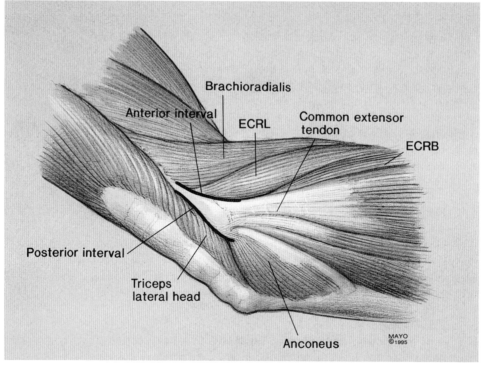

Figure 21-1. A: The concept of the column procedure. Identify the supracondylar ridge and approach the anterior and posterior aspects of the capsule as necessary. Osteophytes are readily removed from the coronoid process or the olecranon. **B:** Relevant anatomy of the "column." The anterior and posterior aspects of the lateral column are identified (*solid lines*). (Abbreviations: ECRL, extensor carpi radialis longus; ECRB, extensor carpi radialis brevis.)

PREOPERATIVE PLANNING

The column release is indicated in those with extrinsic pathology (i.e., extrinsic to the joint surface). This is determined in my practice by a simple lateral radiograph. This is the least expensive and the most accurate manner of evaluating the joint before surgery. There is no indication for an MR or a CT scan in treating patients with capsular contracture or post-traumatic loss of motion.

The second consideration before surgery is whether there are both flexion and extension elements to the contracture. If the patient has normal or near normal flexion, then the dissection may be limited to the anterior capsule with the simple elevation of the common extensor tendon and exposure of the anterior capsule. If the patient has limitation of flexion, then elevation of the triceps and removal of the posterior capsule are necessary. Although the determination of the extent of such resection is obviously done at the time of surgery, it is important to discuss the nature of the surgery preoperatively with the patient in the context of the anticipated rehabilitation and ultimate result.

Since the first edition we have become increasingly aware of the implications of ulnar nerve irritation before surgery. This aspect is carefully sought and discussed. If present, a posterior incision is made and the ulnar nerve is explored. If it is injured before or after capsule release, the nerve is decompressed or translocated.

If the pathology suggests that there is intrinsic involvement or that a release of the collateral ligament is necessary to obtain adequate exposure, then the surgeon should be prepared to apply the distraction device protecting the collateral ligament repair and separating the joint surfaces for approximately 3 weeks after surgery (see Chapters 8 and 22). It is uncommon to be faced with this option if the proper determination of the nature of the contracture and adequate imaging and assessment of the joint surface have occurred before the surgery as discussed earlier.

Finally, it is important for the patient to have a clear understanding of the time commitment that is required after such surgery. The emphasis on the maintenance of the splinting program for several weeks or even months following the procedure is quite important, particularly depending upon the type of occupation and the expectations that the patient may hold.

Either general or regional anesthesia may be used. The column procedure consists of arthrotomy, release of the anterior and posterior capsule if needed, and excision of osteophytes through a limited lateral approach (Fig. 21-1).

TECHNIQUE

The patient is placed supine with a sandbag under the ipsilateral extremity and the arm draped free and brought across the chest. The proximal one-half of a Kocher incision, which extends 6 cm proximal to and 3 cm distal to the epicondyle, is used if there is no previous incision and if there are no symptoms related to the ulnar nerve (Fig. 21-2). If there are symptoms related to the ulnar nerve, a midline posterior incision is made so that the nerve can be explored. If there is gross evidence of impingement before or after the capsular release, the nerve is decompressed as necessary.

To release the anterior aspect of the capsule with minimum disruption of normal tissue, the fleshy origin of the extensor carpi radialis longus and the distal fibers of the brachioradialis are identified (Fig. 21-3). Release of the origin of these muscles from the humerus provides direct access to the superolateral aspect of the capsule (Fig. 21-4). The brachialis is swept from the anterior aspect of the capsule with a periosteal elevator. The capsule is entered anteriorly at the radiohumeral joint to allow assessment of the thickness of the capsule (Fig. 21-5A). A modified knee retractor (V. Muller and Co., St. Louis, MO) with a blade-shaft angle of 130 degrees (Fig. 21-5B) protects the brachialis, the radial nerve, and the brachial artery. The anterior aspect of the capsule is grasped, and the lateral half is ex-

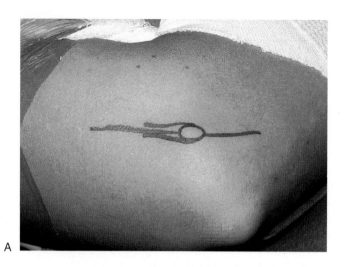

A

Figure 21-2. A,B: If a simple "column" release is anticipated a limited incision measuring 6 to 8 cm in length is made over the lateral column, ending 2 cm distal to the lateral epicondyle as shown in this right elbow.

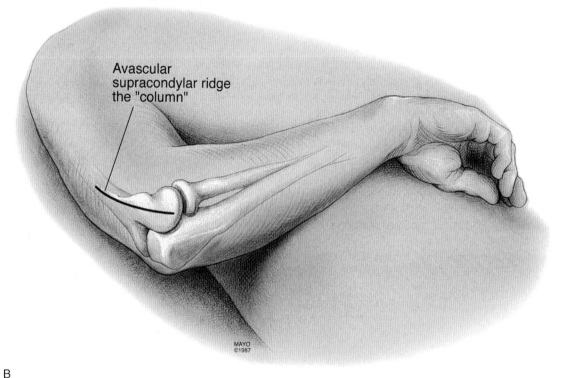

Avascular
supracondylar ridge
the "column"

MAYO
©1987

B

cised to at least the level of the coronoid. The most medial aspect of the capsule, which can sometimes be difficult to visualize but can be palpated, is incised to complete the release (Fig. 21-6). The elbow is extended, and any remnant adhesion is gently lysed. At this time, if there is full extension or if extension is within 10 degrees of normal and there are no radiographically evident spurs on the olecranon, no additional release is needed. The capsule is left open, and the wound is closed.

If flexion is limited or if extension is not complete, this is probably the result of extensive scarring and adhesions involving the posterior aspect of the capsule. If this is the case, the triceps is elevated from the posterior aspect of the humerus, the posterior aspect of the capsule is released, and the olecranon fossa is cleaned of soft tissue. The tip of the olecranon is removed with an osteotome if there are osteophytes (Fig. 21-7). The amount of flex-

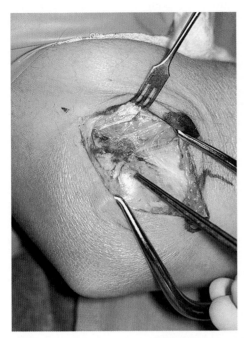

Figure 21-3. The proximal most muscular attachment to the common extensor tendon defines the origin of the extensor carpi radialis longus. The forceps are on the lateral epicondyle.

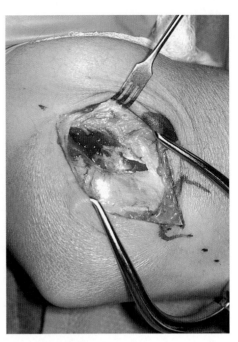

Figure 21-4. With the elbow at 90 degrees of flexion, the fibers of the extensor carpi radialis longus are followed down to the capsule. The brachialis is elevated from the anterior capsule.

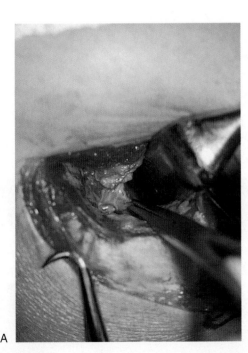

A

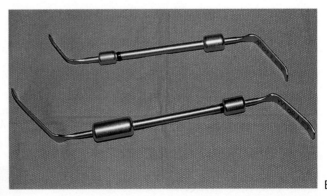

B

Figure 21-5. A: Elevation of the extensor carpi radialis longus (ECRL) and the distal fibers of the brachioradialis. The anterior aspect of the capsule is isolated from the brachialis and is identified with an arthrotomy at the anterior aspect of the radiohumeral joint. **B:** Special retractors (available from Müeller, in two sizes) facilitate exposure and protection of the anterior structures.

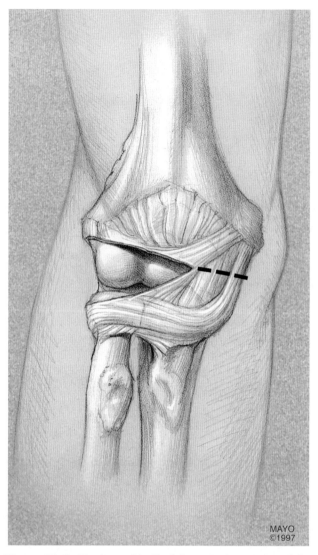

Figure 21-6. The lateral half of the anterior aspect of the capsule is excised as widely as possible, and the remaining medial half is incised (*dotted line*).

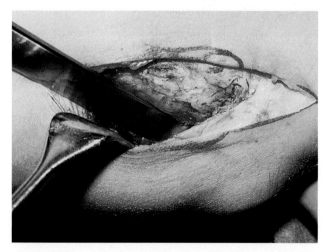

Figure 21-7. In those instances in which there is also loss of flexion, the triceps is elevated from the posterolateral column and the posterior capsule is also excised. If an osteophyte is present, it is removed with an osteotome.

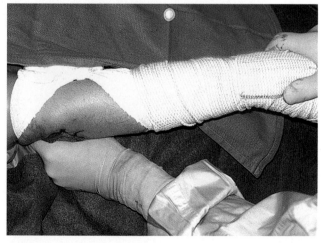

Figure 21-8. As the joint tends to "rebound" about 15 to 20 degrees from the amount of extension gained at surgery, full extension at the time of surgery is considered a must with this type of procedure.

ion and extension of the elbow is assessed. Typically, full extension is readily attained (Fig. 21-8). If there is at least 130 degrees of flexion, nothing more needs to be done posteriorly. If flexion is limited, the coronoid is inspected and any osteophytes are removed.

If there is evidence of irritation of the ulnar nerve, which is defined as a subjective alteration in sensation without objective sensory or motor changes or atrophy, a posterior incision is used to allow assessment of the lateral and medial aspects of the elbow through the same skin incision. The ulnar nerve is inspected, and occasionally it is translocated, but more often it is simply decompressed *in situ.*

POSTOPERATIVE MANAGEMENT

If the neurologic examination in the recovery room reveals normal findings, a catheter is inserted percutaneously for a brachial plexus block, which is maintained with a continuous pump (2). The arm is elevated as much as possible, and continuous passive motion is begun on the day of the operation (1,9). The machine is adjusted to provide as much motion as pain or the machine itself allows. The block is discontinued 2 days postoperatively, and continuous passive motion is discontinued 3 days postoperatively, at which time the patient is dismissed.

Physical therapy is not used, but a detailed program of therapy with adjustable splints, which depends on the motion before and after the procedure, is prescribed. The splints include a hyperextension or hyperflexion brace, or both. The splint program usually begins with 20 hours/day for 3 weeks (see Chapter 9).

RESULTS

The Mayo experience with 38 column procedures has been reported by Mansat and Morrey (6).

The mean preoperative arc of flexion of 49 degrees (from 52 to 101 degrees) improved postoperatively to a mean arc of 94 degrees (from 27 to 121 degrees) (Fig. 21-9). The mean total gain in the arc of flexion-extension was 45 degrees. Overall, 31 elbows (82%) had a satisfactory result. Greater improvement was obtained in elbows that had had the more severe stiffness. Others have reported similar results with the more limited exposure and release (4,12).

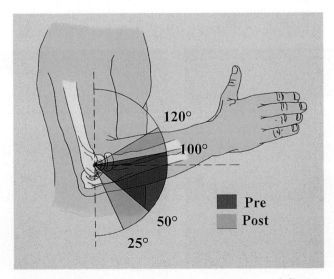

Figure 21-9. The overall gain in extension and flexion from 52–101 to 27–121 degrees.

COMPLICATIONS

No more complications have been associated with the technique described. To date no patients have permanent neurologic deficiency, but two have ulnar nerve irritation. Infection, ectopic bone, or increased pain, although a possibility, have not been recorded.

ILLUSTRATIVE CASE

A 28-year-old male sustained an elbow dislocation and was treated in a cast for 3 weeks and developed a contracture from 70 to 100 degrees (Fig. 21-10). After release the arc im-

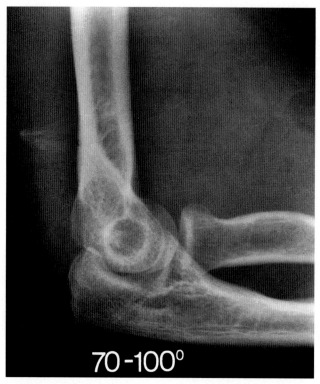

Figure 21-10. Marked contracture developed after 3 weeks immobilization for "simple" dislocation. The joint is intact.

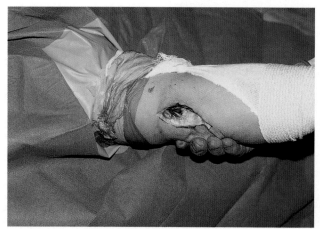
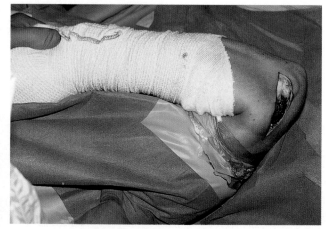

Figure 21-11. A,B: Near normal motion of 0 to 135 degrees was obtained at the time of surgery after anterior/posterior capsular release.

proved from 20 to 125 degrees (Fig. 21-11). There was no pain and the patient was pleased with the outcome.

RECOMMENDED READINGS

1. Breen TF, Gelberman RH, Ackerman GN. Elbow flexion contractures: treatment by anterior release and continuous passive motion. *J Hand Surg* 1988;13B:286–287.
2. Gaumann DM, Lennon RL, Wedel DJ. Continuous axillary block for postoperative pain management. *Reg Anaesth* 1988;13:77–81.
3. Gates HS III, Sullivan FL, Urbaniak JR. Anterior capsulotomy and continuous passive motion in the treatment of post-traumatic flexion contracture of the elbow: a prospective study. *J Bone Joint Surg* 1992;74A:1229–1234.
4. Husband JB, Hastings H. The lateral approach for operative release of post-traumatic contracture of the elbow. *J Bone Joint Surg* 1990;72A:1353–1358.
5. Jones GS, Savoie FH III. Arthroscopic capsular release of flexion contractures (arthrofibrosis) of the elbow. *Arthroscopy* 1993;9:277–283.
6. Mansat P, Morrey BF. The column procedure: a limited lateral approach for extrinsic contracture of the elbow. *J Bone Joint Surg* 1998;80A:1603–1615.
7. Morrey BF. Post-traumatic contracture of the elbow. *J Bone Joint Surg* 1990;72A:601–618.
8. Richards RR, Beaton D, Bechard M. Restoration of elbow motion by anterior capsular release of post-traumatic flexion contractures. *J Bone Joint Surg* 1991;73B(Suppl II):107.
9. Salter RB, Hamilton HW, Wedge JH, et al. Clinical application of basic research on continuous passive motion for disorders of injuries of synovial joints. *J Orthop Res* 1984;1:325.
10. Urbaniak JR, Hansen PE, Beissinger SF, et al. Correction of post-traumatic flexion contracture of the elbow by anterior capsulotomy. *J Bone Joint Surg* 1985;67A:1160–1164.
11. Tsuge K, Mizueki T. Debridement arthroplasty for advanced primary osteoarthritis of the elbow: results of a new technique used for 29 elbows. *J Bone Joint Surg* 1994;76B:641–646.
12. Weiss AP, Sachar K. Soft tissue contractures about the elbow. *Hand Clin* 1994;10:439–451.

22

Interposition Arthroplasty of the Elbow

Avrum I. Froimson and Bernard F. Morrey

Although a number of reconstructive options are available for elbow arthritis, one of the oldest reconstructive procedures (2), interposition arthroplasty, continues to be a viable reconstructive option in all practice, particularly in the young patient (5,13).

INDICATIONS/CONTRAINDICATIONS

Fascial interposition elbow arthroplasty is indicated in the relatively young adult patient. Although there have been significant advances in total elbow arthroplasty in recent years, the ongoing need to address severe arthritis in a patient in the third, fourth, or fifth decade of life continues to warrant consideration of this alternative procedure to restore motion and relieve discomfort.

In these instances in which the elbow later becomes painful or unstable, total elbow replacement may be performed with minimal technical difficulty, inserting the prosthetic stems into intact medullary canals of humerus and ulna (3). Specifically, (a) interposition arthroplasty is especially attractive in the management of posttraumatic ankylosis of the elbow (14). The anatomic requisite is that the broad contour of the distal humerus has not been significantly disrupted (Fig. 22-1). For those in whom the prosthesis is to be avoided, usually due to a very young patient, less than 40 years of age, reconstruction of the distal humerus may precede the interposition procedure. (b) In those less than 40 to 50 years of age with severe pain but with good motion, interposition may be considered instead of prosthetic replacement (5). (c) A third indication for this procedure is the young adult with stage I or II rheumatoid arthritis where the elbow is stiff and/or painful but the osseous architecture is reasonably intact. Resurfacing this elbow with an interposed membrane has been found to be successful in alleviating crepitus and pain, and provides a very satisfactory range of function (12).

A.I. Froimson, M.D.: Department of Orthopaedics, Case Western Reserve University, Cleveland Clinic, Cleveland, Ohio.

B.F. Morrey, M.D.: Mayo Medical School and Department of Orthopaedics, Mayo Clinic and Mayo Foundation, Rochester, Minnesota.

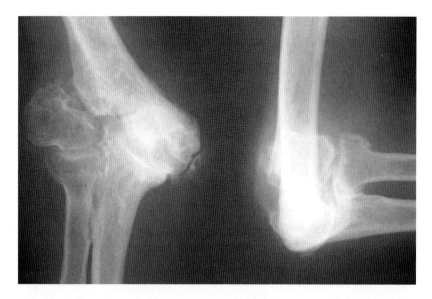

Figure 22-1. The lateral condylar nonunion narrows the distal humeral articulation and thus is a contraindication for interposition arthroplasty.

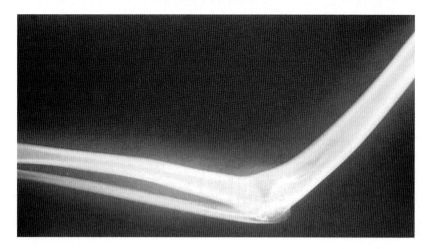

Figure 22-2. It is important to recognize that conditions such as congenital ankylosis are also associated with a significant deprivation of soft tissue. Absence of collateral ligaments such as occurs in this condition is a contraindication to interposition arthroplasty.

Arthroplasty procedures are contraindicated in the presence of active infection. The grossly unstable rheumatoid or posttraumatic elbow cannot be adequately stabilized by a fascial interposition procedure. Congenital ankylosis of the elbow joint (Fig. 22-2) lacks the necessary soft-tissue ligamentous and muscular support to allow soft-tissue interposition. Attempts to use this procedure for this indication have been abandoned intraoperatively and total elbow replacement has been substituted, even in the adolescent. As with other elbow arthroplasty techniques, the patient's need to use the upper extremities in ambulation or transfer from bed to chair is a relative contraindication, since excessive loading of the elbow will destabilize the joint. The noncompliant patient should be identified and avoided.

PREOPERATIVE PLANNING

The presence of ulnar nerve symptoms should be carefully assessed before surgery with the intention of addressing this at the time of the interposition procedure.

Plain radiographs of the elbow should include lateral films in maximum possible flexion and extension. If there are associated signs or symptoms of compromise of the ipsilateral shoulder and wrist, they should also be included in the radiographic studies.

For the cutis procedure the prospective skin graft donor site should be selected by examination of the lower abdomen or lateral thigh. Hairy donor sites should be avoided, since the presence of numerous large hair follicles in the cutis graft may theoretically predispose to increased incidence of epidermoid inclusion cysts. Since harvest of the cutis graft will leave a significant postoperative scar, the patient should participate in the selection of the most suitable donor site. Because the procedure is done under tourniquet control, blood loss is not excessive and transfusion is not anticipated.

The cutis is the material of choice of one of us (AF) for fascial interposition arthroplasty of the elbow. This is the most commonly used tissue reported in the recent literature (1,4,6–9). This is the thick dermal layer of skin that remains after a superficial epidermal layer of 0.0010 to 0.0012 inch has been peeled back with a dermatome. Cutis is a very tough and durable but flexible material that, when attached to the cut surface of the distal humerus, rapidly adheres to the bone. Cutis has been used by various authors as an interposing membrane in resection arthroplasties of various joints since 1913. It has been used in the elbow successfully in many instances in various centers. One of us prefers the achilles tendon allograft (BFM). If an achilles tendon allograft is to be used, availability of this material must, of course, be determine before surgery.

SURGERY

The patient is placed supine on the operating table with a large pillow or bolster under the ipsilateral shoulder, allowing the operated extremity to rest across the trunk for the procedure (Fig. 22-3). For a cutis interposition the skin graft donor site that has been selected, either abdomen or thigh, is prepared and draped and then covered until needed. The entire upper extremity is prepared and draped with stockinette, venous blood is expressed with an elastic bandage, and a pneumatic tourniquet is applied as proximally as possible on the upper arm and inflated for the duration of the procedure (Fig. 22-3).

CUTIS ARTHROPLASTY

Technique

A posterior skin incision is used. If the ulnar nerve is symptomatic, it is exposed and decompressed past the level of constriction. The extensile Kocher deep lateral approach to the joint is preferred, and a flap of tissue is elevated laterally to identify Kocher's interval (Fig. 22-4). It proceeds down the supracondylar ridge of the humerus between extensor carpi ul-

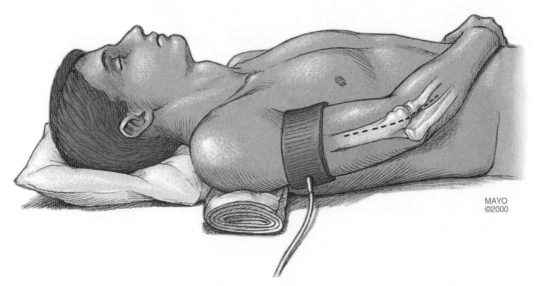

Figure 22-3. An extensile Kocher approach to the posterolateral aspect of the elbow is preferred.

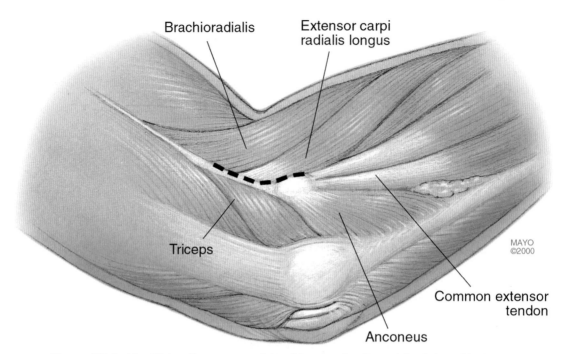

Figure 22-4. Identifying the supracondylar ridge proximally and the interval between the extensor carpi ulnaris and the anconeus muscle distally allows entry into the posterolateral, lateral, and anterolateral aspect of the joint.

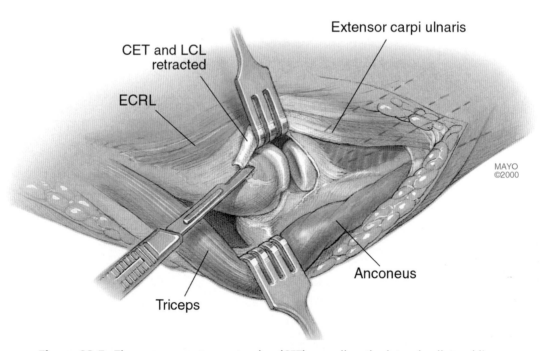

Figure 22-5. The common extensor tendon (CET) as well as the lateral collateral ligament (LCL) are taken off as a single layer. Occasionally, the collateral ligament can be isolated from the extensor origin and released separately. (Abbreviation: ECRL, extensor carpi radialis longus.)

naris and anconeus muscles. The extensor mass, lateral collateral ligament origin, and periosteum are dissected off of the lateral condyle and distal humerus (Fig. 22-5). Further release of the capsule exposes the medial collateral ligaments. If necessary, these are sectioned from within (Fig. 22-6), although one of us (BFM) preserves the medial ligament. If sectioned, this is most safely performed by release from the ulna. Varus stress allows the joint to dislocate and exposes the distal humerus and proximal ulna (Fig. 22-7). We do not

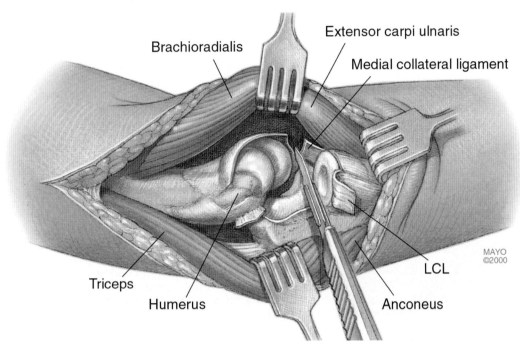

Figure 22-6. The anterior and posterior capsules are then released, and the anterior bundle of the medial collateral ligament is sectioned from the ulnar aspect of the medial aspect of the joint.

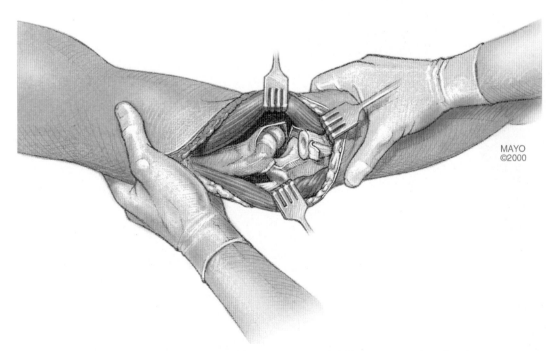

Figure 22-7. A varus stress allows the elbow to open and dislocate, exposing the distal humerus and proximal ulna.

routinely expose or transpose the ulnar nerve unless, as mentioned earlier, the ulnar nerve has been entrapped in posttraumatic scar on the medial side of the elbow, in which case a medial approach may be selected to perform the entire procedure. If the patient has cubital tunnel syndrome with ulnar nerve compromise, the ulnar nerve is transposed at this point in the procedure.

After dislocating the elbow, the distal end of the humerus is prepared by excising osteophytes, removing all articular cartilage and ununited bone fragments and fibrous debris (Fig. 22-8). That should yield a smooth, rounded surface 4 or 5 cm wide and approximately 2 cm from anterior to posterior. This prepared cancellous surface is the tissue to which the

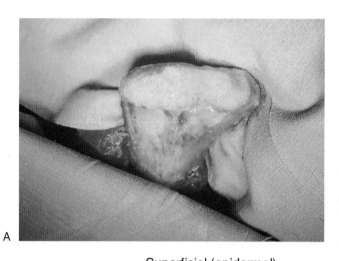

A

Figure 22-8. A: The distal humerus is freed of the articular debris and osteophytes, providing a smooth, round surface on which the dermal graft will be applied. **B:** The dimensions of the distal humerus are typically approximately 4 to 5 cm wide and about 2 cm from anterior to posterior.

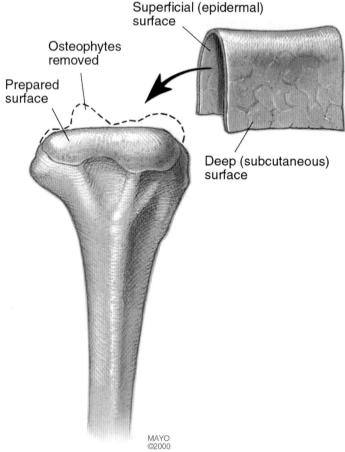

Superficial (epidermal) surface

Osteophytes removed

Prepared surface

Deep (subcutaneous) surface

MAYO
©2000

B

cutis graft will be attached. On average. only about 1 to 1.5 cm of the distal humerus is re-sected. Where possible the articular surfaces of the proximal radius and ulna are disturbed as little as possible. If those joint surfaces are irregular, they are simply smoothed down with bur or rasp before reducing the elbow. We prefer to debride the radial head if neces-sary to restore pronation and supination. An intact radial head provides a much broader dis-tal half of the articulation, resulting in better postoperative stability.

As I have become more experienced with this procedure, I have tended to remove a smaller amount of bone from the distal humerus than I did earlier in the series. This yields a higher degree of stability but necessitates that the surgeon, after having reduced the el-bow, ensure that there is a satisfactory range of movement and that the elbow is not overly tight, since the patient will not regain any more motion in the postoperative period of reha-bilitation than was present at the completion of the procedure.

After completing the preparatory stage of the elbow procedure, the surgeon determines how large a cutis graft is needed and then, using a hand-held or motorized dermatome, takes a thin (10 to 12 mils) split-thickness skin graft from the donor site (Fig. 22-9). The bed of the donor site then has the typical appearance with punctate bleeding. The surgeon then ex-cises this deep dermal layer of skin, cutting it off of the subcutaneous fat by scalpel dis-section (Fig. 22-10), thus harvesting the cutis graft (Fig. 22-11). After securing hemostasis with electrocautery, the split-thickness graft is then reapplied over the donor site and held in place with sutures (Fig. 22-12) and a stent (Fig. 22-13).

One of us (BFM) has altered this technique. An ellipse of skin measuring about 4 × 10 cm is outlined in the groin or bikini line. Strips of dermis 3 to 4 mm wide are sharply re-moved, leaving the cutis (Fig. 22-14). The cutis is then sharply excised and the wound is closed with a vertical mattress suture (Fig. 22-15).

The cutis graft is then draped over the prepared distal end of humerus, applying the su-perficial cut surface of dermis to bone (Fig. 22-16). This ensures that vascularization of the skin graft and healing to the cancellous bone surface will be optimized. The surgeon drills

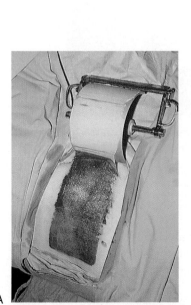

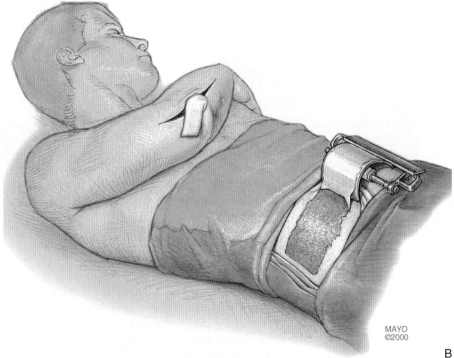

MAYO
©2000

A   B

Figure 22-9. A,B: The ipsilateral anterolateral aspect of the abdomen is exposed and a motorized dermatome removes a thin, 10- to 12-mil split-thickness skin graft.

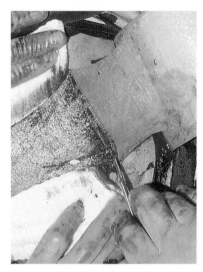

Figure 22-10. The dermis layer is harvested by sharp dissection from the subcutaneous bed immediately below the dermal layer.

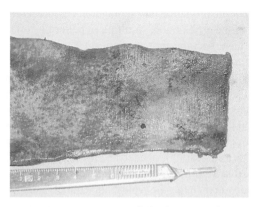

Figure 22-11. Appearance of the harvested cutis graft.

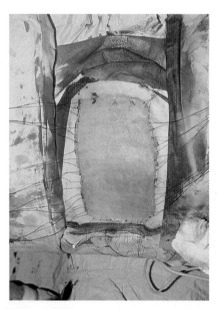

Figure 22-12. The epidermis is then reapplied as a split-thickness skin graft to the donor site and is held in place with sutures.

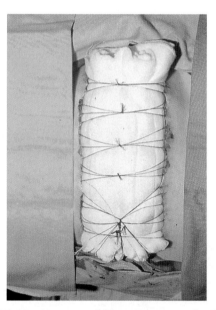

Figure 22-13. A stent stabilizes the reattached dermis.

several small holes through the medial and lateral epicondylar ridges and to these the dermal graft is sutured, thus covering the distal end of the humerus in a manner that resembles a stocking covering a foot (Fig. 22-17). The deep surface of the cutis graft containing some adipose tissue faces the new joint space.

The elbow is then reduced, the extensor musculature is reapproximated with nonabsorbable suture (Fig. 22-18), and a compression dressing is applied, followed by a posterior plaster splint at 90 degrees of flexion.

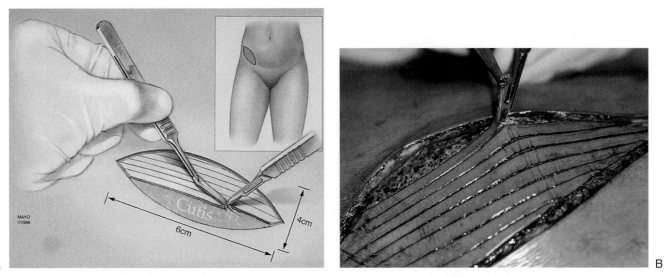

Figure 22-14. A,B: Strips of epidermis are removed sharply from an ellipse of skin taken from the groin region.

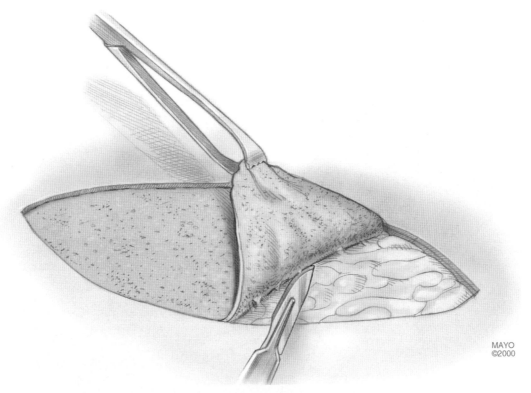

Figure 22-15. The cutis is then harvested and the incision is closed.

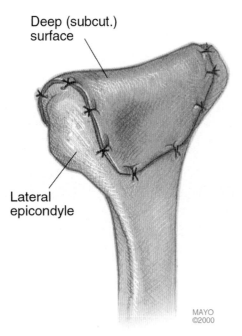

Deep (subcut.)
surface

Lateral
epicondyle

MAYO
©2000

Figure 22-16. The cutis graft is then applied to the distal humerus with the superficial aspect of the dermis applied to bone and the deep or subcutaneous surface exposed to the proximal ulna. The graft is held in place with multiple sutures placed through bone.

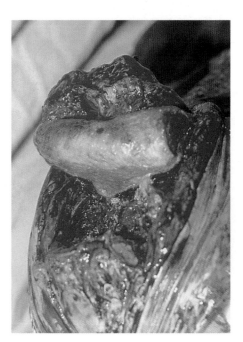

Figure 22-17. The graft completely covers the distal humerus.

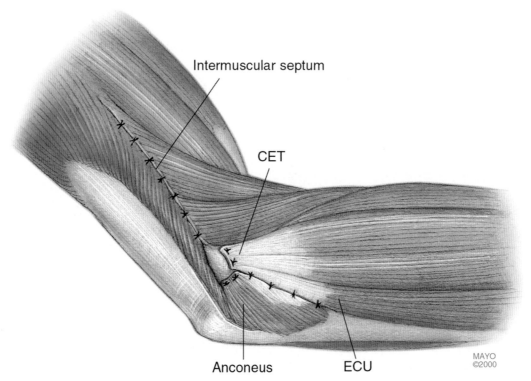

Intermuscular septum

CET

Anconeus   ECU

MAYO
©2000

Figure 22-18. The elbow is reduced without taking particular care to reattach the collateral ligaments. Nonabsorbable sutures are used to close the extensor mechanism and common extensor intervals. (Abbreviation: ECU, extensor carpi ulnaris.)

POSTOPERATIVE MANAGEMENT

Cutis Arthroplasty

Postsurgical drains are not usually used. The initial splint and dressing are not disturbed for approximately 2 weeks, at which time the sutures are removed. During the first 2 weeks the patient is seen by the upper-extremity therapist for shoulder range of movement, hand and wrist motion, and instructions in activities of daily living. When the first postoperative dressing and splint are removed, many patients are fitted with a hinged cast brace or splint, allowing freedom of flexion and extension but protecting the arthroplasty from excessive medial and lateral stresses as the soft tissues are maturing. By 1 month, resistive flexion exercises are started, and at 6 weeks extension strengthening exercises are added. The articulated splint or cast brace is usually discarded at 6 weeks, but an elastic elbow support may be used for added comfort and reassurance for another month.

Since soft-tissue interposition arthroplasty of the elbow does not provide the same fixed axis of rotation as does a total elbow replacement device, some degree of medial/lateral laxity must be accepted. In those elbows without serious bony deficiency in which the radial head has been preserved, no more than 15 to 20 degrees of medial/lateral laxity occurs.

ACHILLES TENDON ALLOGRAFT

For Achilles tendon allograft, the patient is supine and the arm is brought across the chest.

We prefer a posterior incision, as we always expose the ulnar nerve. The elbow is then addressed as described previously with an extensile Kocher exposure, occasionally releasing a small portion of the lateral triceps attachment to improve the exposure. The lateral collateral ligament is released and the anterior and posterior capsules are excised. The radial head is preserved if at all possible. Pronation of the articulating surfaces is quite important, removing bone and deformity to balance the ulnohumeral articulation. Care is taken to remove the ridge (incisura) of the olecranon to allow a flat articulation on the humerus. It is important to remove enough bone for the trochlea and capitellum to accommodate the tendon graft and also to allow a few millimeters of laxity to ensure adequate motion. We also attempt to leave a slight ridge of bone medially and laterally on the humerus to help stabilize the construction (Fig. 22-19). The distal humerus is prepared by three or four drill holes

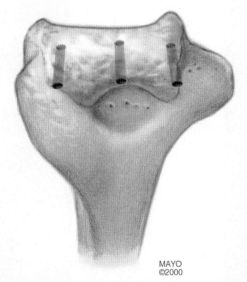

MAYO
©2000

Figure 22-19. Distal humeral preparation develops bones ridges medially and laterally to help enhance stability.

from posterior to anterior and covering the full width of the humerus. The Achilles tendon is assessed to determine the width required to cover the full dimension of the distal humerus (Fig. 22-20). The tendon portion is generally placed anteriorly, and the broad fascial portion is directed posteriorly. This provides the maximum graft thickness anteriorly and makes tissue available for ligament reconstruction posteriorly. The tendon is then situated over the humerus and the best portion of the graft needed to cover the humerus is defined. The anterior excess of the graft is defined and transected. Using No. 1 nonabsorbable sutures, the anterior graft is sewn to the anterior humerus, the graft is pulled taut and the posterior flap is secured (Fig. 22-21). At this juncture the determination is made of whether the ligament tissue is adequate for repair. If not, a strip of Achilles graft is taken medially, laterally, or both, measuring about 0.5×6 cm.

For lateral reconstruction two drill holes are placed from anterior to posterior, originating at the axis of rotation. The graft is rotated around the lateral epicondyle and secured with the suture (Fig. 22-22). A similar technique may be used medially, but the graft is brought under and secured to the medial epicondyle. If both ligaments are to be reconstructed, a hole is placed between the sublime tubercle and the crista supernatoris. Once the ligaments have been secured, this construct is usually protected with a half-frame DJDII™ external fixator (Fig. 22-23). Before application of the external fixator, the tourniquet is released, hemostasis is obtained, the triceps is reattached as described in Chapter 1, and the extensor muscle mass is reattached as well. The ulnar nerve is again inspected and if it is subluxing or constricted with flexion, it is translocated into a subcutaneous pocket. Closure is then routine.

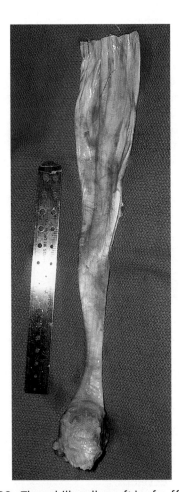

Figure 22-20. The achilles allograft is of sufficient size to allow easy coverage of the distal humerus.

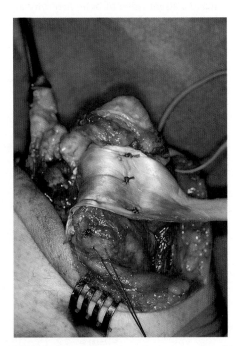

Figure 22-21. The graft is placed over the distal humerus and secured.

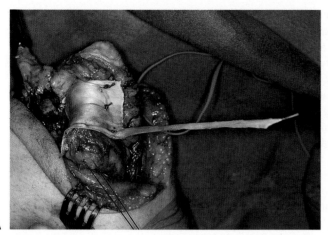
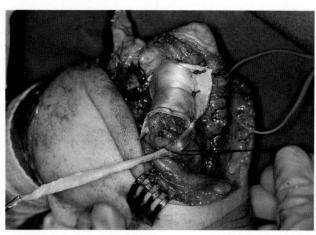

Figure 22-22. A: The posterior proximal aspect of the graft is prepared in 3- to 5-mm strips to use as collateral ligament reconstruction. **B:** The graft is secured laterally and medially at the anatomic site of ligament origins medially and laterally.

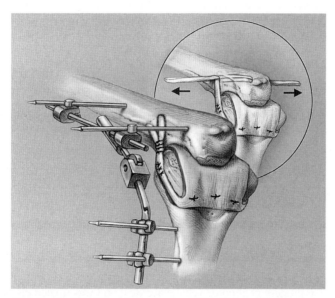

Figure 22-23. The hinge fixator (DJD II) is applied to protect the reconstruction.

Aftercare   Motion is begun on the first day with a continuous motion machine and maintained for 3 to 4 weeks. The fixator is removed under anesthesia and elbow motion and stability are examined. Activity is begun and, if the joint is stiff, static splints are prescribed.

RESULTS

Although both rheumatoid and traumatic conditions are amenable to interposition arthroplasty if the proper indications are met (1,6,9–11,15), there are little data regarding the outcome in the nonrheumatoid patient.

One recent review of 37 fascial arthroplasties for rheumatoid arthritis (12) revealed that 26 patients (70%) had excellent or good results. There is only a single report regarding the outcome for painful, nonankylosis posttraumatic arthritis. When used to treat the stiff joint with intrinsic pathology, a satisfactory rate of 80% was reported. This reflected an improvement-of-motion arc from 30 to 100 degrees and minimal pain in 88% (16). Of 13 patients with traumatic arthritis, Cheng and Morrey (5) documented 75% satisfactory results using fascia lata, a mean of 5 (range, 2 to 12) years after surgery. It is of note that those without preexisting instability revealed 80% satisfactory outcomes.

Complications of this procedure included bone resorption, heterotopic bone formation, triceps rupture, medial and lateral subluxation, infection, and seroma formation in the fascial graft donor site, and long-term failure.

Bone resorption occasionally occurs at the distal humeral condyles and often causes no difficulty. If significant instability develops as a late sequela, ligamentous reconstruction may be beneficial. I (BFM) have successfully avoided instability by repairing or reconstructing the collateral ligaments and applying a distraction device as mentioned earlier (14).

Triceps rupture is an uncommon complication that is related to the surgical exposure rather than to the procedure itself. This can be minimized by using the exposure described subsequently or by elevating the triceps in continuity.

Infection following fascial arthroplasty should be managed promptly and aggressively. For superficial infections and cellulitis, the part should be placed at rest, elevated, and immobilized in a long-arm posterior splint while appropriate antibiotics are administered. If the infection involves the deep structures, open drainage and excision of the fascial graft may be required. If bony infection occurs, removal of the implant and osseous debridement is required. Although this will leave the elbow more unstable, a useful limb often can be salvaged. Salvage with prosthetic replacement is out of the question.

If a hematoma or seroma forms at the fascial donor, it will usually resolve over a period of weeks. These collections rarely require drainage. If such an accumulation persists or is unusually large, drainage, if undertaken, must be done with strict aseptic technique. Needle aspiration should be attempted first.

Failure of the procedure due to pain, reankylosis, or instability may occur. The result can deteriorate with time, especially in the active individual. Typically, prosthetic replacement is the salvage procedure of choice and is readily performed and has recently been shown to be more than 90% successful in a series of 13 patients so treated at the Mayo Clinic (3).

ILLUSTRATIVE CASES

Case 1

A 43-year-old right-handed electrician sustained a comminuted fracture of the left olecranon process in a motor vehicle accident and was treated elsewhere with screw fixation of the olecranon and long-arm cast immobilization for 1 month. He presented 6 months later with ankylosis of the left elbow at 75 degrees of flexion with the radiograph showing

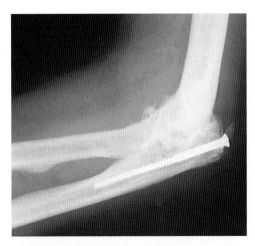

Figure 22-24. Posttraumatic arthrosis in a 43-year-old right-handed electrician.

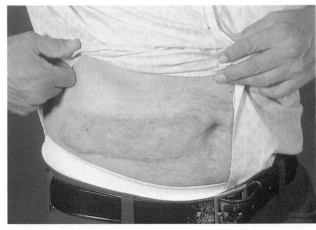

Figure 22-25. A cutis arthroplasty was performed with a lower abdominal donor site.

marked narrowing of the elbow joint (Fig. 22-24). Cutis arthroplasty was performed with a lower abdominal donor site (Fig. 22-25). Postoperative management was routine, with a rigid postoperative plaster splint worn for 2 weeks, followed by a cast brace for 4 more weeks, followed by a vigorous resistive exercise therapy program.

He returned to his work as an electrician 3 months following surgery and, as shown here, 2 years later has range of elbow motion of from 15 to 115 degrees with full pronation and supination (Fig. 22-26). Medial/lateral stability was excellent, with 15 degrees of deviation on stress testing. He has been followed at intervals and has recently retired from his work at age 61; a recent radiograph 18 years after surgery shows preservation of excellent flexion and extension (Fig. 22-27).

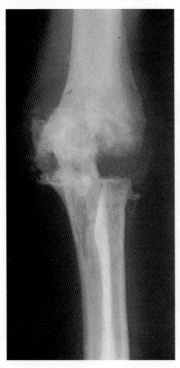

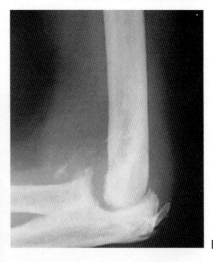

Figure 22-26. A: After surgery the patient has an arc of motion of 15 to 115 degrees. **B:** Normal pronation and supination.

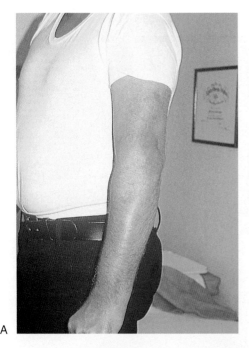

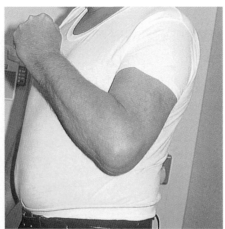

Figure 22-27. A,B: Radiographs 18 years after surgery show preservation of excellent joint surface, and the patient is pleased with the result.

Case 2

This 28-year-old male had a fracture dislocation of the elbow and after radial head excision developed arthrodesis and an unstable joint (Fig. 22-28). At surgery the lateral ligament was dysfunctional scar tissue, so an interposition arthroplasty with ligament reconstruction was carried out (Fig. 22-29). The reconstruction was protected with a hinged external fixator (Fig. 22-30A,B). A satisfactory outcome, including adequate motion of 25 to 120 degrees (Fig. 22-31A,B) and minimal pain, was attained at 3 years (Fig. 22-31C).

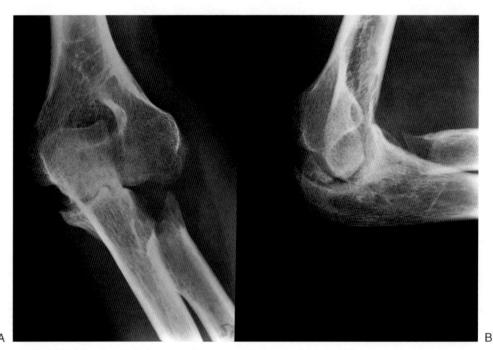

A   B

Figure 22-28. A,B: Extensive posttrauma arthrosis with instability and radial head excision.

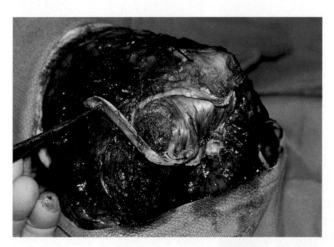

Figure 22-29. An achilles tendon allograft interposition ligament reconstruction was performed.

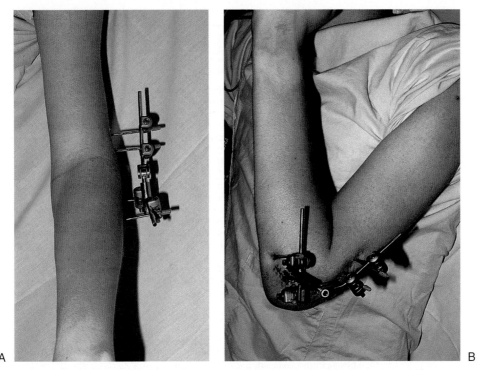

Figure 22-30. A,B: The reconstruction was protected with the external fixator.

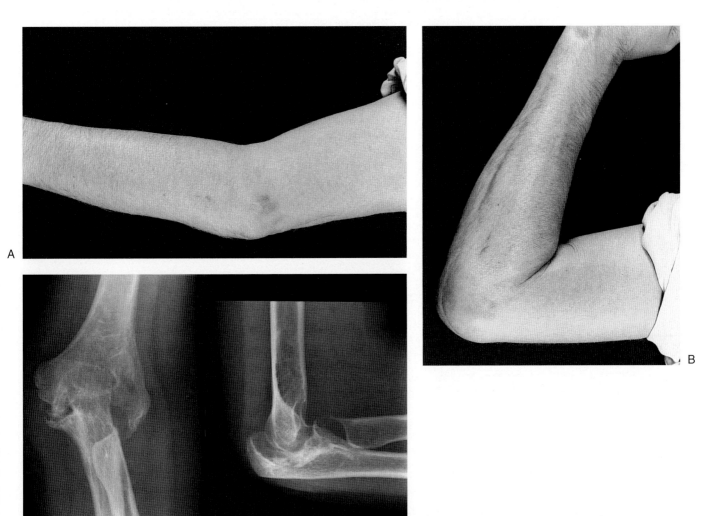

Figure 22-31. Satisfactory results at 3 years, both clinically (**A,B**) and radiographically (**C**).

RECOMMENDED READINGS

1. Agrifoglio E, DeBenedetti M. Artroplastica con interposizione di lembo cutaneo nelle rigidita e anchilosi del gomito. *Arch Orthop* 1959;72:603–614.
2. Barton JR. On the treatment of ankylosis by the formation of artificial joints. *North Am Med Surg J* 1827;3:279, 400.
3. Blaine T, Morrey BF. The salvage of failed interposition arthroplasty by total joint replacement. (Submitted for publication.)
4. Brown JE, McGaw WH, Shaw DT. Use of cutis as an interposing membrane in arthroplasty of the knee. *J Bone Joint Surg* 1958;40A:1003–1018.
5. Cheng SL, Morrey BF. The treatment of the none-stiff, painful arthritic elbow by distraction interposition arthroplasty. *Br J Bone Joint Surg.* 2000;82B:233–238.
6. Froimson AI, Silva JE, Richey D. Cutis arthroplasty of the elbow joint. *J Bone Joint Surg* 1976;58A:863–865.
7. Grishin IG, Goncharenko IV, Kozhin NP, et al. Restoration of the function of the cubital joint in extensive defects of bones and soft tissues using endoprosthesis and free skin grafts. *Acta Chir Plast* 1989;31:143–147.
8. Gui L. La cura chirurgica delle rigidita post-traumatiche del gomito e del ginocchio. *Arch Putti* 1953;3:390–412.
9. Hamalainen MMJ, Kataoka Y. Late radiographic results after resection skin interposition arthroplasty of the elbow in rheumatoid arthritis. *Rheumatology* 1991;15:42–46.
10. Hurri L, Pulkki T, Vainio K. Arthroplasty of the elbow in rheumatoid arthritis. *Acta Chir Scand* 1964;127:459.
11. Kimura C, Vainio K. Arthroplasty of the elbow in rheumatoid arthritis. *Arch Orthop Unfallchir* 1976;84:339–348.
12. Ljung P, Jonsson K, Larsson K, et al. Interposition arthroplasty of the elbow with rheumatoid arthritis. *J Shoulder Elbow Surg* 1996;5(Part I):81.
13. Mills K, Rush J. Skin arthroplasty of the elbow. *Aust N Z J Surg* 1971;41:179–181.
14. Morrey BF. Post-traumatic contracture of the elbow: operative treatment including distraction arthroplasty. *J Bone Joint Surg* 1990;72A:601.
15. Uuspaa V. Anatomical interposition arthroplasty with dermal graft. A study of 51 elbow arthroplasties on 48 rheumatoid patients. *Z Rheumatol* 1987;46:132–135.

23

Anconeus Arthroplasty

Bernard F. Morrey and Alberto G. Schneeberger

The management of posttraumatic proximal radiohumeral and radioulnar dysfunction, pain, or instability is a challenging problem without well-documented solutions. The unreliability or unsuitability of prosthetic replacement and lack of an alternate solution has prompted the development of a proximally based soft-tissue rotational arthroplasty procedure employing the anconeus muscle. The attractiveness of this procedure is that the muscle is innervated and vascularized from distinct vascular pedicles originating from the recurrent posterior interosseous artery and from the medial collateral artery (3). This allows the entire muscle to be mobilized, leaving it attached to the triceps fascial expansion, preserving its viability. Cadaver dissections have demonstrated a mean length of approximately 9 to 10 cm and a width of about 3 cm (2) (Fig. 23-1), sufficient to allow several variations of interposition procedures. Furthermore, the absence of this muscle from its anatomic location does not result in any measurable dysfunction or morbidity from a recovery or functional perspective.

The procedure was first performed approximately 10 years ago. Although there are few data regarding the long-term value of the method (2), it is included here for the purpose of introducing the concept as a potential but not necessarily a proven or definitive solution for difficult reconstructive problems for which reliable alternatives do not exist.

INDICATIONS/CONTRAINDICATIONS

In general, this technique is employed in instances when proximal radioulnar or radiohumeral dysfunction occurs following trauma. The three primary indications for the procedure are:

1. Radiohumeral impingement in which the interposition is principally directed at the proximal radiocapitellar articulation.

B.F. Morrey, M.D.: Mayo Medical School and Department of Orthopaedics, Mayo Clinic and Mayo Foundation, Rochester, Minnesota.

A.G. Schneeberger, M.D.: Department of Orthopedic Surgery, Balgrist, University of Zurich, Zurich, Switzerland.

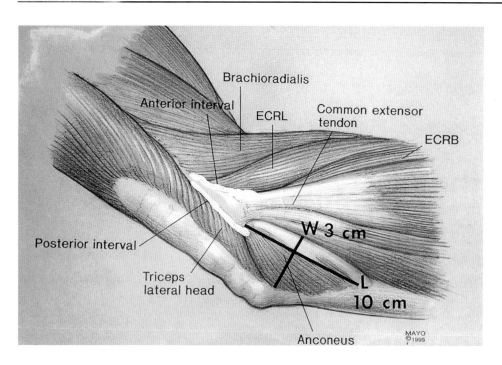

Figure 23-1. The mean dimensions of the anconeus muscle are 9 to 10 cm in length and 3 to 3.5 cm in width at its fascial attachment to the triceps.

2. Proximal radioulnar impingement with or without radiohumeral impingement.
3. Limitation of forearm rotation due to synostosis or fibrosis of the proximal radioulnar relationship in which an interposition material is desired to eliminate recurrence or impingement following resection (1,2).

The primary contraindication to this procedure is an absent or devitalized anconeus muscle. A condition requiring a procedure that resists high axial load along the radius would also rule out use of an anconeus arthroplasty. Lastly, a deficient lateral ulnar collateral ligament that cannot be reconstructed prohibits use of this procedure.

SURGERY

Several variations of the interposition have been used and are classified as follows: type I, radiohumeral "roll-up" interposition; type II, radiohumeral/radioulnar interposition; type III, proximal radial "wrap" (Fig. 23-2). The specific pathoanatomy determines which of the three types of interposition is appropriate. The method of harvest is common for all these applications.

Anconeus Harvest

The patient is placed supine with the forearm brought across the chest. Any previous incision in the region is entered, or a Kocher's-type skin incision is made (Fig. 23-3). The interval between the anconeus and extensor carpi ulnaris is entered and expanded to expose the anconeus muscle (Fig. 23-4). The dissection must be carried distally approximately 10 cm from the lateral epicondyle to expose the distal-most aspect of this muscle insertion. The tip of the anconeus is identified. The muscle is then reflected from the ulna and from the common retinaculum (Fig. 23-5). The dissection is carried proximal to the point of origin from the fascial expansion and attachment to the triceps, retaining its innervation and vascularity (Fig. 23-6).

The lateral joint is entered anterior to the collateral ligament and the relevant pathology is identified. The posterior margin of the ligament is then identified. As in all instances, the transposed muscle is placed under the lateral ulnar collateral ligament (Fig. 23-7).

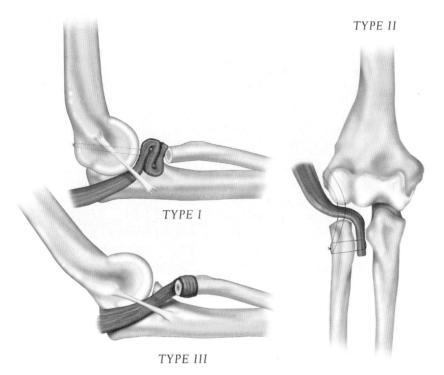

Figure 23-2. Variations of anconeus rotation/interposition arthroplasty: type I, radio-humeral; type II, radiohumeral/radioulnar; type III, radial "wrap."

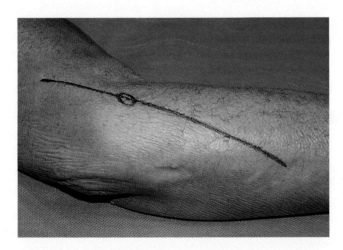

Figure 23-3. A Kocher skin incision is made.

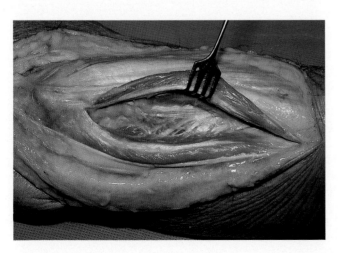

Figure 23-4. The interval between the anconeus and extensor carpi ulnaris is identified and developed.

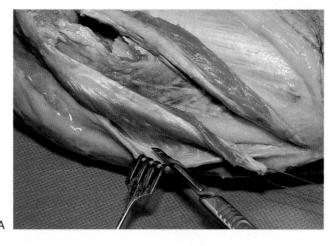

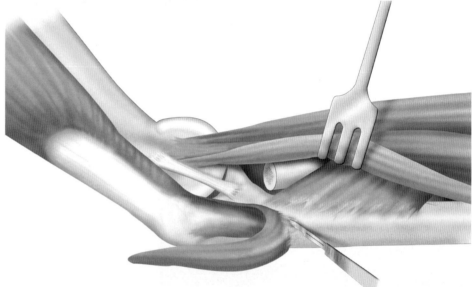

Figure 23-5. A,B: The distal aspect of the anconeus is isolated and the muscle is elevated from its bed and from the forearm fascia.

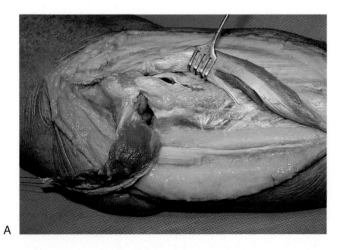

Figure 23-6. A,B: The anconeus is reflected proximally on its pedicle attachment to the triceps.

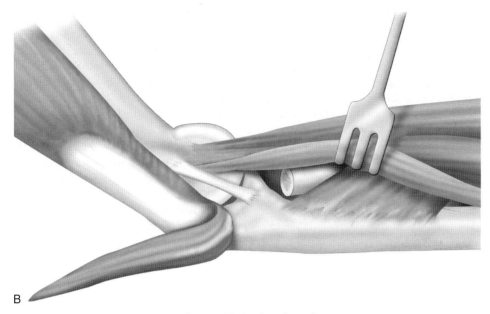

B

Figure 23-6. *Continued.*

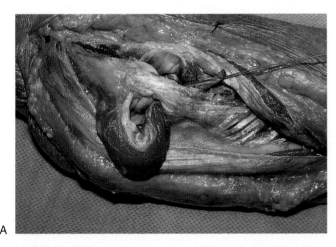

A

Figure 23-7. A,B: In all instances, the muscle is inserted into the joint under the lateral ulnar collateral ligament.

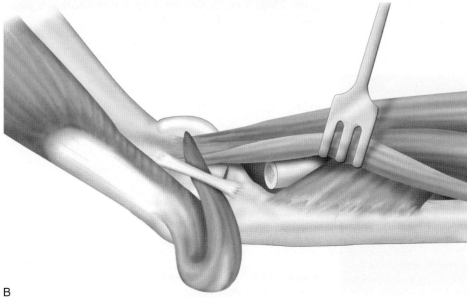

B

Type I: Interposition at the Radiohumeral Joint

The integrity of the lateral collateral ligament is assessed. If this is inadequate, it is reconstructed as described in Chapter 15 or is reinforced with a No. 5 nonabsorbable suture as described in Chapters 5 and 7. If reconstructed, the graft is usually positioned first and then secured at the conclusion of the anconeus reconstructive procedure. Two drill holes are placed from posterior to anterior through the midportion of the capitellum approximately 5 to 7 mm apart (Fig. 23-8), and the anconeus is brought under the intact or reconstructed lateral ulnar collateral ligament (Fig. 23-9). A nonabsorbable suture is passed through one of the two drill holes, then into the anconeus from proximal to distal in such a way as to allow the anconeus to fold on itself when tension is placed on the suture (Fig. 23-10). The suture then passes through the second drill hole in the capitellum and is pulled taut, allowing the anconeus to fold on itself and fill the space created by the absent radial head (Fig. 23-11). The remnants of the collateral ligament are repaired or reinforced. The fascia is approximated to the posterior aspect of the extensor carpi ulnaris (see Fig. 23-22). The remainder of the closure is routine.

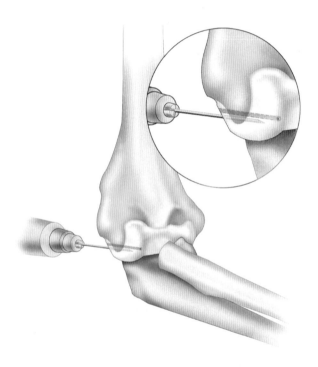

Figure 23-8. Two drill holes 5 to 7 mm apart are placed through the center of the capitellum.

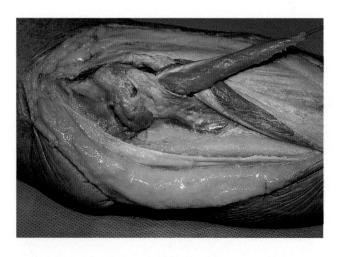

Figure 23-9. The anconeus is brought under the lateral ulnar collateral ligament.

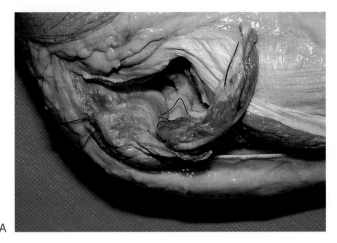

A

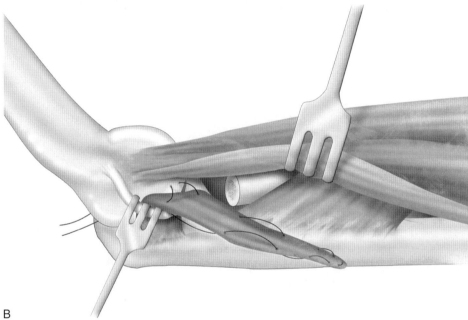

B

Figure 23-10. A,B: A looping-type stitch proceeding from proximal to distal, then distal to proximal in a parallel fashion is used to collapse the anconeus on itself.

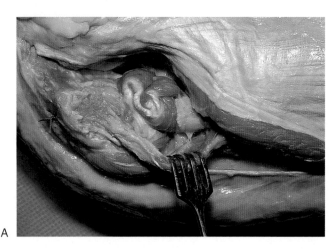

A

Figure 23-11. A,B: By tightening the suture the anconeus is folded on itself and interposed between the proximal radius and capitellum.

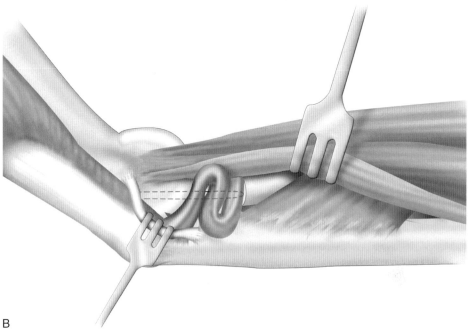

B

Type II: Radiohumeral/Radioulnar Interposition

The goal of the procedure is to interpose the anconeus between the proximal radius and between the capitellum and ulna. The lateral collateral ligament is managed as described earlier. The interval between the proximal radius and the ulna is developed. If capitellar fixation is desired, two drill holes are placed in the capitellum approximately 5 to 7 mm apart, as earlier. A drill hole is then placed across both cortices of the resected proximal radius from lateral to medial with the forearm in neutral rotation (Fig. 23-12). The anconeus is brought posterior to the lateral ulnar collateral ligament. If capitellar approximation is sought, a No. 1 nonabsorbable suture is placed through the capitellum to fix the interposed muscle between the capitellum and proximal radius. A suture is then placed in the margin of the anconeus that passes through the proximal radius (Fig. 23-13). The suture then passes through the free portion of the anconeus and is tied (Fig. 23-14). The excessive distal aspect of the anconeus is excised (Fig. 23-15). Finally, the free margin is secured with the original suture (Fig. 23-16). The closure is as described earlier.

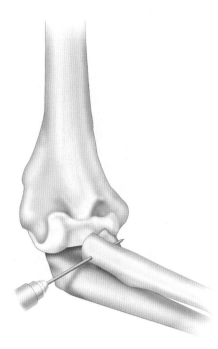

Figure 23-12. A through-and-through drill hole is placed in the proximal radius.

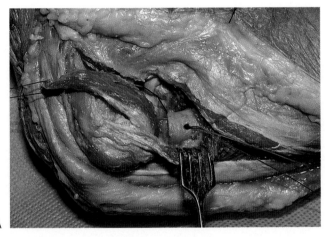

Figure 23-13. A,B: The anconeus is brought under the lateral collateral ligament and a suture is placed in such a manner as to draw the muscle between the ulna and radius, and is threaded through the holes in the proximal radius.

A

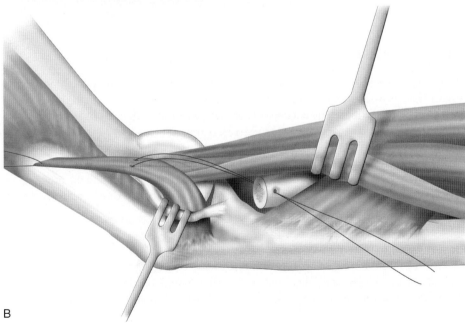

B

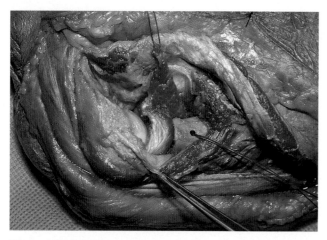

Figure 23-14. The anconeus is secured to the proximal radius by the nonabsorbable through-and-through suture.

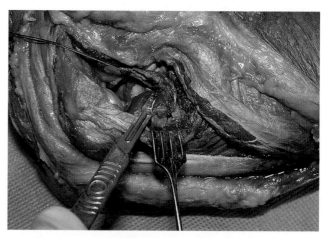

Figure 23-15. The free margin of the anconeus is then brought over the radius and secured with the original suture while the excess is removed.

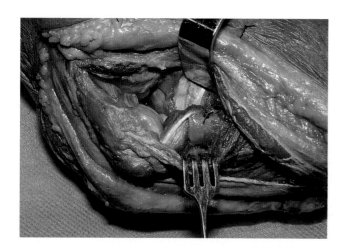

Figure 23-16. The completed interposition rests between the radius and ulna and between the radius and capitellum.

Type III: Wrap of the Proximal Radius

The radius is exposed and freed from the proximal ulna. The site of resection of the synostosis or fibrosis is identified. A through-and-through drill hole is placed in the proximal radius, as earlier described. The anconeus is brought under the collateral ligament and a suture is placed in the medial margin (Fig. 23-17). A free suture is looped through one of the arms of the suture that has been placed in the anconeus. The muscle is drawn between the proximal radius and ulna, and the free suture is brought under the radius (Fig. 23-18). The second suture is used to wrap the proximal portion of the anconeus around the proximal radius, (Fig. 23-19) resulting in a circumferential "wrap" of the proximal radius by the anconeus (Fig. 23-20).

Closure

In all instances the capsule is closed and the fascia is approximated to the posterior aspect of the extensor carpi ulnaris and closed with a running, absorbable suture (Figs. 23-21 and 23-22).

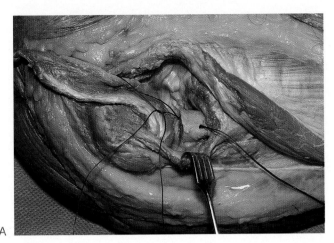

A

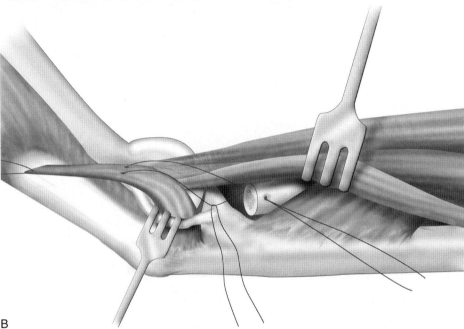

B

Figure 23-17. A,B: The anconeus is inserted into the joint and a suture is placed into its margin so as to draw the muscle between the radius and ulna. A second free suture is looped over one of the sutures at the site of emergence from the anconeus.

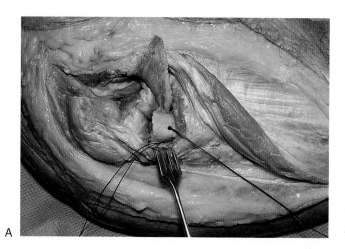

A

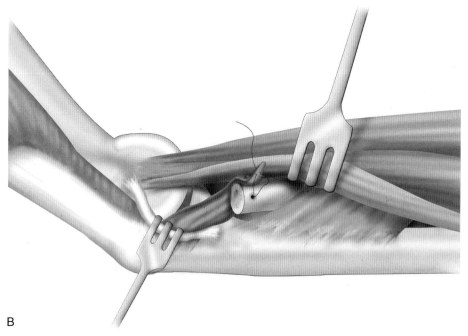

B

Figure 23-18. A,B: The through-and-through suture is used to secure the anconeus muscle to the ulnar aspect of the proximal radius.

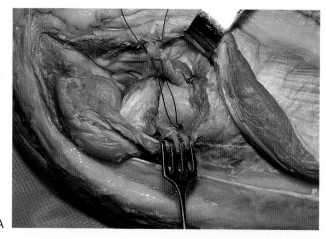

A

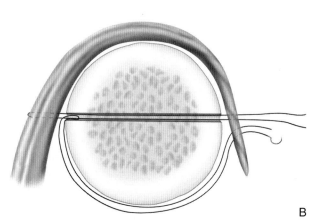

B

Figure 23-19. A,B: The free suture is passed through the distal free end of the anconeus. The free suture is drawn into the hole on the ulnar aspect of the radius and brought under the proximal radius.

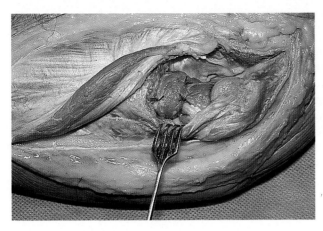

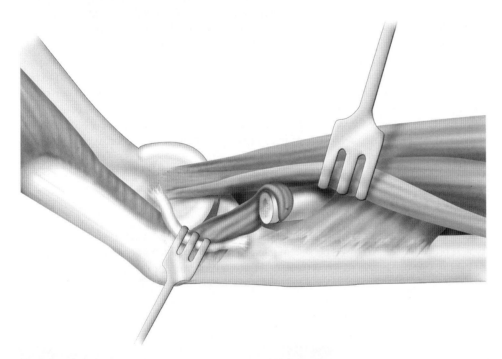

Figure 23-20. The completed "wrap."

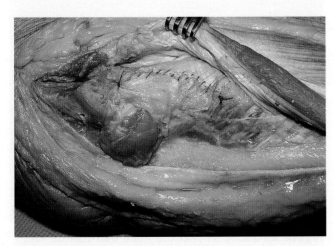

Figure 23-21. The capsule is cased and the collateral lig-ament is reinforced if necessary.

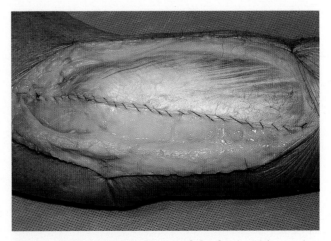

Figure 23-22. Routine closure of the fascia with running absorbable sutures.

POSTOPERATIVE MANAGEMENT

The postoperative management is predicated on the features of the underlying pathology. The anconeus interposition itself prompts immobilization for 5 to 7 days. Passive motion is then preferred for 2 to 3 weeks. Active and full motion is encouraged a month after surgery. Typically, a concurrent reconstruction or reinforcement of the lateral collateral ligament is also carried out during the surgery. If this has been done because of demonstrated instability, the forearm is placed in full pronation and protected for about 6 weeks in a hinged splint. Flexion and extension are encouraged. Carefully controlled pronation and supination are begun on the sixth to eighth day.

RESULTS

Limited results are available. Our assessment of the initial 10 procedures demonstrated that four patients received a type I or type II and that two received a type III interposition. Eight of the 10 patients expressed subjective satisfaction with the procedure, primarily because of reduced pain. Using the Mayo Elbow Performance Score (MEPS), seven were rated satisfactory. Bell has reported three cases in which the distal anconeus was interposed to prevent recurrence of radioulnar synostosis, all with a satisfactory outcome (1). In our series, ulnar shortening was performed in three, and two of the three described minimal, if any, wrist pain. Two patients indicated that elbow pain persisted with no benefit from the surgery. There were no incidences of instability. The value of this procedure continues to be observed and investigated.

COMPLICATIONS

There were no specific complications with the procedure. One patient who underwent a type II procedure experienced persistent pain, so re-exploration was conducted. At the time of exploration the anconeus was viable, and the interposition appeared to be functioning as

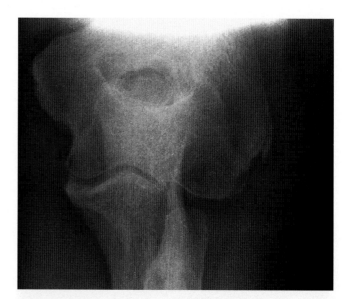

Figure 23-23. A 33-year-old male had painful radio-humeral symptoms after fracture dislocation with radial head excision.

desired. As workers' compensation issues are being debated, the patient continues to complain of pain after reexploration and ligament imbrication.

ILLUSTRATIVE CASE

A 33-year-old man had persistent radiocapitellar pain with an associated radioulnar impingement (Fig. 23-23) after radial head excision and distal radioulnar symptoms from an ulna plus deformity from the Essex-Lopresti lesion. From radial shortening (Fig. 23-24) the anconeus is brought under the collateral ligament (Fig. 23-25), which, because it was insufficient, required further stabilization by reinforcement with a Krachow stitch; an ulnar-shortening procedure was also completed (Fig. 23-26). The patient had minimal pain at the wrist and elbow, and no symptoms of impingement at the elbow at 1 year (Fig. 23-27).

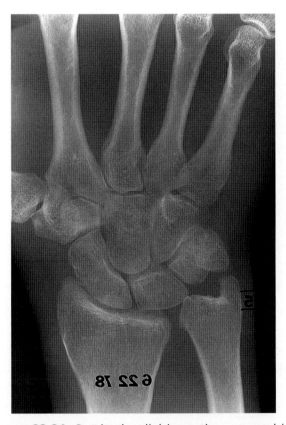

Figure 23-24. Proximal radial impaction occurred because of description of the distal radioulnar stabilizers.

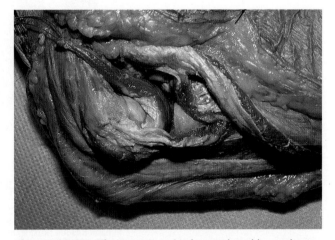

Figure 23-25. The anconeus is elevated and brought under a lax lateral ulnar collateral ligament for a type I repair.

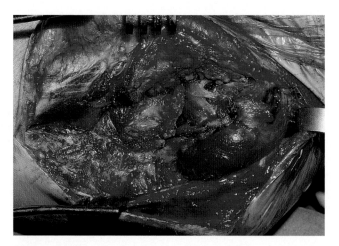

Figure 23-26. The lax lateral collateral ligament is reinforced with a Krachow stitch.

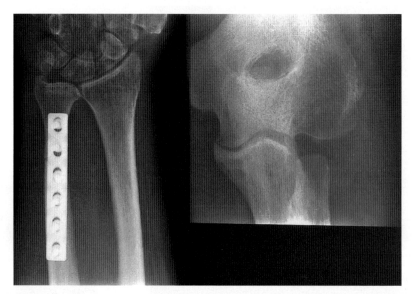

Figure 23-27. The patient had minimal pain and a stable elbow at 1 year.

RECOMMENDED READINGS

1. Bell SN, Benger D. Management of radioulnar synostosis with mobilization, anconeus interposition, and a forearm rotation assist splint. *J Should Elbow Surg* 1999;8:621–624.
2. Morrey BF, Schneeberger A. Anconeus arthroplasty: an anatomical study and clinical experience with a new technique for reconstruction of the radiohumeral/radioulnar joints. Submitted for publication.
3. Schmidt CC, Kohut GN, Greenberg JA, et al. The anconeus muscle flap: its anatomy and clinical application. *J Hand Surg* 1999;24A:359–369.

Index